Pediatric Gastroenterology and Hepatology

DEDICATION

To Eoin, Lochlinn, Chloe, Alex, and Georgia Rae

PEDIATRIC GASTROENTEROLOGY AND HEPATOLOGY

DEIRDRE A KELLY
MD, FRCP
Consultant Paediatric Hepatologist
The Liver Unit
The Children's Hospital
Birmingham, UK

IAN W BOOTH
MD, FRCP
Professor of Paediatric Gastroenterology and Nutrition
Institute of Child Health
The Nuffield Building
Birmingham, UK

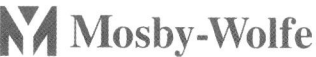 Mosby-Wolfe

London Baltimore Barcelona Bogotá Boston Buenos Aires Carlsbad, CA Chicago Madrid Mexico City Milan Naples, FL New York
Philadelphia St. Louis Seoul Singapore Sydney Taipei Tokyo Toronto Wiesbaden

Publisher	Richard Furn
Development Editor	Jennifer Prast
Project Manager	Dave Burin
Cover Design	Lara Last
Layout	John Ormiston
Illustration Manager	Lynda Payne
Production	Gudrun Hughes
Index	Nina Boyd

Copyright © 1996 Times Mirror International Publishers Limited

Published in 1996 by Mosby–Wolfe, an imprint of Times Mirror International Publishers Limited

Printed in Spain by Grafos S.A. Arte sobre papel, Barcelona, Spain

ISBN 07234 1966 3

All rights reserved. No part of this publication may be reproduced, stored in a retrieval system, copied or transmitted, in any form or by any means, electronic, mechanical, photocopying, recording or otherwise without written permission from the Publisher or in accordance with the provisions of the Copyright Act 1988, or under the terms of any licence permitting limited copying issued by the Copyright Licensing Agency, 33–34 Alfred Place, London, WC1E 7DP, UK.

Any person who does any unauthorised act in relation to this publication may be liable to criminal prosecution and civil claims for damages.

Permission to photocopy or reproduce solely for internal or personal use is permitted for libraries or other users registered with the Copyright Clearance Center, provided that the base fee of $4.00 per chapter plus $.10 per page is paid directly to the Copyright Clearance Center, 21 Congress Street, Salem, MA 01970, USA. This consent does not extend to other kinds of copying, such as copying for general distribution, for advertising or promotional purposes, for creating new collected works, or for resale.

For full details of all Times Mirror International Publishers Limited titles, please write to Times Mirror International Publishers Limited, Lynton House, 7–12 Tavistock Square, London WC1H 9LB, UK.

A CIP catalogue record for this book is available from the British Library.

Library of Congress Cataloging-in-Publication Data applied for.

Contents

Preface 7

Acknowledgements 8

Chapter 1
Congenital and Neonatal Conditions 9

Chapter 2
Oesophagus 19

Chapter 3
Stomach and Duodenum 27

Chapter 4
Small Intestine Diseases 33

Chapter 5
Gastrointestinal Infections 49

Chapter 6
Inflammatory Bowel Disease 57

Chapter 7
Motility and Constipation 69

Chapter 8
General and Abdominal Pain 71

Chapter 9
Gastrointestinal Tumours 75

Chapter 10
Pancreatic and Gallbladder Disease 79

Chapter 11
Neonatal Liver Disease 89

Chapter 12
Inherited Metabolic Disease   99

Chapter 13
Chronic Liver Disease in Childhood   113

Chapter 14
Hepatic Tumours   125

Chapter 15
Acute Liver Disease   131

Chapter 16
Liver Transplantation   137

Chapter 17
Nutrition   149

Index   171

Preface

It is frequently said of clinical diagnosis that if there is no differential diagnosis in the mind of the doctor by the end of history-taking it is very rare to make a diagnosis after examining the patient. Whilst this is as true of paediatric gastroenterology and hepatology as of most other clinical disciplines, it is also clear that correctly identifying physical and radiological signs is of crucial importance.

The purpose of this atlas is to provide an accessible source of reference for both common and rare disorders of the gut and liver for the non-specialist paediatrician and the paediatric trainee, but we hope that it will also be of value to other medical and paramedical disciplines.

Clinical problems are presented highlighting relevant physical signs and appropriate diagnostic investigations with information about management and outcome. Although endoscopy plays an increasingly important part in diagnosis, it is well covered in other atlases and consequently we have limited the number of endoscopy pictures.

The importance of malnutrition secondary to gastrointestinal and liver disease has been emphasised as this is perhaps one of the most neglected elements in the care of sick children for which there are now effective strategies.

The increasing success of transplantation as therapy for children with gut or liver disease has encouraged us to include a section on the indications and outcome for both liver and bowel transplantation.

We are indebted to many colleagues who have generously provided pictures for this atlas—a reflection of the multidisciplinary nature of our specialty. In this context we are particularly grateful to Faro Raafat, Stefan Hubscher, Philip John and Steve Chapman from the Children's Hospital.

Deirdre A Kelly
Ian W Booth

Acknowledgements

We would like to acknowledge the help of our colleagues both at the Children's Hospital and the Queen Elizabeth Hospital.

Many thanks for radiological slides and advice:
Dr Kish Shah
Dr Helen Alton
Dr Steve Chapman
Dr Philip John

Many thanks for pathology slides and interpretation:
Dr Faro Raafat
Dr Gill Douce
Mr Alan Brownhill
Dr Stefan Hubscher
Dr Steven Mills

Many thanks to colleagues at the Children's Hospital who provided us with clinical slides and information:
Dr Susan Beath
Dr Stephen Murphy
Dr Tawny Southwood
Staff of Microbiology and Virology Departments
Dr Amanda Goldstein
Dr Patrick McKiernan

Many thanks to colleagues elsewhere:
Dr Ahmed
Dr M. Baraitser
Dr Huw Jenkins
Professor JA Walker-Smith
Dr John Puntis
Professor Brian Lake
Professor B Nelson
Dr M Rawasdeh
Dr Antony Oakhill
Dr Habib
Dr Graham Clayden
Dr Martin Ament
Professor David Candy
Dr Peter Daish
Professor Ken Setchell
Dr DPR Miller
Professor L Spitz
Dr Clive Ryder

And a very special thank you to Mrs Tracy Ellis and Mrs Jenny Target for secretarial help and assistance.

Sources of other illustrations are:
Smith, Kline and French for **2.13**, **2.14**, **2.15**, **2.18**, from the Tagamet slide atlas, 1981; Dr JJ Misiewicz for **3.8**, which is Figure 24 from the *Glaxo/Gower Slide Atlas of Gastroenterology: Stomach*; Current Science Ltd for **3.9**, which is Slide 1 from the *Slide Atlas of Gastrointestinal Endoscopy, Stomach*; Professor F Silverstein and Professor GNJ Tytgat for **3.10** and **3.11**, which are Figures 12 and 28, respectively, in the *Glaxo/Gower Slide Atlas of Gastroenterology: Stomach*; Churchill Livingstone for **4.36**, which is re-drawn from *Clinical Nutrition in Gastroenterology*, RV Heatley et al.; Professor AG Billoo, University of Karachi for **5.3** and **5.6**, which appeared in *Management of Diarrhoea in Children*; Institute of Child Health for **5.7**, which appeared in *Teaching Aids at Low Cost*; The BMJ Publishing Group for **10.29**, which appeared as Figure 1 in "The Johanson-Blizzard Syndrome", M Baraitser et al., *J. Med. Genetics*; Professor R Hendriksen for **17.3**, which is 27 in *Color Atlas of Nutritional Disorders*, DS McLaren, Wolfe Medical Publications, 1981; Dr DS McLaren for **17.11**, **17.12**, **17.14** and **17.15**, which are **10**, **280**, **50** and **61**, respectively, in *Color Atlas of Nutritional Disorders*; Dr WR Tyldesley for **17.31**, which is **118** in *Color Atlas of Nutritional Disorders*; Dr M Zatouroff for **17.32**, which is **170** in *Color Atlas of Nutritional Disorders*.

Every effort has been made to obtain permission for copyright material used in this book. Where this has not been possible, please contact the publishers, who will ensure that full acknowledgement is made in future editions.

1. Congenital and Neonatal Conditions

CONGENITAL ANOMALIES

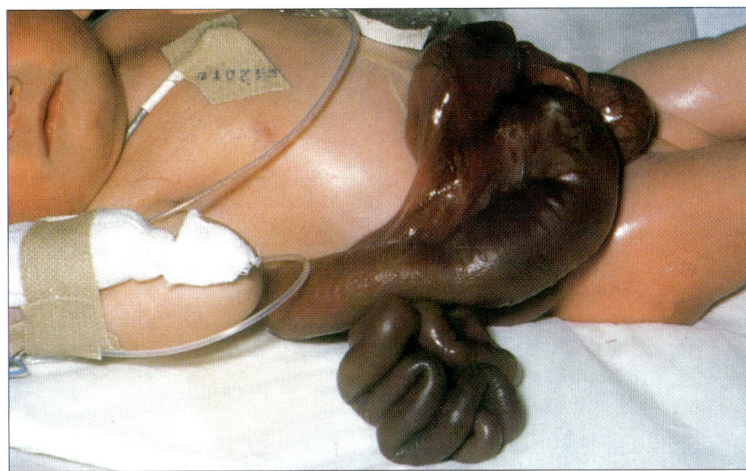

Fig. 1.1 Gastroschisis. Gastroschisis is the herniation of the gut through a narrow opening in the anterior abdominal wall to the right of a normal umbilicus. The cause is unknown. The gut is shortened and thickened, and covered by a fibrinous exudate. Following surgical repair, the gut is often dysmotile, so prolonged parenteral nutrition may be necessary. The herniated gut may become strangulated by a narrow opening in the abdominal wall, leading to infarction (as here). Atretic bowel may be present at the exit and entry sites.

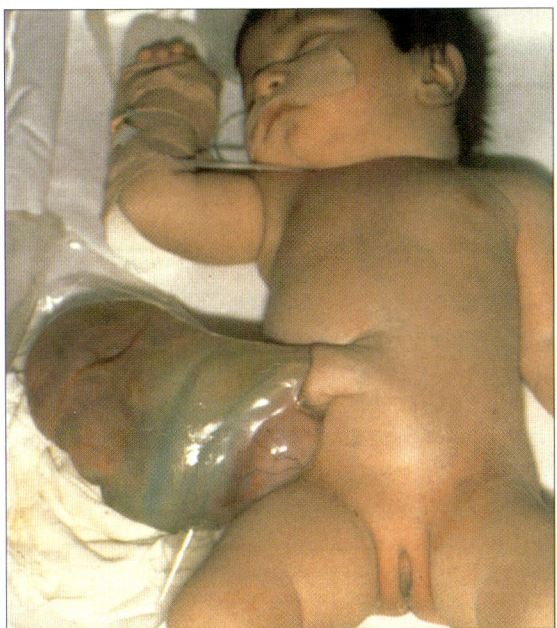

Fig. 1.2 Exomphalos. The abdominal contents are herniated at the umbilicus into a sac comprising peritoneum and amnion. One third of affected infants are born pre-term and other congenital abnormalities may be present, including Beckwith's syndrome (see **Fig. 1.3**).

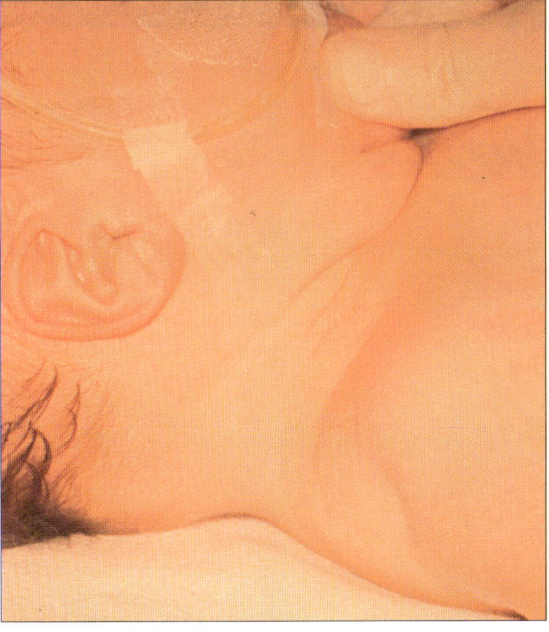

Fig. 1.3 Beckwith's syndrome. These infants are of high birth weight, with macroglossia, exomphalos (see **Fig. 1.2**), and visceromegaly. Characteristic linear creases are present in the ear lobe. Hypoglycaemia is common and may be severe and persistent. Affected children are also at increased risk of developing hepatoblastoma.

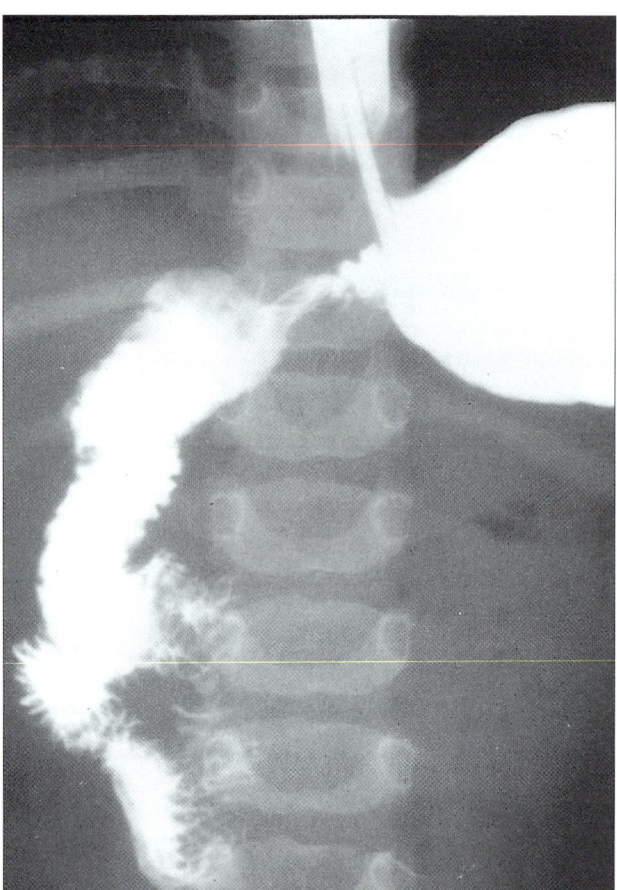

Fig. 1.4 Malrotation. Malrotation usually presents in the newborn period with intestinal obstruction, due to duodenal obstruction by Ladd's bands. In addition, failure of descent of the caecum and terminal ileum leaves the midgut suspended from a narrow pedicle, which renders the midgut liable to volvulus.

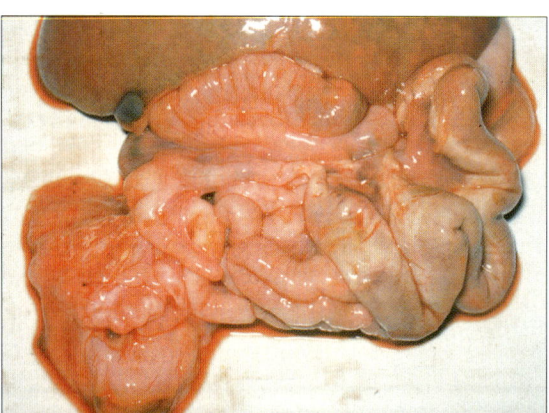

Fig. 1.5 Midgut infarction due to malrotation. The narrow mesenteric pedicle in the malrotated gut is liable to volvulus causing obstruction of the root of the middle mesenteric artery. Midgut infarction then results, leading to loss of the entire small intestine and the right colon. Intestinal obstruction may be incomplete or intermittent, and therefore any bile-stained vomiting in the newborn should be investigated immediately, often by barium meal.

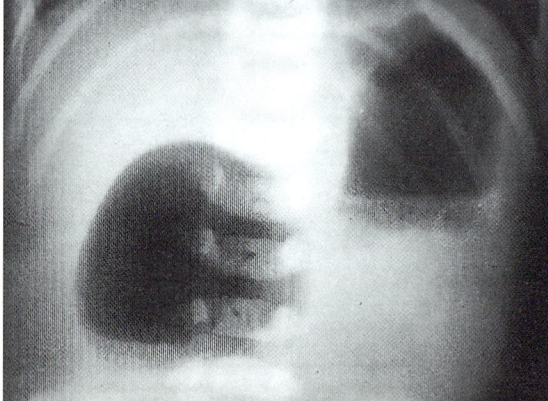

Fig. 1.6 Duodenal atresia. Shown here is the classic 'double bubble' radiological appearance of duodenal atresia, with fluid levels only in the stomach and duodenum. Presentation is with vomiting in the first day or so of life, which in over 75% of cases is bile-tinged. In the remainder, involving the supra-ampullary region of the duodenum, the vomitus is clear. Associated anomalies are frequent, and found in 50% of babies with duodenal atresia – Down's syndrome (30%), malrotation (20%), and cardiac anomalies (10%) are the most common.

Congenital and Neonatal Conditions

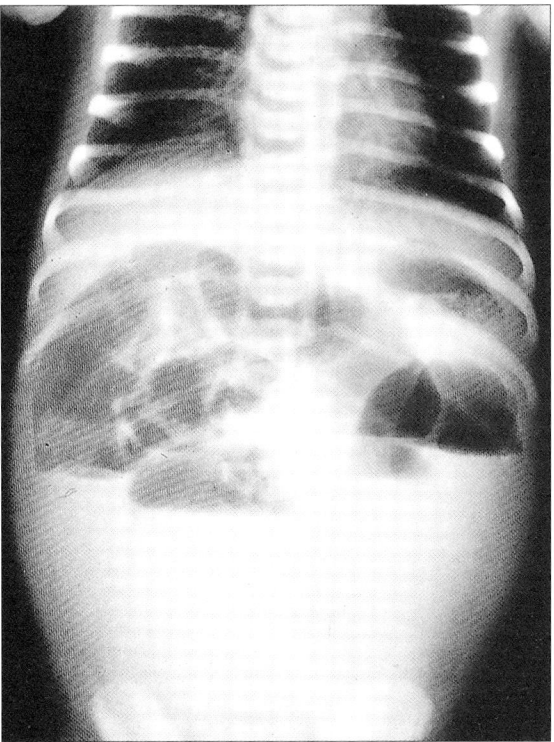

Fig. 1.7 Jejunal atresia. This erect plain abdominal radiograph shows air–fluid levels in the obstructed and dilated proximal bowel, and an absence of gas beyond the atresia in the jejunum. Presentation is with bile-stained vomiting, failure to pass meconium, and abdominal distension.

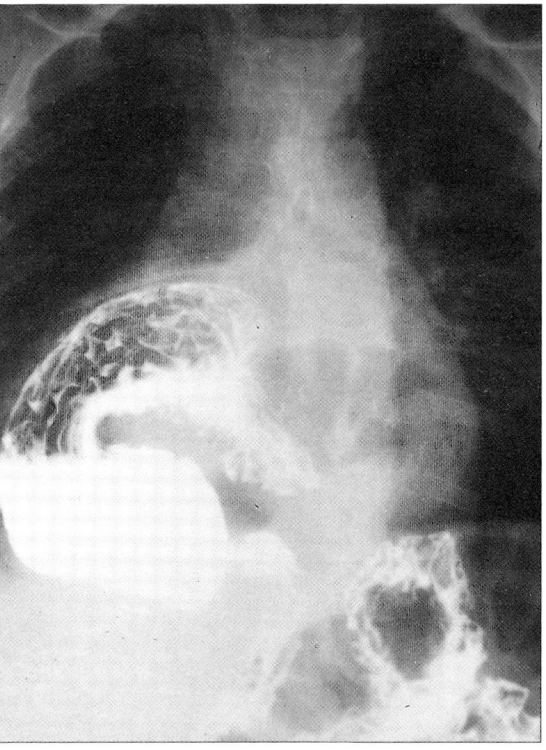

Fig. 1.8 Large congenital diaphragmatic hernia. A defect in the dome of the diaphragm (right-sided in 80% of cases) permits herniation of the stomach (as here), small bowel, spleen, and part of the large bowel into the chest. The lung on the affected side is frequently severely hypoplastic, the contralateral lung less so. Infants present with apparent dextrocardia, cyanosis, and dyspnoea. Cysts of staphylococcal pneumonia may cause similar appearances on a chest radiograph. Extracorporeal membrane oxygenation may salvage some infants with severe pulmonary hypoplasia.

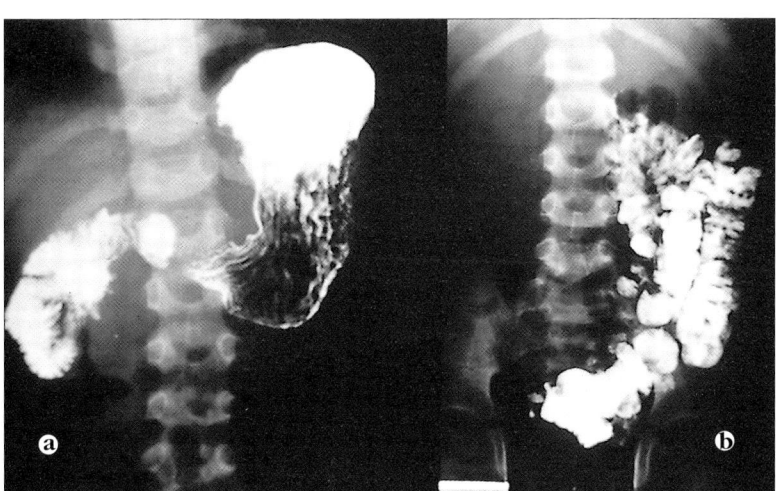

Fig. 1.9 Intestinal non-rotation. Intestinal non-rotation results when the process of midgut rotation, which takes place *in utero* at about the 10th week of gestation, completely fails to occur. The duodenojejunal loop lies on the right of the abdomen (**a**), and the caecum and colon on the left (**b**). The base of the mesentery is fairly broad and the duodenum is separate from the caecum. Consequently, obstruction or volvulus is uncommon. The anomaly is associated with gastroschisis, exomphalos, and diaphragmatic hernia.

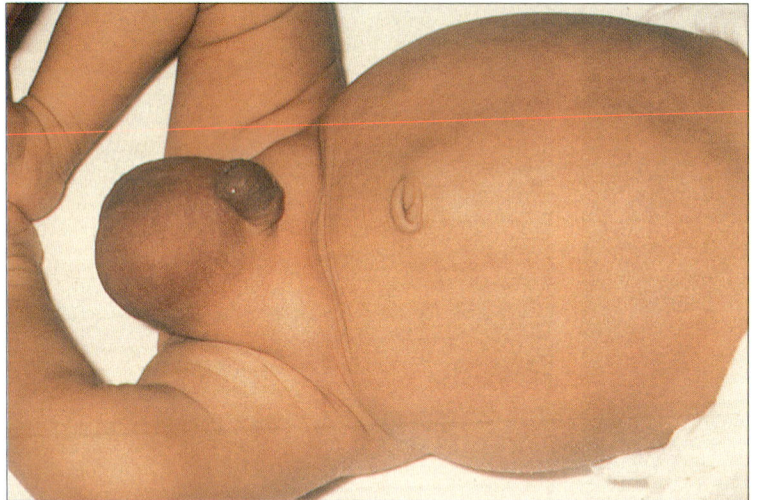

Fig. 1.10 Bilateral inguinal hernia. Bilateral inguinal and scrotal swellings are present as a result of herniation of the abdominal contents along a patent processus vaginalis. Early herniotomy is indicated in all cases. Inguinal hernia in a female suggests possible testicular feminisation syndrome.

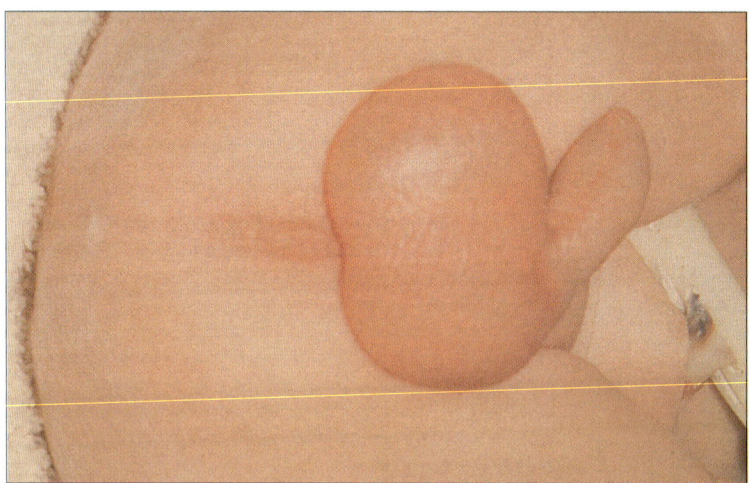

Fig. 1.11 Rectal atresia. The normal anal opening is absent and replaced by a small depression. The rectum ends blindly in the pelvis above the levator ani muscle. Associated anomalies are often present, particularly of the upper urinary tract. A right hydrocoele is also present in this case.

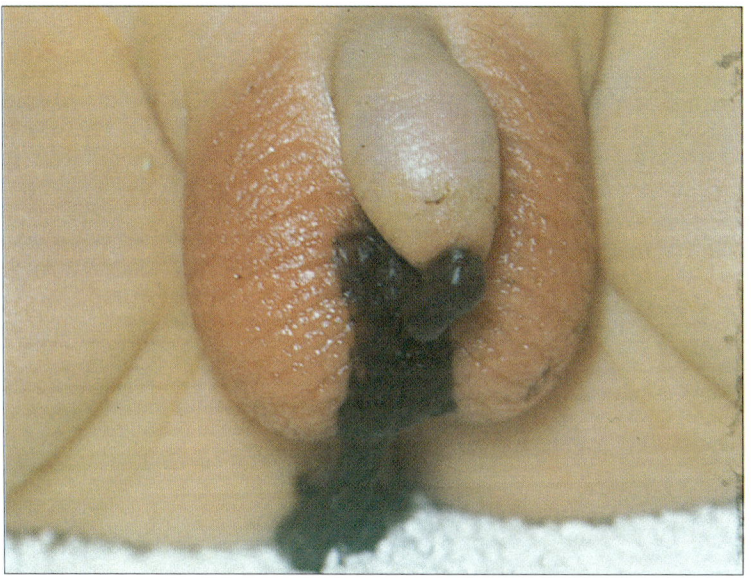

Fig. 1.12 Rectovesical fistula. Meconium has been passed per urethra in this newborn infant, indicating the presence of a rectourinary fistula. Fistulae into the vagina or perineum also occur.

Congenital and Neonatal Conditions

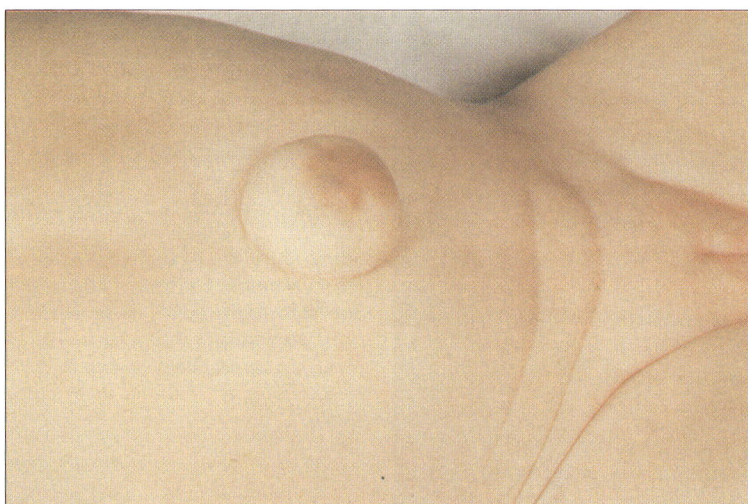

Fig. 1.13 Umbilical hernia. A soft swelling is present at the umbilicus, which enlarges with crying but is fully reducible. Umbilical herniae are particularly common in Afro-Caribbean infants. Most resolve spontaneously by the age of 5 years; only rarely is surgery necessary for persistent herniae or strangulation.

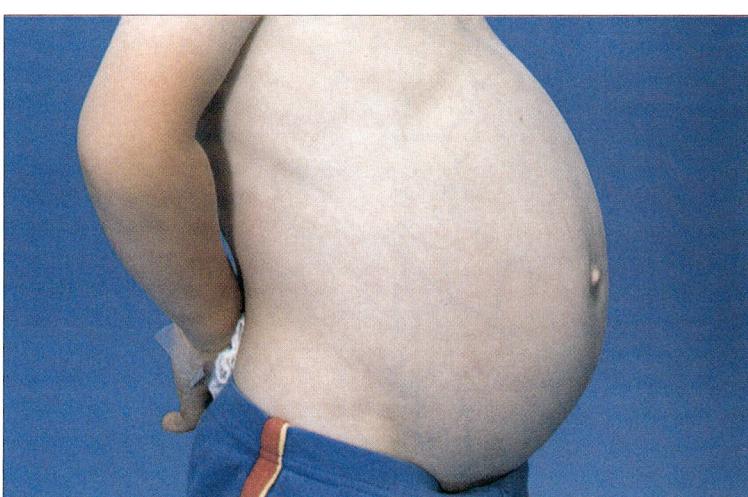

Fig. 1.14 Mesenteric cyst (clinical). This boy presented with painless abdominal swelling of several months' duration. Clinically, the abdominal distension was difficult to distinguish from ascites.

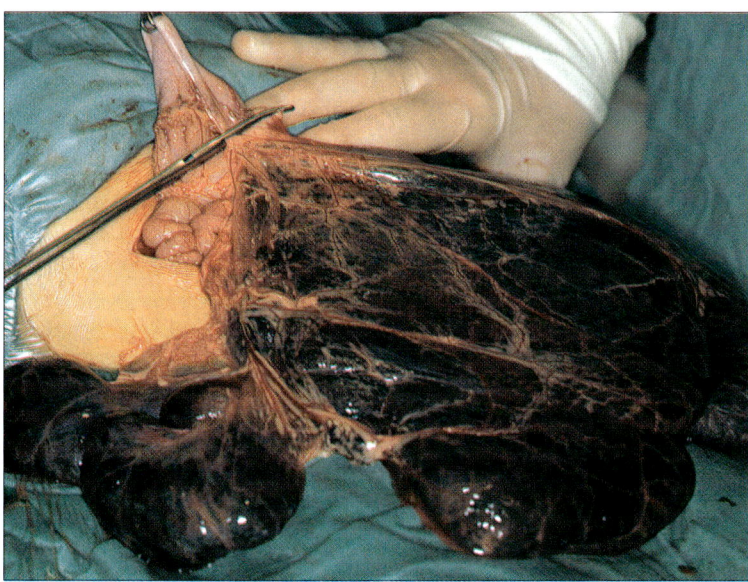

Fig. 1.15 Mesenteric cyst (operative). At operation a large, benign, congenital mesenteric cyst was found and removed uneventfully from the boy shown in **Fig. 1.14**. Mesenteric cysts are rare; they have been reported from the duodenum to the rectal mesentery, but are most common in the ileal mesentery. Less than 3% are malignant.

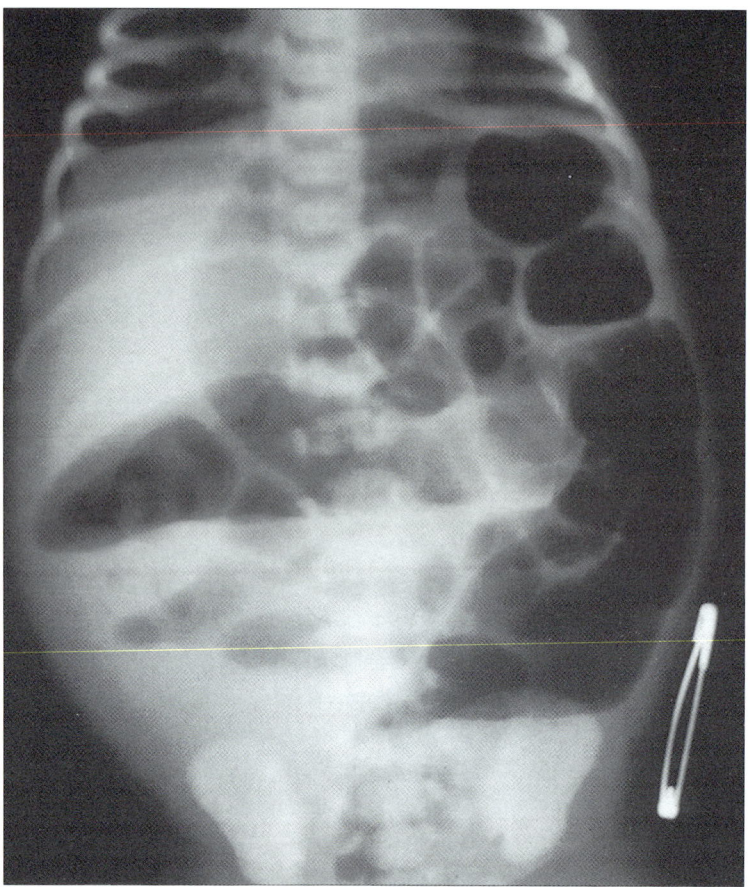

Fig. 1.16 Neonatal intestinal obstruction due to Hirschsprung's disease. An absence of ganglion cells in the distal rectum, extending proximally for a variable distance, is associated with a narrowing and failure of relaxation in the aganglionic segment. Most patients (80–90%) present with intestinal obstruction in the newborn period in association with a history of failure to pass meconium; a plain abdominal film of such a patient is shown here. Small and large bowel dilatation and fluid levels are present, maximal in the distal colon.

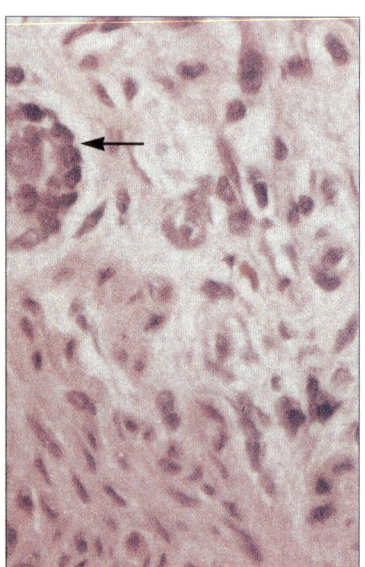 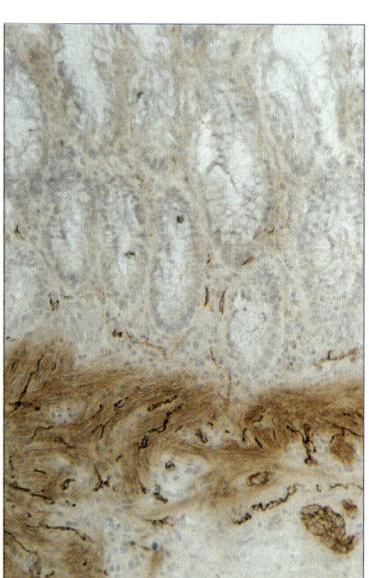 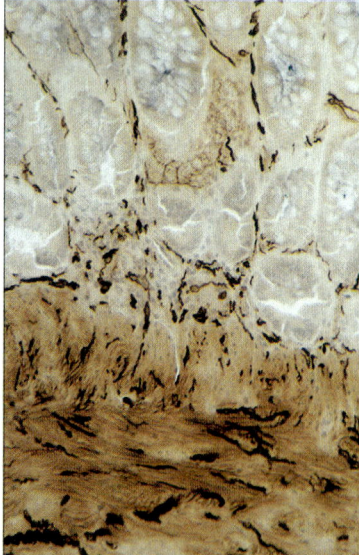

Figs 1.17–1.19 Neonatal intestinal obstruction due to Hirschsprung's disease. The diagnosis for the case shown in **Fig. 1.16** was confirmed by rectal biopsy, which demonstrated the absence of ganglion cells (a ganglionic biopsy is shown in **Fig. 1.17**: the ganglion cells are arrowed). In addition, increased acetylcholinesterase staining was present. Acetylcholinesterase staining is shown in a control biopsy (**Fig. 1.18**) and in a biopsy from this patient (**Fig. 1.19**) in which giant nerve trunks are present. A colostomy was performed followed by a definitive pull-through procedure when the child was 12 months old.

Congenital and Neonatal Conditions

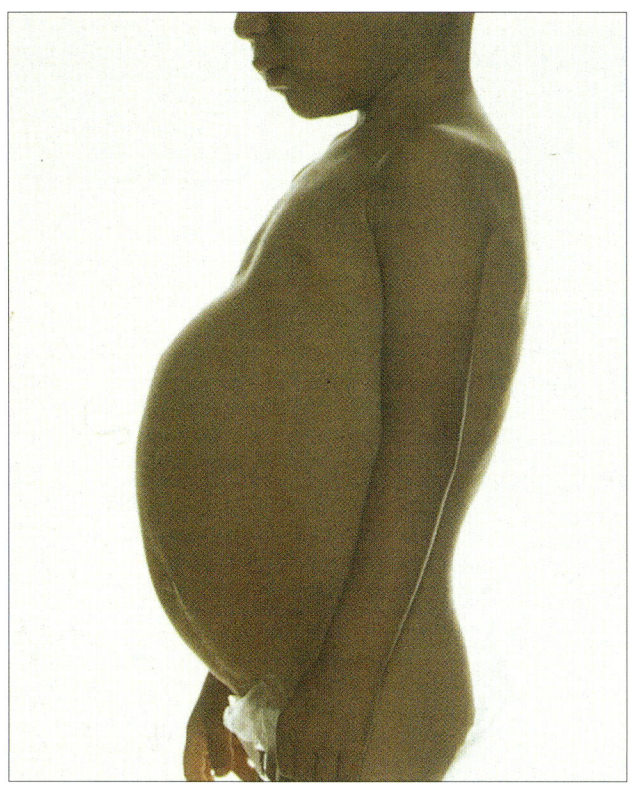

Fig. 1.20 Late-onset Hirschsprung's disease. A few children with Hirschsprung's disease present in later childhood. The lesion is usually of the short-segment type. Affected children may have a history of delay in the passage of meconium, followed usually by a history of severe, early-onset intractable constipation, with little or no soiling. There may be a history of severe, unexplained diarrhoea (enterocolitis), failure to thrive, and marked abdominal distension due to fecal retention, as shown here. The diagnosis is made by rectal biopsy (**Figs 1.17–1.19**). Coeliac disease is the major differential diagnosis.

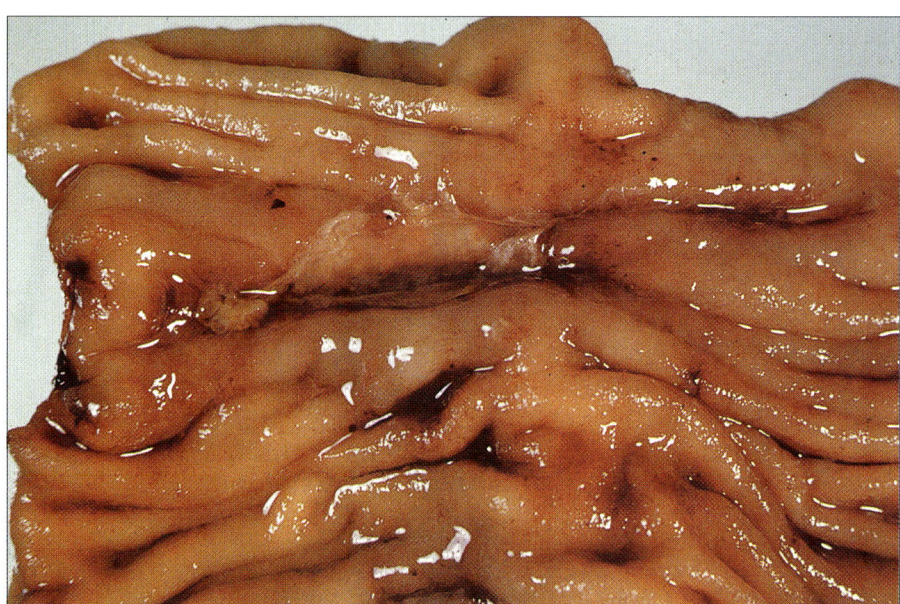

Fig. 1.21 Ileocolic anastomotic bleeding. This patient underwent an ileocolic resection and ileocolic anastomosis because of a gangrenous intussusception at the age of 8 months. He presented again at 4 years of age with a severe iron-deficiency anaemia (haemoglobin, 4 g/dl) and positive tests for fecal occult blood. Colonoscopy revealed a series of small, bleeding anastomotic ulcers which histologically showed non-specific acute on chronic inflammation. Symptoms resolved following revision of the anastomosis, although in some patients, re-ulceration can occur. This complication of ileocolic anastomoses can occur many years after the initial surgery. The cause is not known.

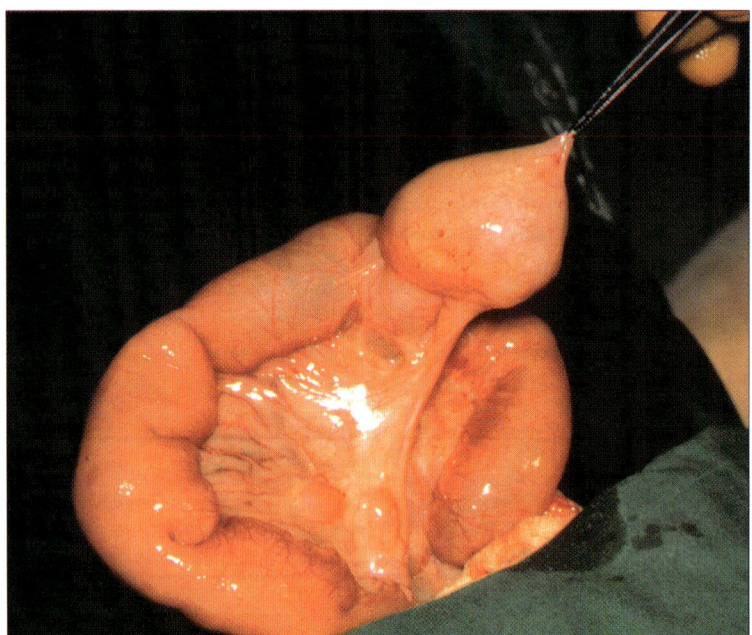

Fig. 1.22 Meckel's diverticulum. This remnant of the vitellointestinal duct is present in 1–2% of the population. Most give no trouble, but they can cause massive rectal haemorrhage (when ectopic gastric mucosa induces ulceration in the adjacent ileal mucosa), obstruction, an umbilical sinus (due to persistence of the vitellointestinal duct), or, less frequently, pain (which frequently mimics appendicitis).

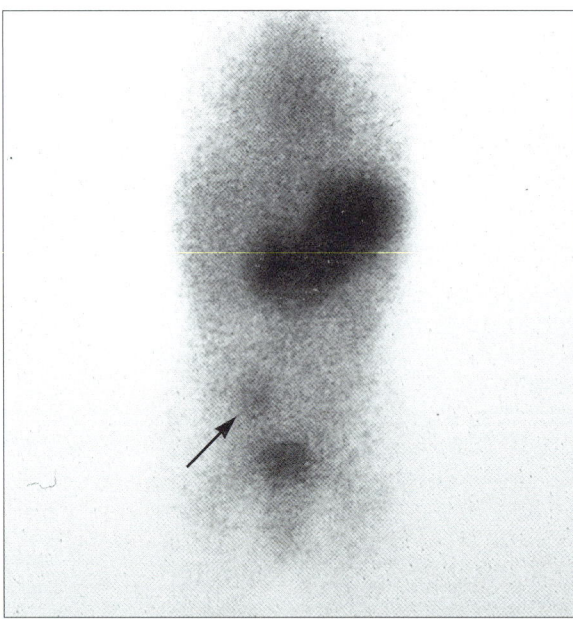

Fig. 1.23 Technetium Meckel's scan. A Meckel's diverticulum cannot usually be demonstrated on contrast study, but ectopic gastric mucosa (present in 30% of cases) excretes technetium. The diverticulum is seen as a hot spot, usually in the right lower quadrant. With the administration of an H_2-antagonist pre-scan, 95% accuracy can be achieved when ectopic gastric mucosa is present. False positives are rare.

Congenital and Neonatal Conditions

NECROTISING ENTEROCOLITIS

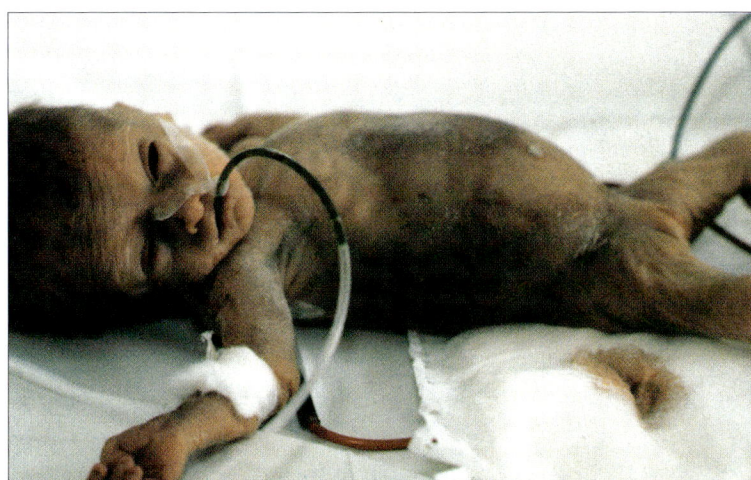

Fig 1.24 Necrotising enterocolitis. NEC occurs almost exclusively in the newborn, and is a focal or diffuse disorder, characterised by ulceration and necrosis of the gut, usually the distal small bowel and colon. Clinically, neonates develop distension, bile-stained vomiting, and blood in the stools. In some babies, like the one shown, the disease runs a fulminant course, and emergency surgery, following resuscitation, is required to save life. The disease affects 2.5% of all infants in neonatal intensive care units. Risk factors include prematurity, asphyxia, exchange transfusion, and intrauterine growth retardation.

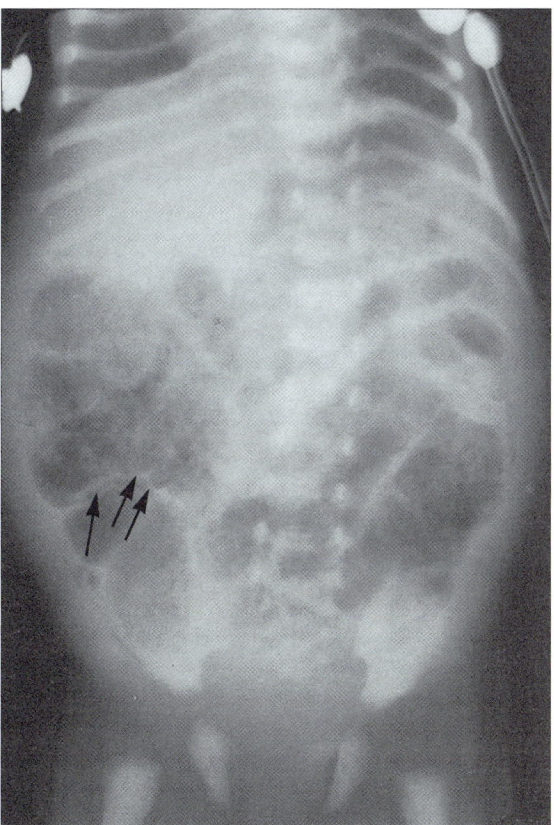

Fig. 1.25 Necrotising enterocolitis: radiology. Pneumatosis intestinalis (intramural gas) is the pathognomonic radiological sign in NEC. Intestinal dilatation, pneumoperitoneum, and intra-abdominal fluid may also be present; the finding of either of the latter two usually indicates the need for surgical intervention.

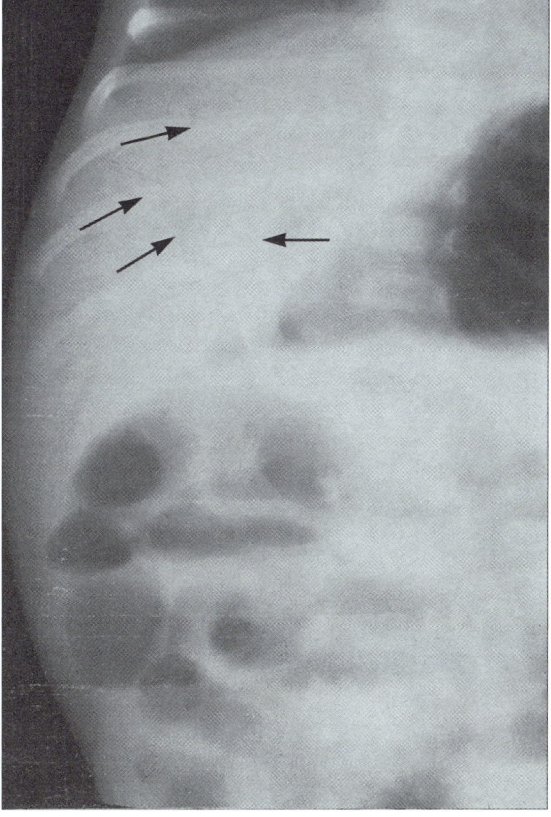

Fig. 1.26 Necrotising enterocolitis: radiology. The invasion of the gut wall by gas-forming organisms may lead, in addition to intramural gas, to gas within the hepatic portal venous system, as shown here.

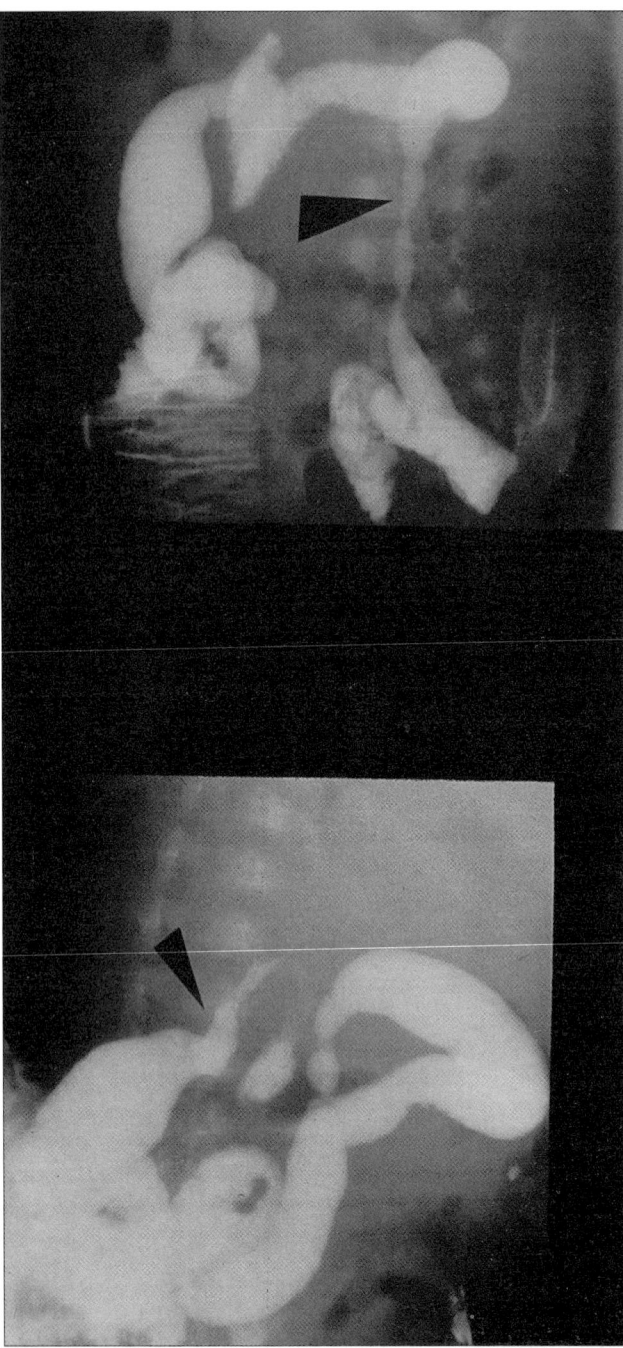

Fig. 1.27 Necrotising enterocolitis: strictures. This complication (arrowed) occurs in up to 15% of cases of NEC. It is therefore essential to investigate radiologically any defunctioned gut before restoring continuity surgically. Most stenoses (80–90%) occur in the colon, particularly in the left colon. Severe NEC is a potent cause of intestinal failure, either as the result of extensive necrosis and/or resection, or because of long-term mucosal dysfunction in the remaining intestine. Long-term parenteral nutrition is often required in such patients.

2. Oesophagus

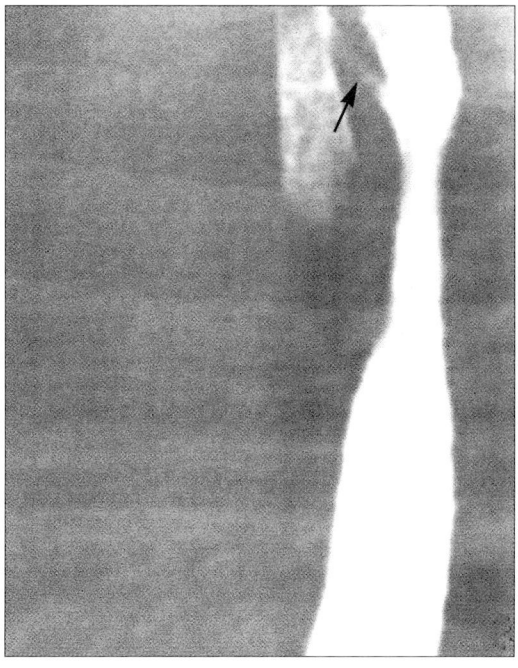

Fig. 2.1 Oesophagus. The oesophagus is the commonest site of atresia in the alimentary tract, caused by failure of canalisation of the alimentary tube. Ninety per cent of cases have an associated distal tracheo-oesophageal fistula. This slide shows an example of the uncommon, H-type fistula. Symptoms include choking associated with feeding and recurrent pneumonia. The diagnosis is made by demonstrating the fistula with Gastrografin.

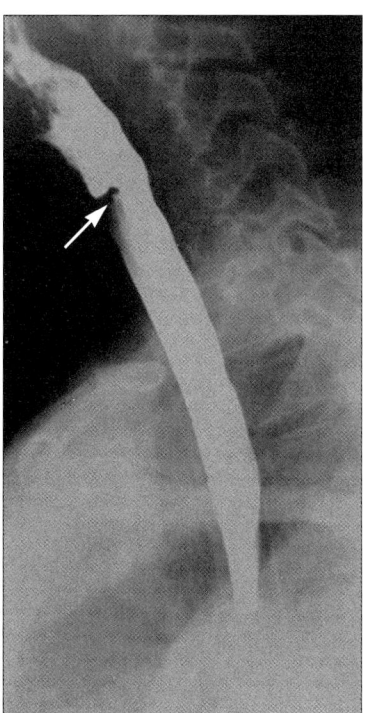
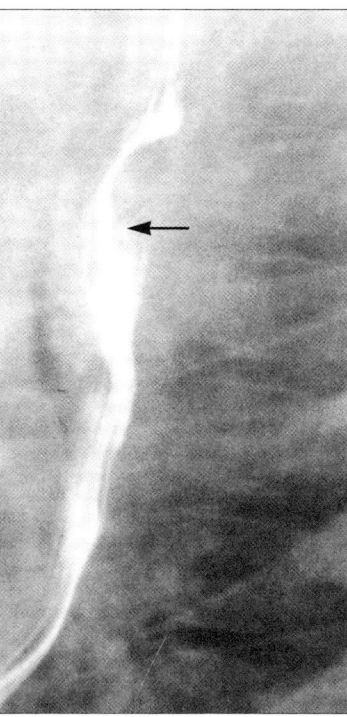

Figs 2.2, 2.3 Dysphagia. Dysphagia may also be caused by an oesophageal web (Plummer–Vinson syndrome) (**2.2**, left) or a vascular ring (**2.3**, right).

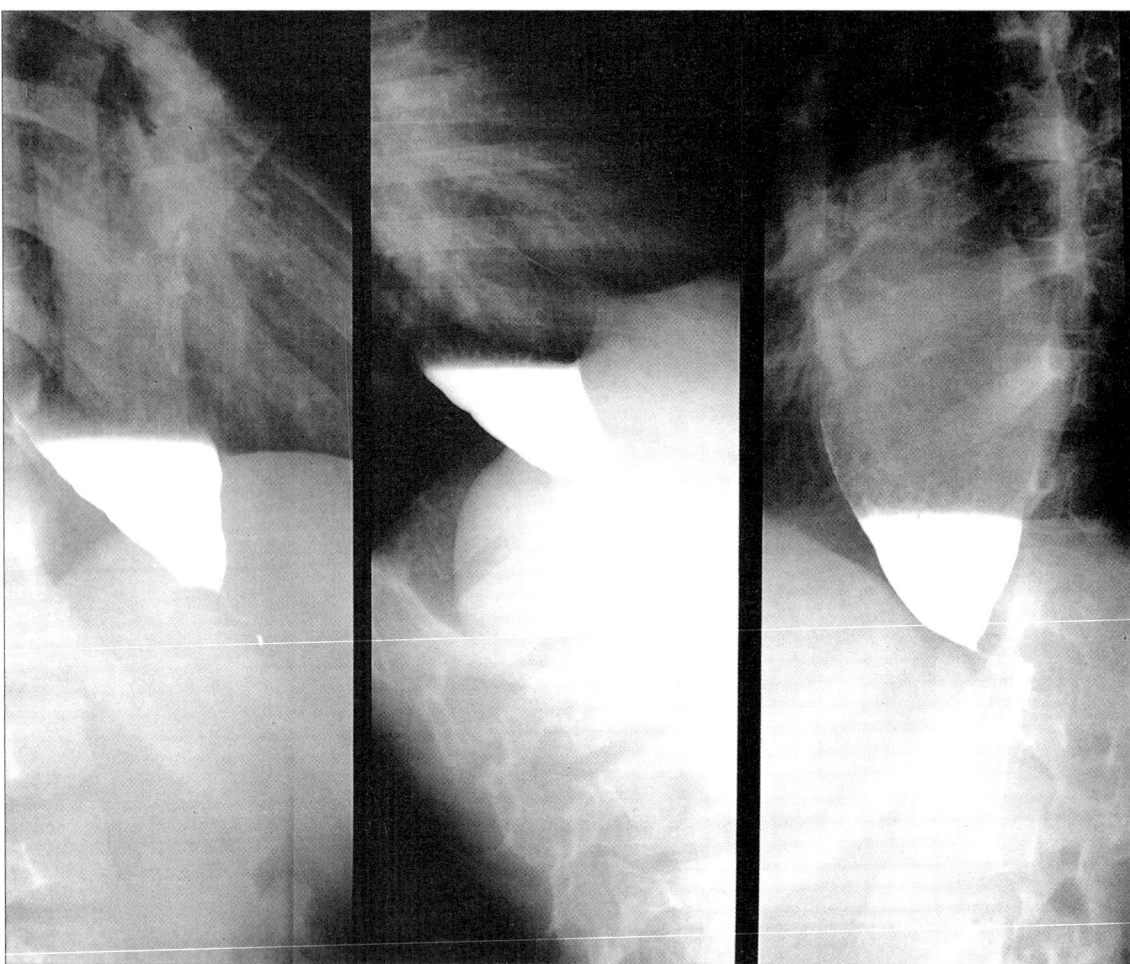

Fig. 2.4 Achalasia. Achalasia of the oesophagus is an uncommon cause of dysphagia and vomiting in childhood. The aetiology is unknown, but it may be secondary to a neuropathic process affecting the myenteric plexus. Motility studies show disturbed peristalsis and the lower oesophageal sphincter has a raised basal pressure and poor relaxation on swallowing. The diagnosis is demonstrated here by a barium swallow, which shows pooling of the barium above the achalasia. It is possible to dilate the constricted lower oesophageal sphincter using a balloon, but a myotomy may be the treatment of choice.

Figs 2.5, 2.6 Gastro-oesophageal reflux. Gastro-oesophageal reflux is a common symptom in infancy. It may be associated with a sliding hiatus hernia (**2.5**, top), which is complicated by pulmonary aspiration in this child (**2.6**, bottom). Note the fluid level in the large hiatus hernia seen behind the heart (**2.6**, bottom).

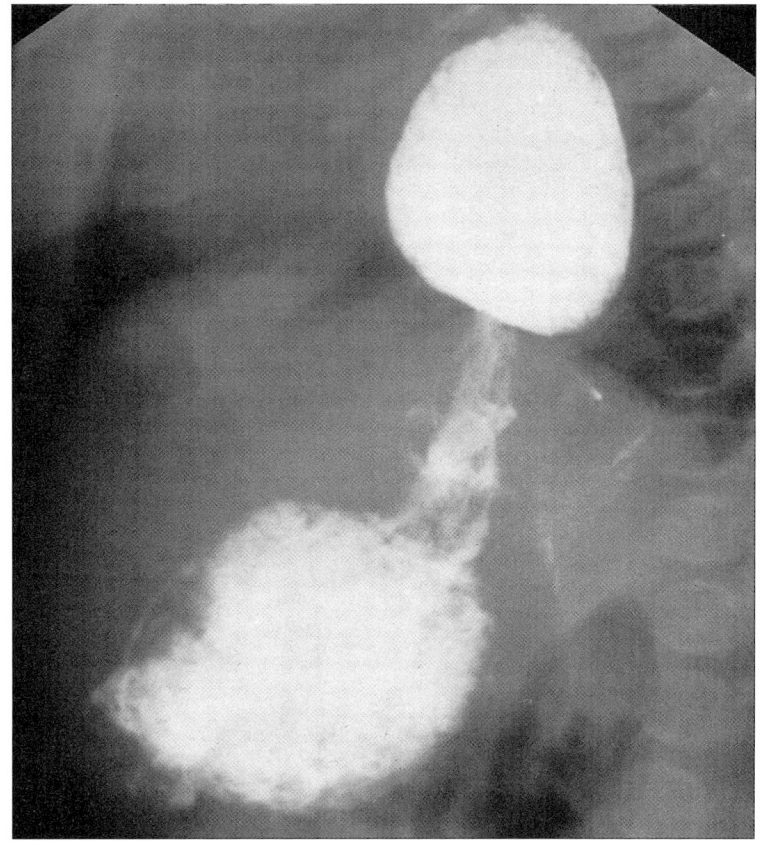

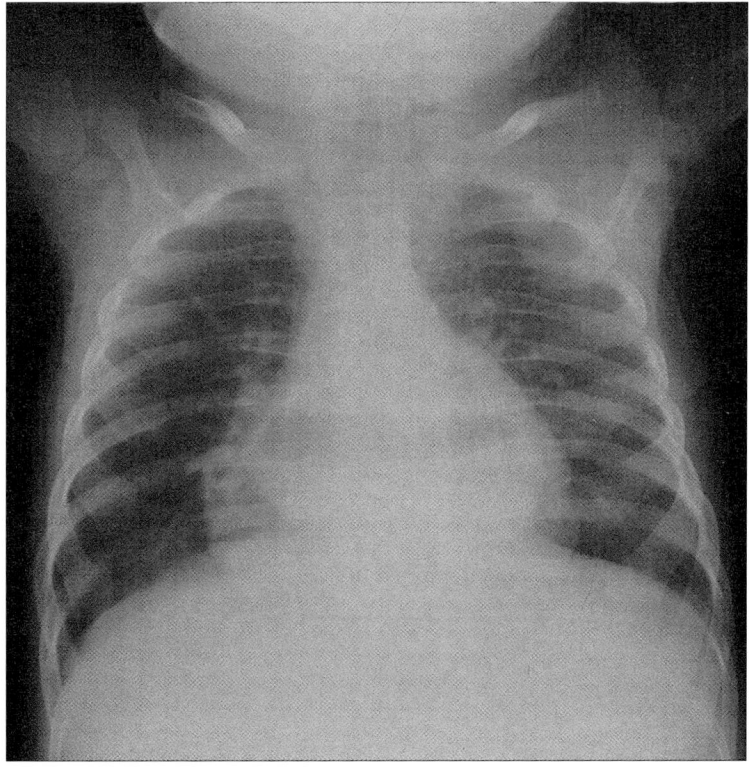

Pediatric Gastroenterology and Hepatology

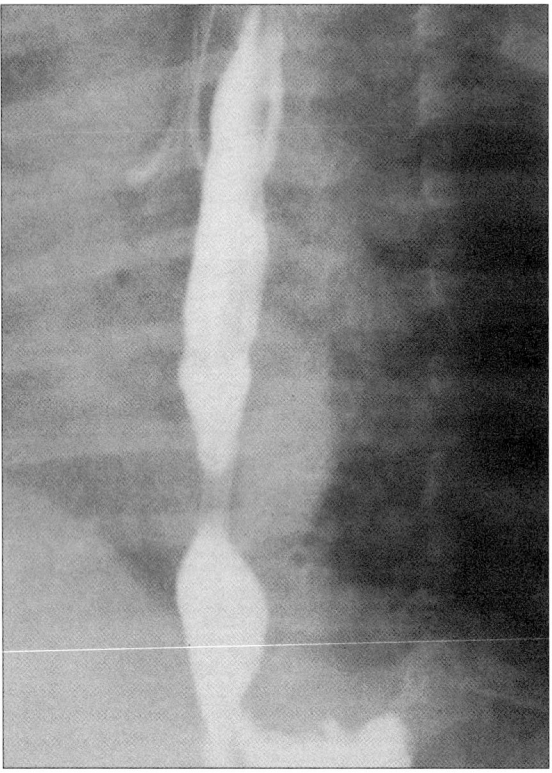

Fig. 2.7 Gastro-oesophageal reflux. Severe gastro-oesophageal reflux may be complicated by recurrent pulmonary aspiration. Reflux of barium to the level of the thoracic inlet and the aspiration of contrast into the trachea are shown here.

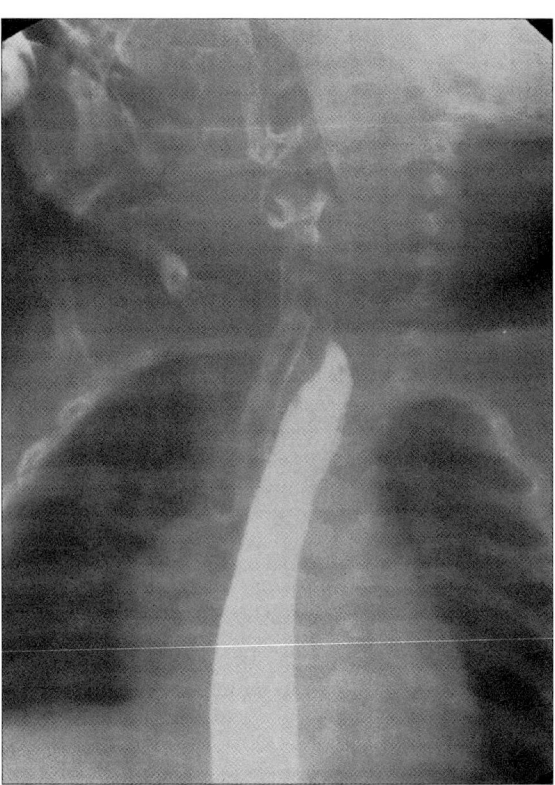

Fig. 2.8 Recurrent pulmonary aspiration. In some patients recurrent pulmonary aspiration may occur as a result of an incoordinated swallow.

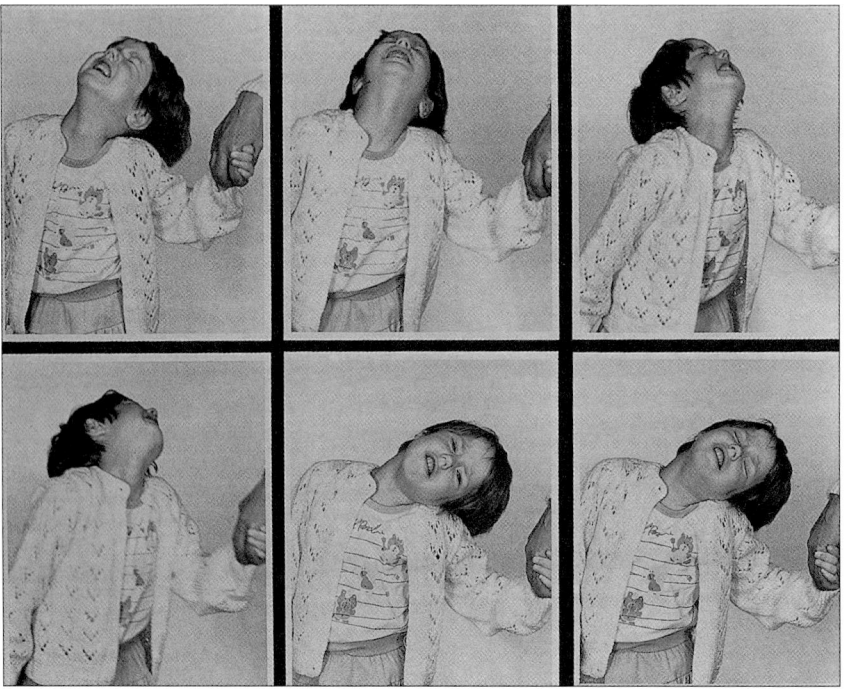

Fig. 2.9 Sandifer's syndrome. Sandifer's syndrome comprises severe gastro-oesophageal reflux and dystonic head posturing. Severe oesophagitis and iron-deficiency anaemia are common, and fundoplication is required. Symptoms disappear completely with successful treatment, usually fundoplication.

Oesophagus

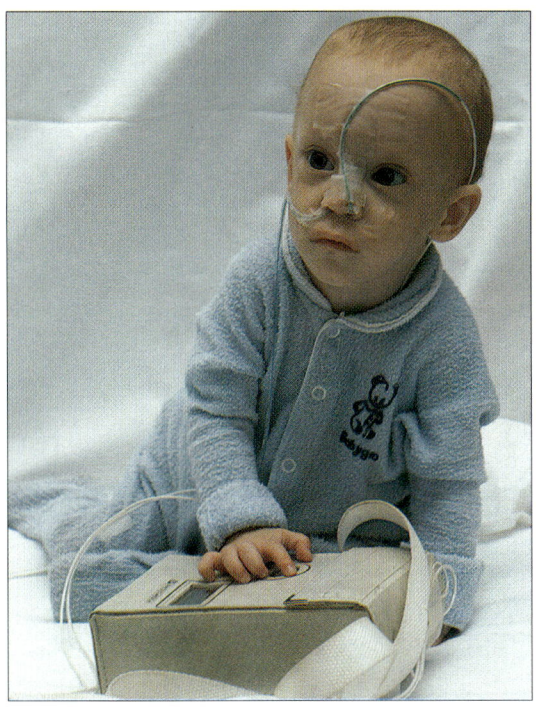

Fig. 2.10 Gastro-oesophageal reflux. The diagnosis of gastro-oesophageal reflux is best made by 24-hour ambulatory oesophageal pH monitoring. This is usually well-tolerated, even in very young patients.

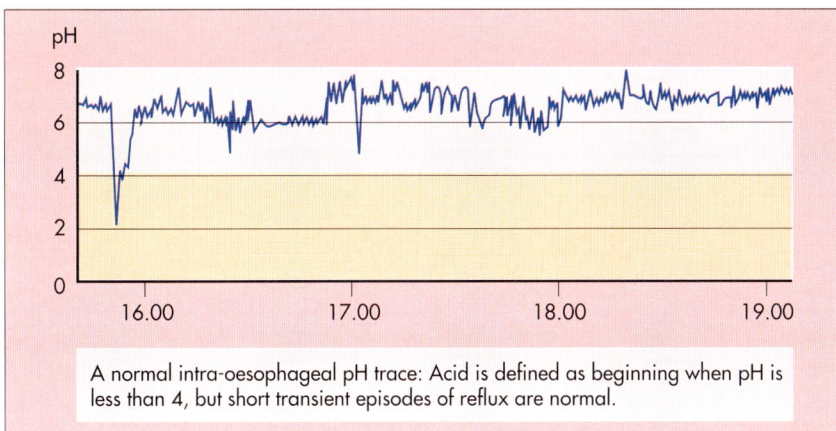

A normal intra-oesophageal pH trace: Acid is defined as beginning when pH is less than 4, but short transient episodes of reflux are normal.

Figs 2.11, 2.12 Oesophageal pH. Acid reflux is defined as beginning when the lower oesophageal pH falls to less than 4. In normal children, the lower oesophageal pH falls below pH 4 only infrequently (**2.11**, top), whereas in pathological reflux the lower oesophageal pH is below 4 for at least 5 % of the recorded time (**2.12**, bottom). (M = meal)

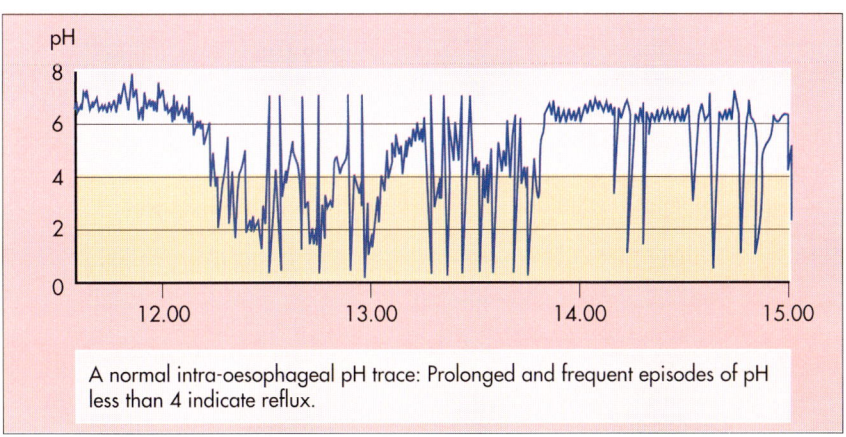

A normal intra-oesophageal pH trace: Prolonged and frequent episodes of pH less than 4 indicate reflux.

Pediatric Gastroenterology and Hepatology

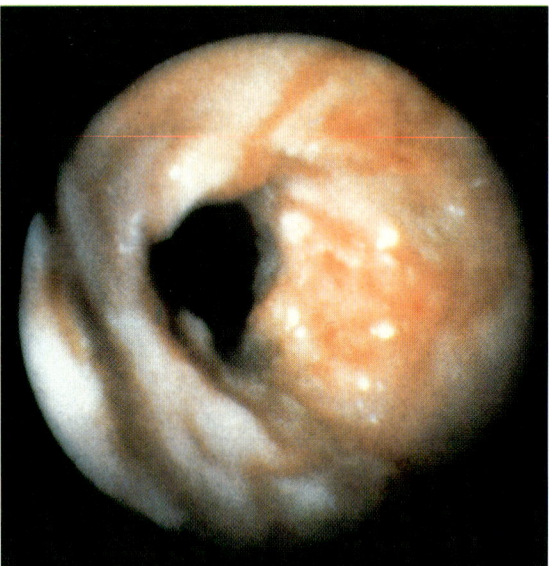 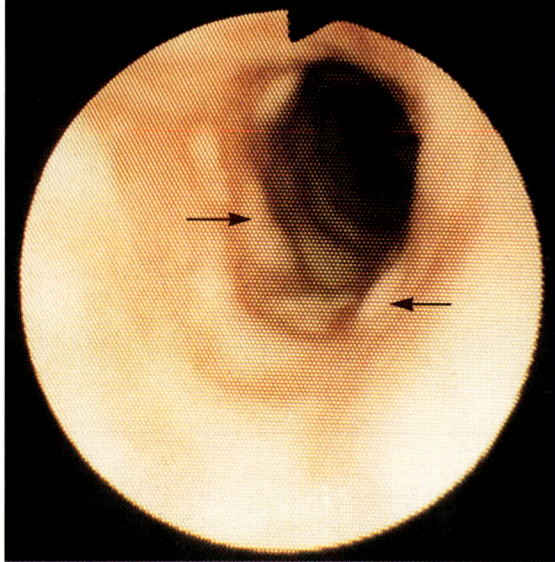

Figs 2.13, 2.14 Oesophagitis. The diagnosis of oesophagitis may be made endoscopically. There may be severe erosions and thickening of the mucosa (**2.13**, left) and occasionally ulceration (**2.14**, right).

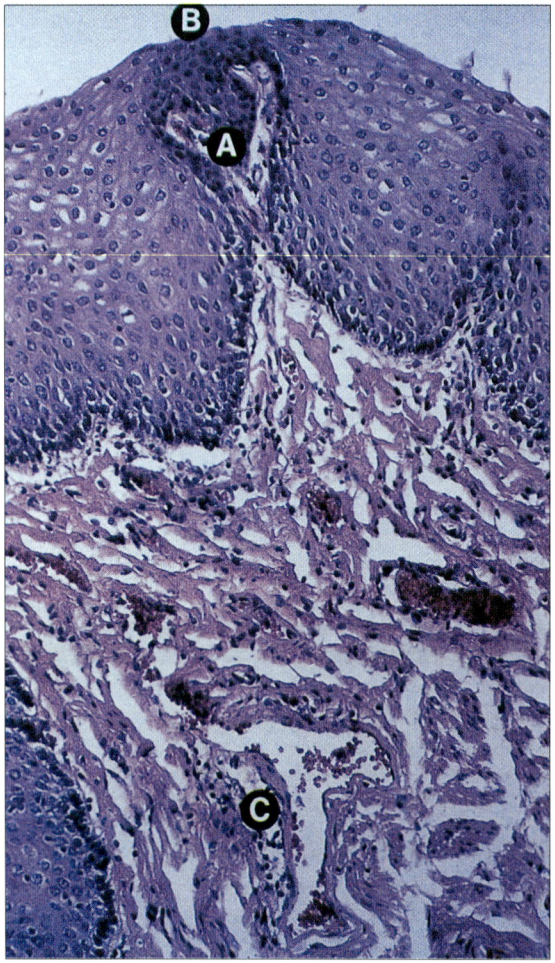

Fig. 2.15 Cellular hyperplasia. The absence of endoscopic abnormalities does not exclude reflux oesophagitis, so it is important to perform biopsies – cellular hyperplasia is noted in 90% of patients with oesophagitis. This biopsy shows basal cell hyperplasia accompanied by an increase in the height of the papillae (A). The superficial squamous cell level (B) is thinned and the lamina propria (C) shows minimal inflammatory cell infiltrate. (Haemotoxylin and Eosin, ×20.)

Oesophagus

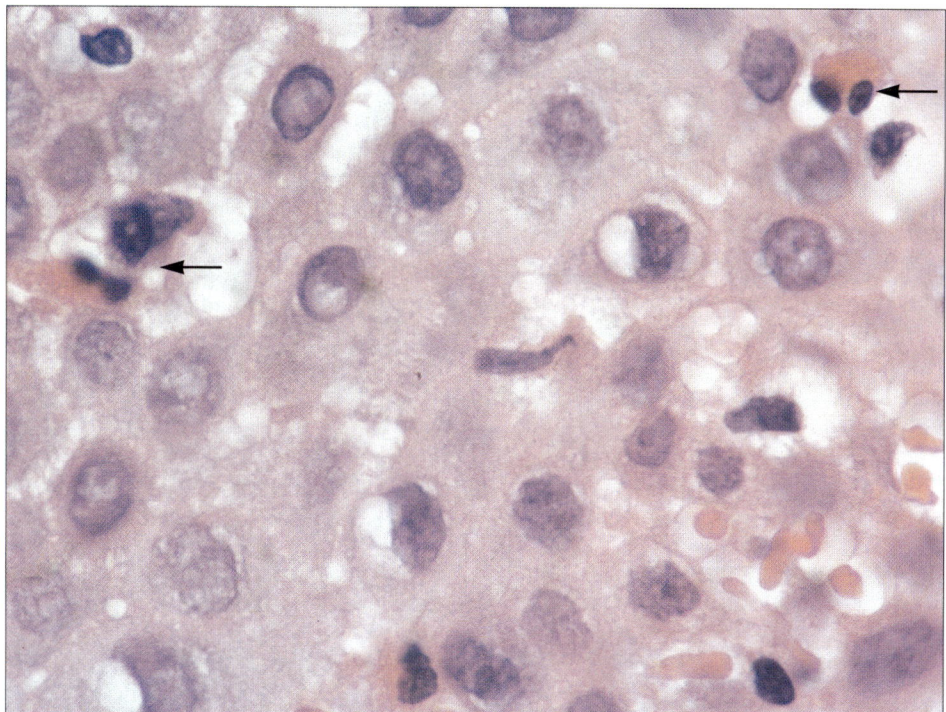

Fig. 2.16 Neutrophils and eosinophils. The presence of intraepithelial neutrophils and eosinophils in an oesophageal biopsy is abnormal and characteristic of reflux oesophagitis (Haemotoxylin and Eosin, ×40.).

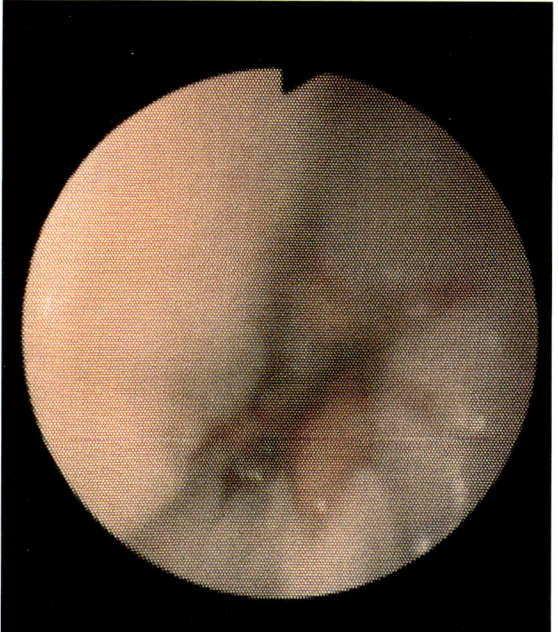 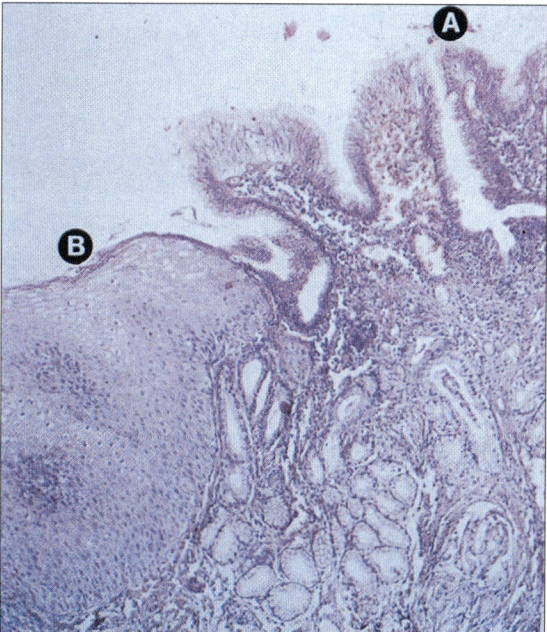

Figs 2.17, 2.18 Barrett's oesophagus. In Barrett's oesophagus (**2.17**, left) the distal part of the oesophagus is not lined by stratified squamous epithelium, but by columnar epithelium similar to that found in the stomach. The aetiology remains obscure, but gastro-oesophageal reflux is thought to be important. The propensity for columnar epithelium in this situation to develop adenocarcinoma is the chief cause for concern. Characteristic histological features (**2.18**, right, Haemotoxylin and Eosin, ×10) of Barrett's oesophagus are that islets of columnar (A), gastric-type mucosa are demonstrated between areas of squamous epithelium (B).

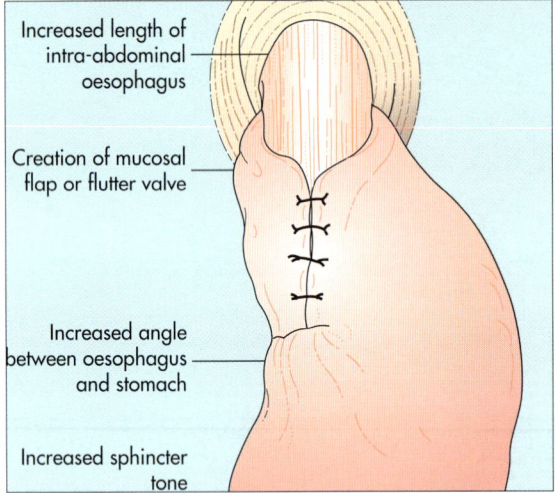

Fig. 2.19 Treatment of gastro-oesophageal reflux. The initial treatment of severe gastro-oesophageal reflux is usually with prokinetic agents (e.g., cisapride) and H$_2$-antagonists or proton pump inhibitors. If medical measures fail, then the treatment of choice is fundoplication, in which the gastric fundus is wrapped around the intra-abdominal portion of the oesophagus.

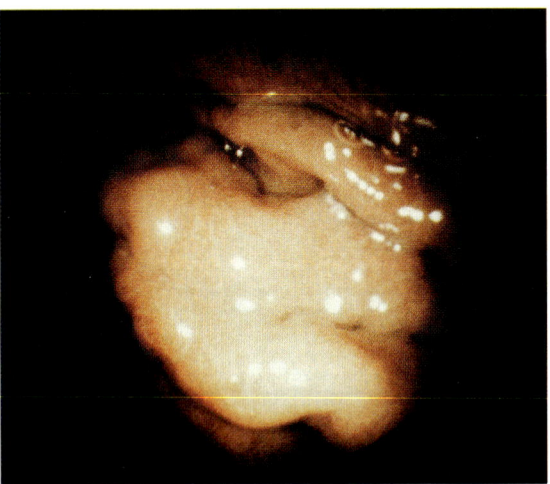
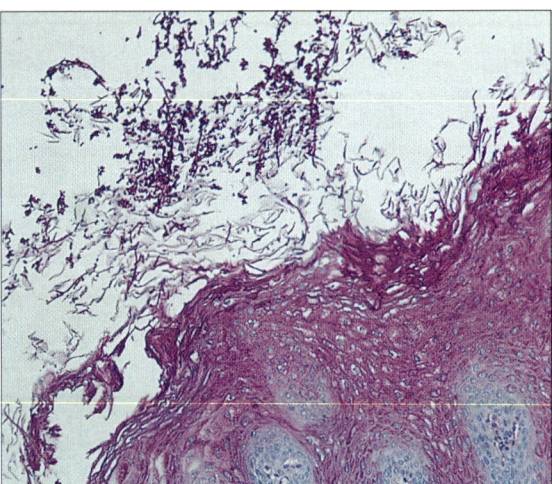

Figs 2.20, 2.21 Candidiasis. In immunosuppressed patients, candidiasis may affect the oesophagus. This may be demonstrated endoscopically (**2.20**, left) and confirmed histologically (**2.21**, right) by establishing the presence of hyphae and yeast on the surface of the epithelial mucosa (Periodic Acid–Schiff, ×10).

3. Stomach and Duodenum

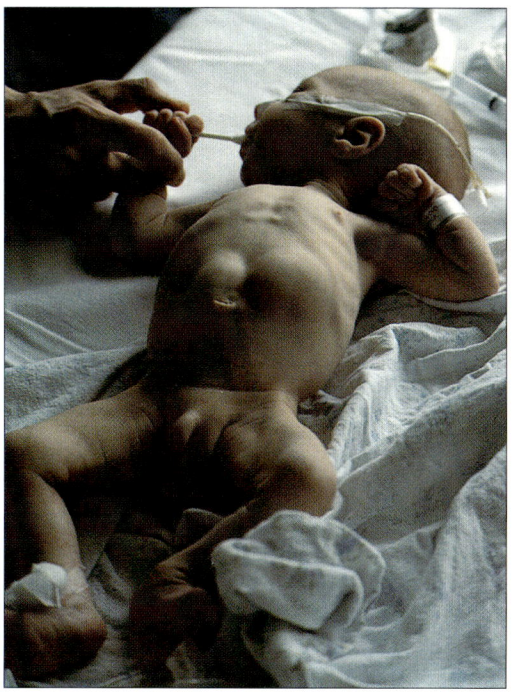

Fig. 3.1 Pyloric stenosis. Pyloric stenosis presents with projectile vomiting at about 4–6 weeks of age. Subsequent electrolyte and fluid imbalance is frequent. Males are affected 4–5 times more commonly than are females, particularly first-born males. Demonstrated here is visible peristalsis in a dehydrated baby who had a 48-hour history of projectile vomiting.

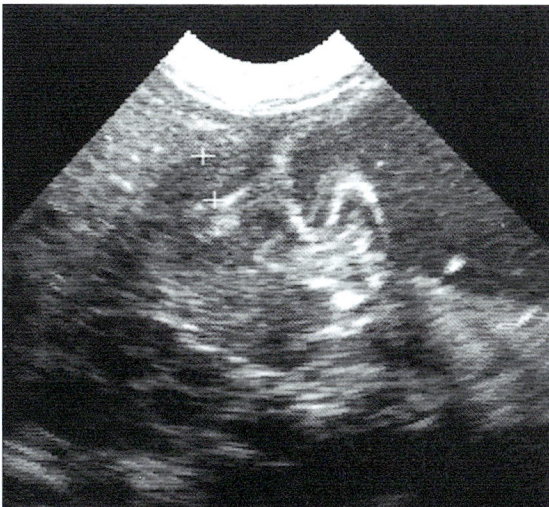

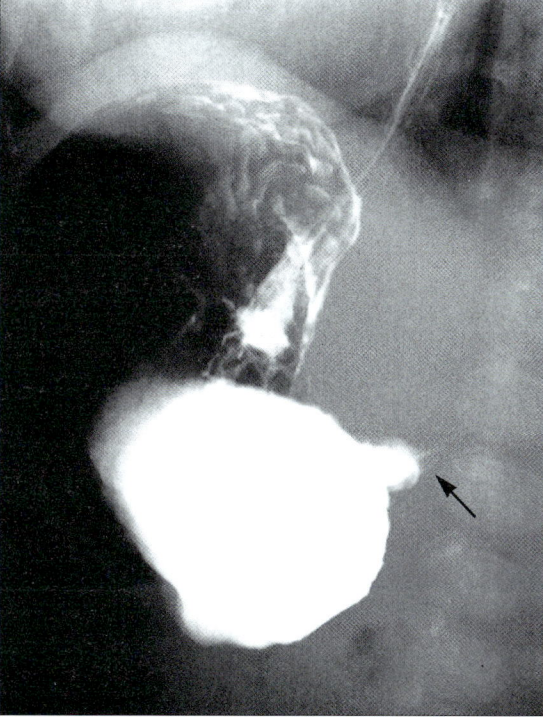

Figs 3.2, 3.3 Pyloric stenosis. The diagnosis may be suggested by ultrasonography, which reveals the thickened muscle as well as lengthening of the pyloric canal (**3.2**, left). If ultrasound is equivocal, the diagnosis may then be confirmed by barium meal, which demonstrates an elongated and narrow pylorus (tramline) (**3.3**, right).

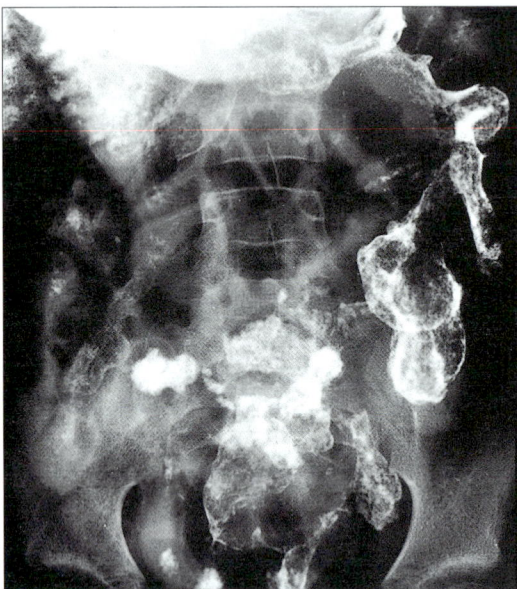
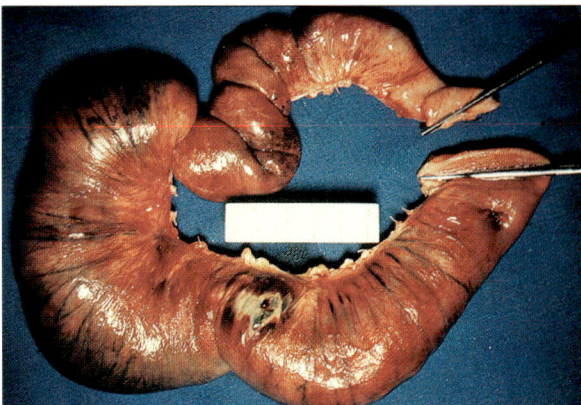
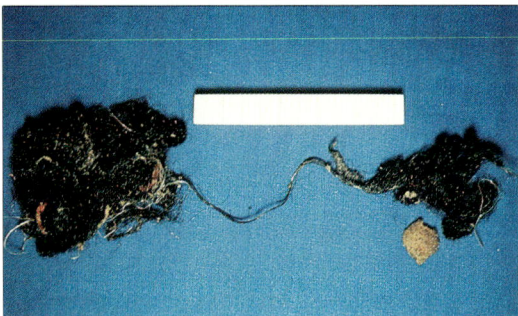

Figs 3.4–3.6 Foreign bodies. Psychologically disturbed children may swallow large numbers of foreign bodies, particularly hair and other non-nutritive material. This patient presented with recurrent abdominal pain and vomiting, and on three occasions with acute intussusception. Barium studies show multiple filling defects, which give rise to a bizarre radiological picture (**3.4**, top left). At laparotomy the gangrenous ileo-ileal intussusception was resected (**3.5**, top right). On opening, this revealed hair, string, foam, and wool (**3.6**, bottom left).

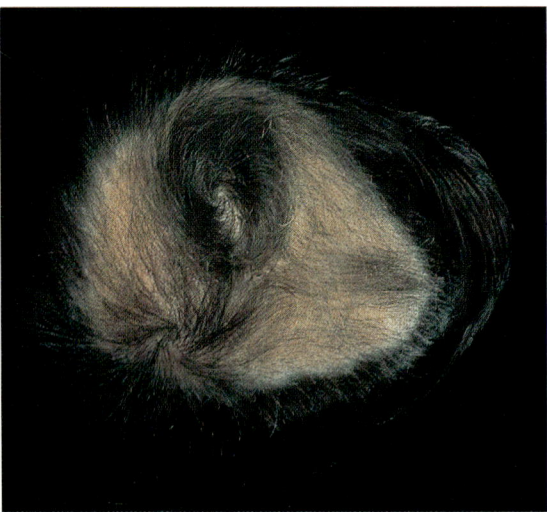

Figs 3.7 Trichotillomania This child's scalp showed evidence of trichotillomania. The area of hair loss was irregular and tended to migrate, with stubble growing at the edges. This was produced by repetitive twisting and pulling of hair which was then ingested.

Stomach and Duodenum

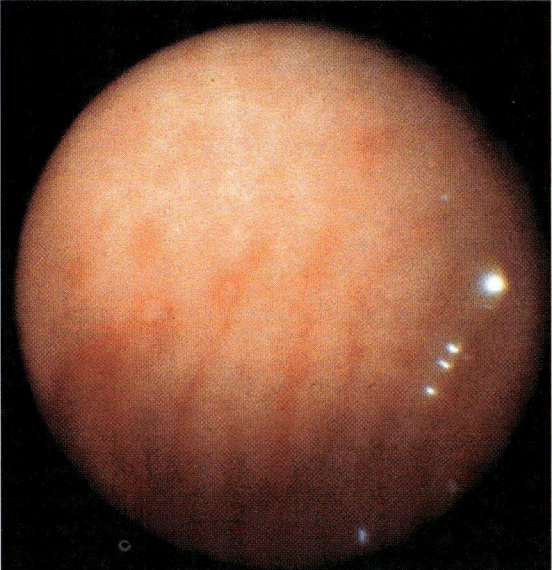 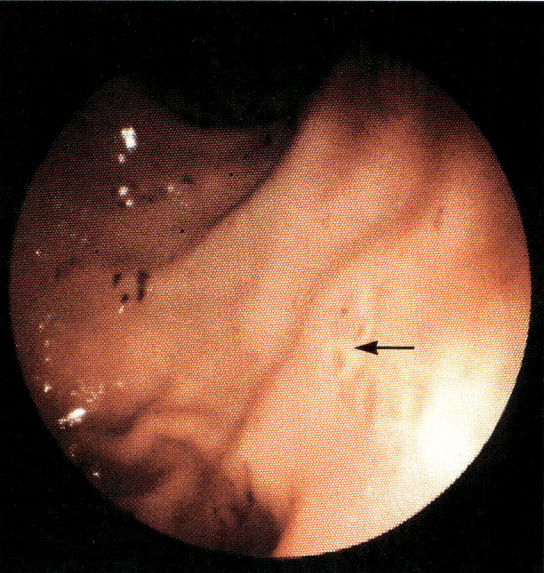

Figs 3.8, 3.9 Stress ulceration. The commonest disorders to affect the stomach are related to acid peptic disease. Gastric ulcers are rare in children under 6 years of age, but duodenal ulcers have been detected in children of all ages. Stress ulceration accounts for at least 80% of peptic disease in infancy and early childhood and is associated with shock, respiratory failure, sepsis, hypoglycaemia, intracranial lesions, burns, and liver disease (**3.8**, left). Stress ulceration may also be secondary to the use of aspirin or other non-steroidal anti-inflammatory agents (**3.9**, right). Symptoms include vomiting, abdominal discomfort, and haematemesis.

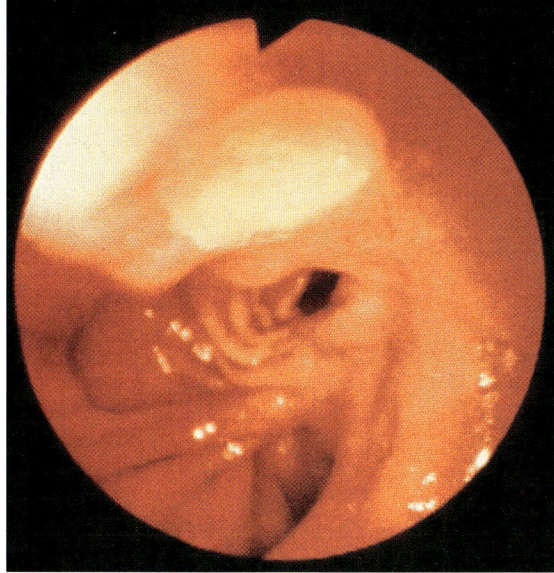

Fig. 3.10 Gastric ulcers. Gastric ulceration is rare in childhood. When it occurs, the ulcers are usually detected in the gastric antrum and may be diagnosed endoscopically. There is good response to H_2-antagonists or proton pump inhibitors. Recurrence is rare.

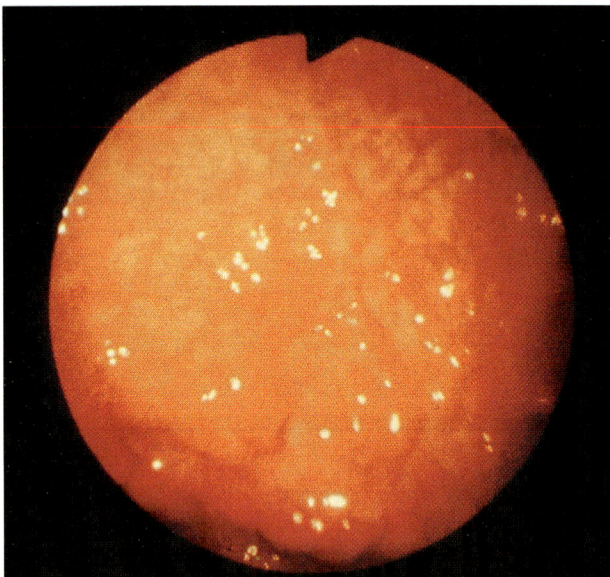

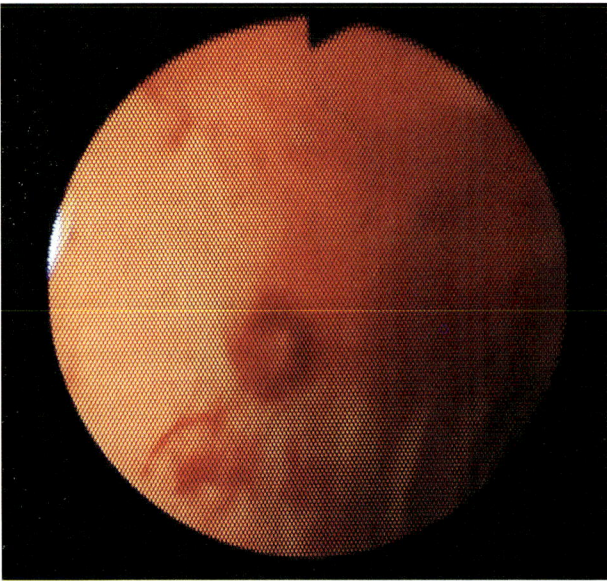

Figs 3.11, 3.12 *Helicobacter pylori* infection.
H. pylori may be associated with an antral gastritis (**3.11**, top) or with a bleeding duodenal ulcer (**3.12**, bottom). The diagnosis of *H. pylori* infection may be made serologically or histologically. Treatment is with antibiotics and H_2-antagonists or proton pump inhibitors.

Stomach and Duodenum

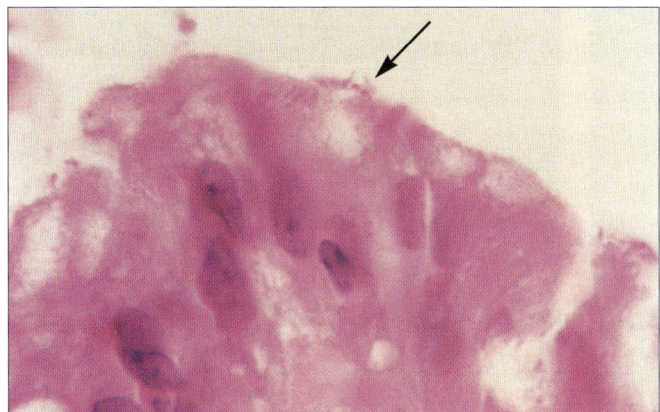

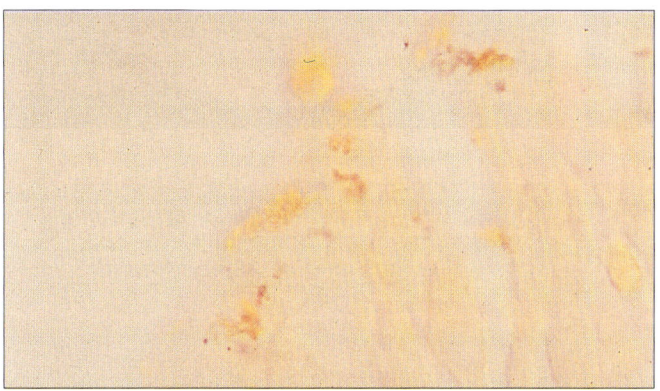

Figs 3.13, 3.14 xHelicobacter pylori. This biopsy demonstrates helicobacter on the surface of the gastric mucosa (**3.13**, top). The bacteria may also be demonstrated using a silver stain (**3.14**, bottom). (**3.13**, Haematoxylin and Eosin ×40; **3.14**, silver stain ×40).

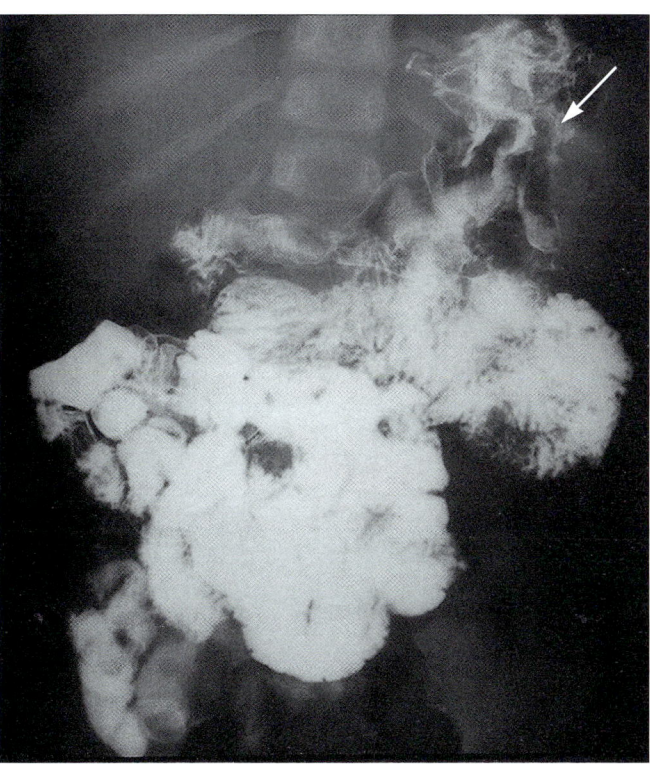

Fig. 3.15 Ménétrier's disease. Ménétrier's disease, or hypertrophic gastropathy, may produce severe protein loss in an otherwise asymptomatic child. This barium study indicates hypertrophic gastric folds with increased gastric residue. The cause is unknown, although cytomegalovirus infection has been described in some cases.

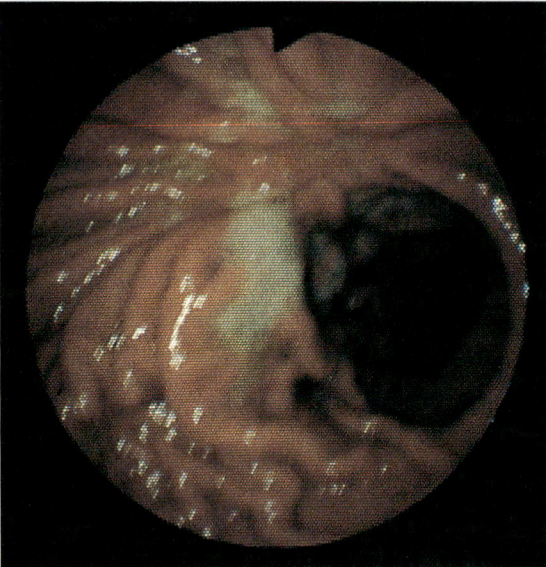

Fig. 3.16 Carcinoma. Carcinoma of the stomach is extremely rare in childhood. However, the stomach may be involved with lymphoma, which may present as a gastric ulcer.

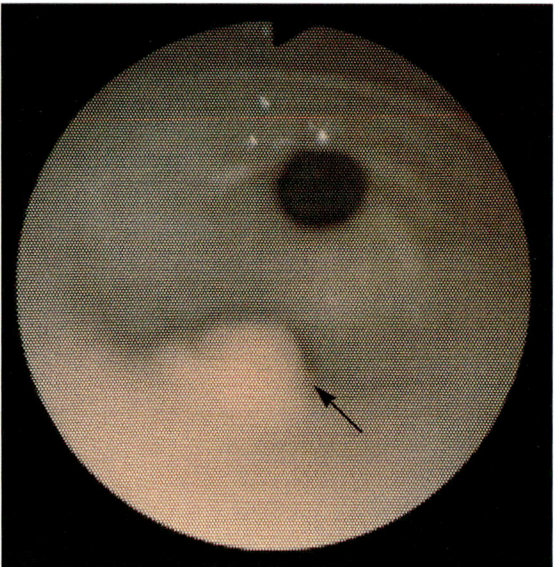

Fig. 3.17 Pancreatic rest. Ectopic pancreatic tissue within the submucosa of the stomach is an uncommon coincidental finding in children undergoing endoscopy; central umbilication is characteristic. The lesion may occasionally ulcerate, bleed, or produce obstruction.

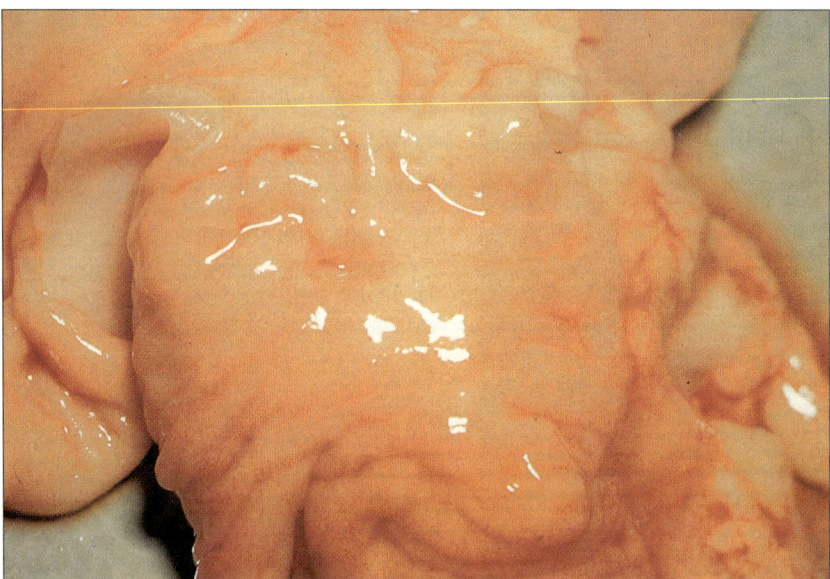

Fig. 3.18 Duodenal ulceration. Although duodenal ulceration is less common in children than in adults, difficulties in diagnosis may lead to perforation, as in this 5-year-old boy.

4. Small Intestine Diseases

COELIAC DISEASE

In contrast to other dietary protein intolerances, intolerance to gluten in coeliac disease is life-long. The proximal small intestinal mucosa is abnormal, and removal of gluten from the diet leads to clinical and histological resolution. The incidence of malignancy in later life is increased, but is probably normal in those patients who adhere strictly to a gluten-free diet.

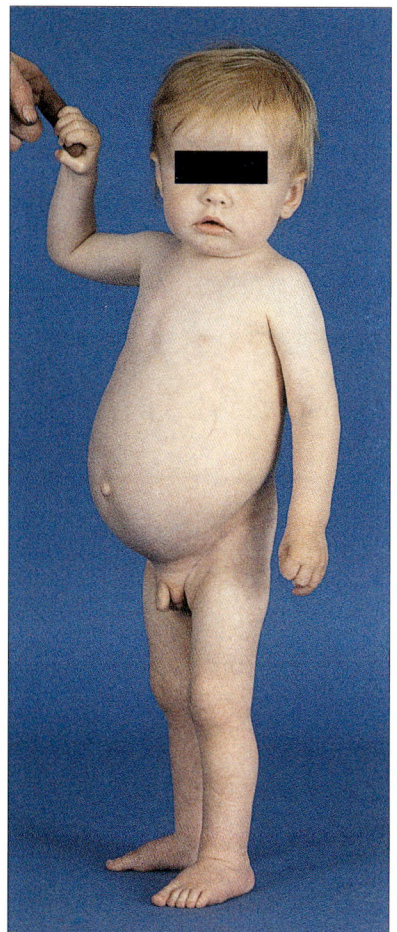

Fig. 4.1 Coeliac disease in a toddler. This 24-month-old child presented with a history of several months diarrhoea and failure to thrive. The abdomen is markedly distended and the child looks miserable. Muscle wasting is present and the child was hypotonic with delayed motor milestones. These classic appearances are often much less marked.

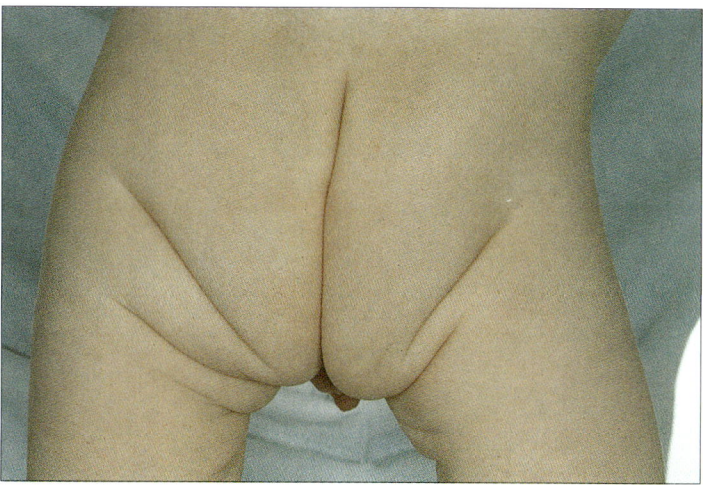

Fig. 4.2 Buttock wasting. Buttock wasting is marked in this child with coeliac disease. Redundant skin over the buttocks leads to the production of abnormal skin creases.

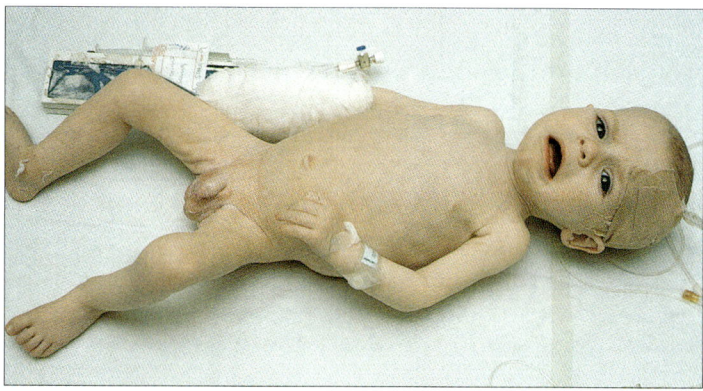

Fig. 4.3 Coeliac crisis. This boy presented at 7 months of age with severe protracted diarrhoea, malnutrition, and electrolyte disturbance. He required intravenous fluids, but failed to improve despite the removal of gluten from his diet. He responded quickly to corticosteroids and enteral nutrition. This presentation of coeliac disease is now fortunately rare, and tends to be confined to young patients less than 2 years of age.

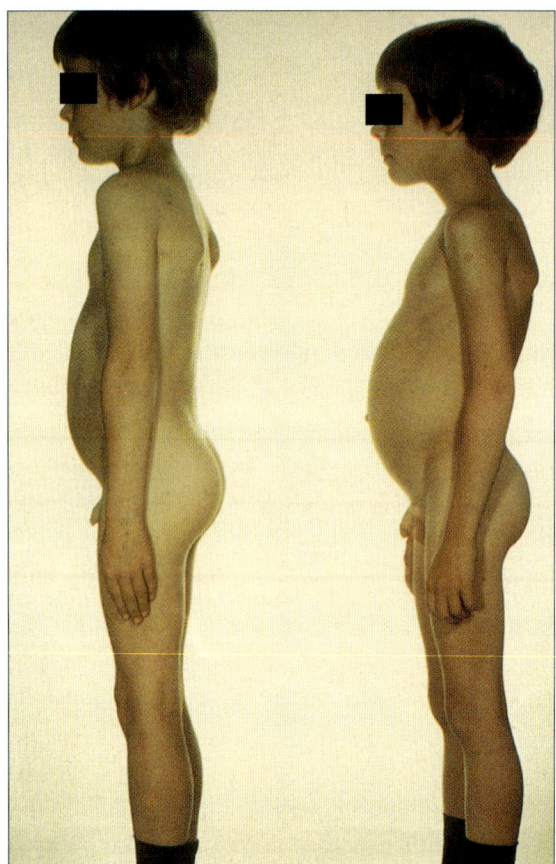

Fig. 4.4 Growth failure. Patients with coeliac disease may present with growth failure, but without gastrointestinal symptoms. The shorter of these identical twins was referred from the growth clinic, after tests for growth hormone deficiency proved normal. Crohn's disease may present in a similar way.

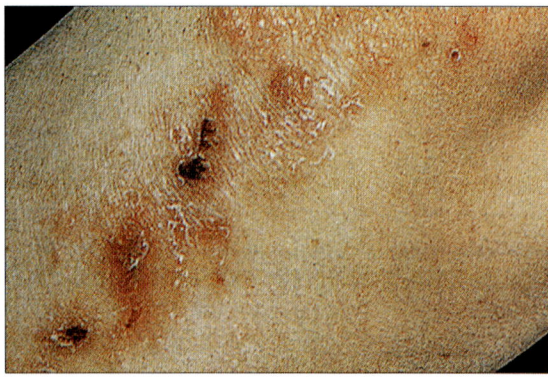

Fig. 4.6. Dermatitis herpetiformis. Shown here is the intensely itchy and vascular skin rash of dermatitis herpetiformis. The disease is associated with a lesion in the jejunal mucosa in over 80% of cases; the lesion is histologically identical to that in coeliac disease. Gluten withdrawal generally leads to resolution of both the rash and the intestinal lesion.

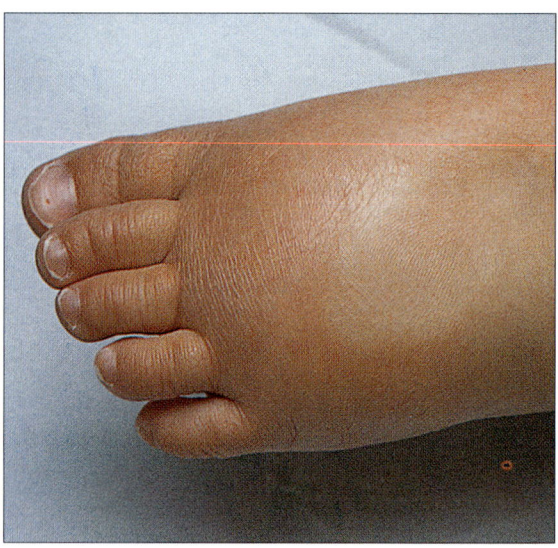

Fig. 4.5 Hypoalbuminaemic oedema in coeliac disease. Presentation in some patients with coeliac disease may be dominated by the sequelae of malabsorption, such as anaemia. Oedema due to hypoalbuminaemia may be the dominating feature in about 15% of patients. Hypoalbuminaemia results from a combination of maldigestion, malabsorption, and protein-losing enteropathy.

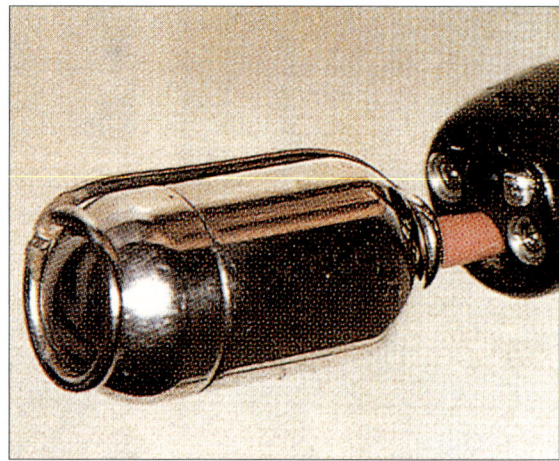

Fig. 4.7 Jejunal biopsy. Despite the high diagnostic sensitivity and specificity of anti-gliadin and anti-endomyseal antibody assays in combination, jejunal biopsy remains an essential part of the diagnosis of coeliac disease. A characteristically abnormal biopsy, with typical clinical and anthropometric responses, is required in children over 2 years of age. A later gluten challenge is also required in the presence of atypical features or an early presentation below 2 years of age (when transient gluten intolerance is possible). The classic jejunal biopsy capsule provides excellent biopsies, but may be time-consuming, can fail to deliver a biopsy, and involves exposure to irradiation. Endoscopy biopsies with forceps are quicker, but the biopsies are smaller. 'Muzzle loading' the capsule into an endoscope is felt by some to be the best compromise.

Small Intestine Diseases

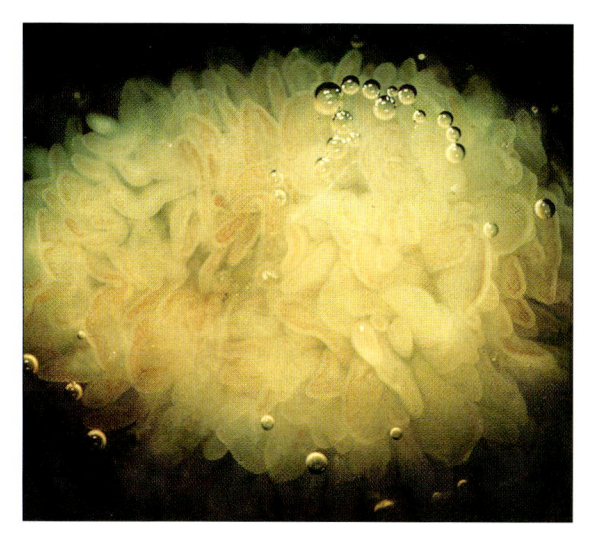

Fig. 4.8 Normal jejunal mucosa. The dissecting microscope appearances of normal jejunal mucosa. Multiple, finger, and leaf-like villi are present.

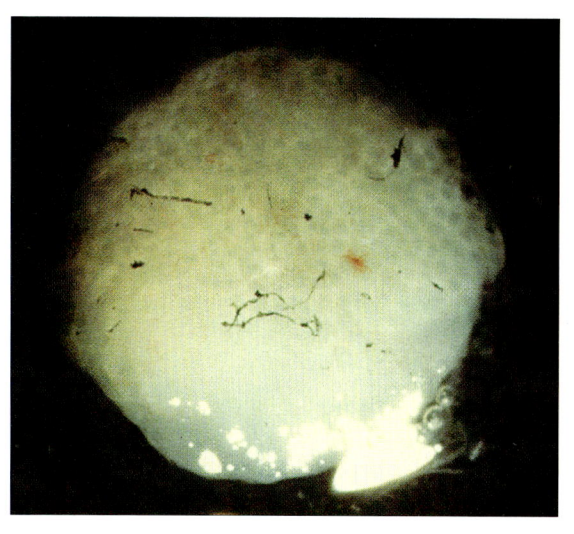

Fig. 4.9 Flat jejunal mucosa. In children with coeliac disease, the dissecting microscope appearances of the jejunum show that the villi are almost completely absent, with a consequent loss of absorptive surface area. The surface has a mosaic appearance due to the presence of hyperplastic crypts.

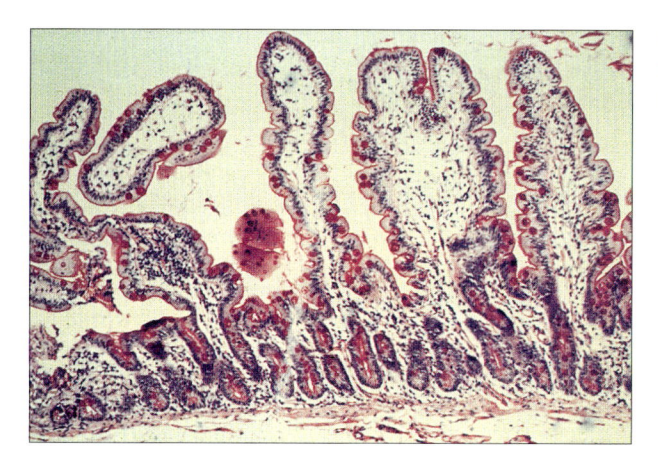

Fig. 4.10 Normal jejunal mucosa on light microscopy. On light microscopy, normal villi are present, with a villus:crypt ratio of at least 2:1.

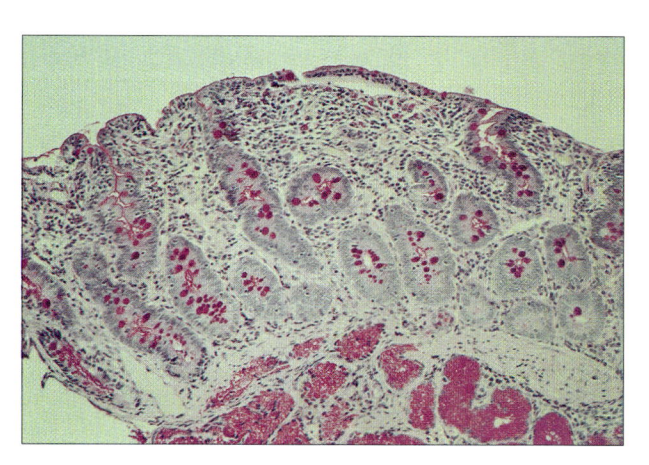

Fig. 4.11 Flat jejunal mucosa in untreated coeliac disease. The villi are almost completely lost (sub-total villous atrophy) and the crypts are elongated and hyperplastic. The lamina propria is infiltrated by plasma cells and lymphocytes, and intraepithelial lymphocytes are increased. The normal columnar epithelial cells are cuboidal.

35

Pediatric Gastroenterology and Hepatology

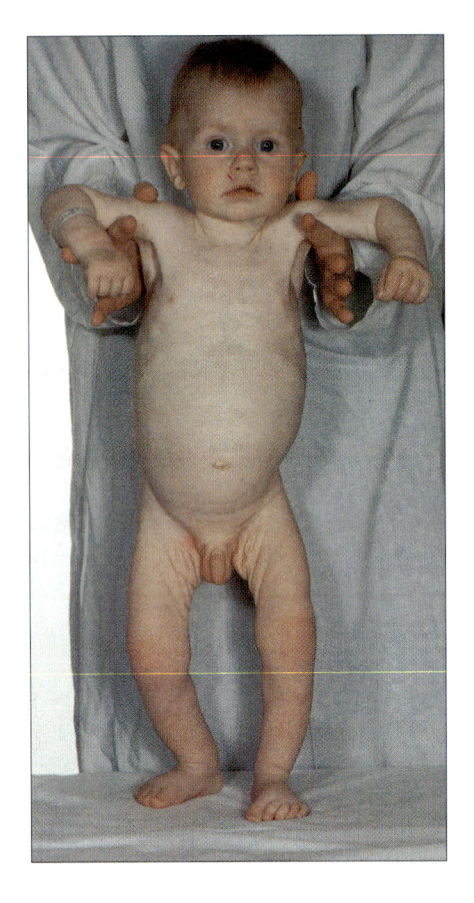

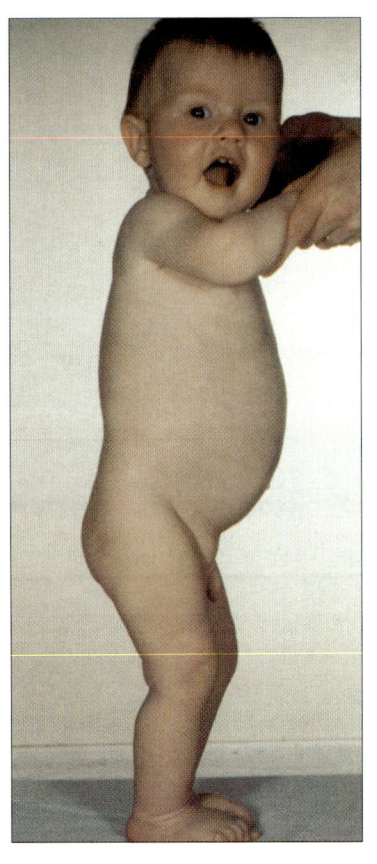

Figs 4.12, 4.13 Response to gluten withdrawal. At presentation, this toddler (**4.12**) was wasted, pot-bellied, apathetic, and miserable. Within a few weeks of gluten withdrawal (**4.13**), his parents described him as a 'different child'. He was happier and playful, and rapid weight gain followed. Catch-up in weight is normally complete 6–12 months after starting the diet, but height does not catch up for 2 years. Abnormal distension is often the final abnormal clinical sign to resolve.

COWS' MILK INTOLERANCE

In contrast to coeliac disease, cows' milk intolerance is transient, and about 70–90% of affected patients have outgrown their intolerance by the age of 2 years. Dietary challenge (which should be done in hospital) is therefore appropriate after this age.

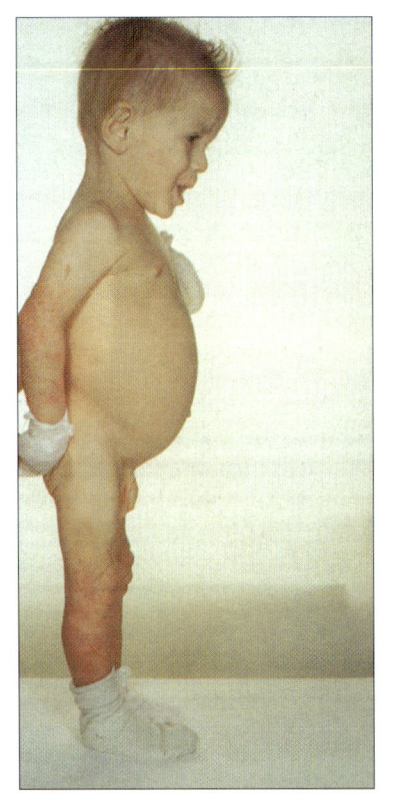

Fig. 4.14 Cows' milk protein intolerance. This toddler developed diarrhoea, vomiting, failure to thrive, and eczema following the introduction of cows' milk formula into the diet at 6 months of age. The patient is malnourished, has abdominal distension, and a jejunal biopsy showed a patchy villous atrophy with an eosinophilic infiltrate. Symptoms resolved rapidly following withdrawal of cows' milk from the diet and its replacement by a cows' milk substitute. Gastro-oesophageal reflux, without diarrhoea, may be an additional or alternative presenting symptom of cows' milk protein intolerance.

Small Intestine Diseases

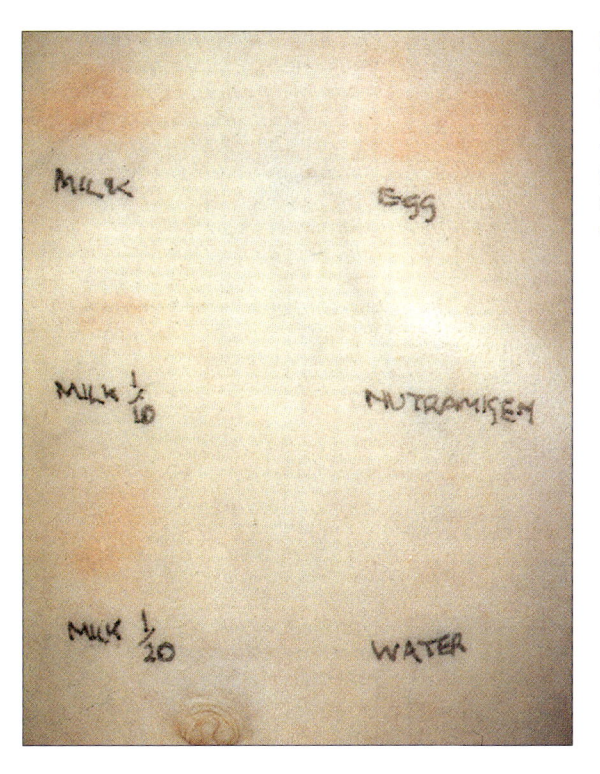

Fig. 4.15 Skin prick tests. Positive skin prick tests have no part to play in the diagnosis; they merely indicate that the patient is atopic. The diagnosis of cows' milk protein intolerance is based on the resolution of symptoms following withdrawal of cows' milk from the diet, and demonstrating the return of symptoms after a subsequent challenge. Tests for specific circulating antibodies to cows' milk (and other dietary antigens) have high specificity, but low sensitivity.

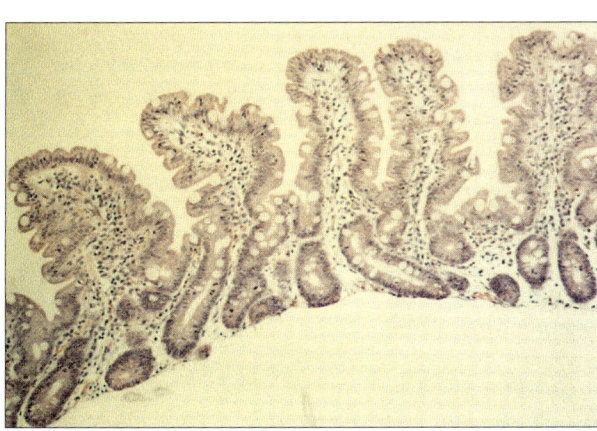

Fig. 4.16 Cows' milk protein intolerance (jejunal biopsy). Cows' milk protein intolerance can sometimes be associated with an enteropathy, leading to diarrhoea and failure to thrive. The lesion is often patchy, with some villi obviously shortened and others essentially normal. Histologically, the lesion is usually mild to moderate in severity; however, a flat biopsy can occur in this disorder.

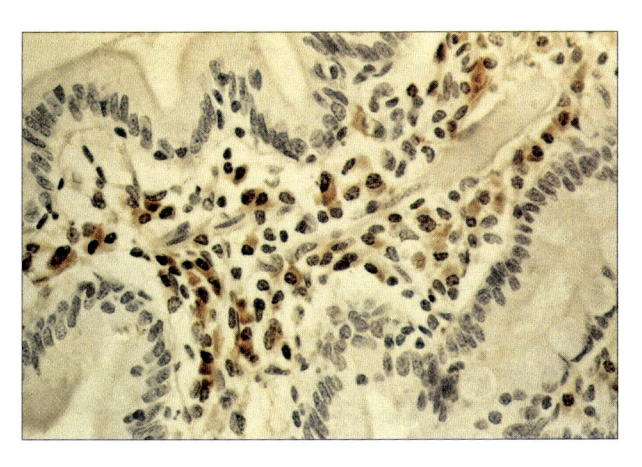

Fig. 4.17 Cows' milk protein intolerance (jejunal biopsy). An increase in eosinophils is sometimes found in the lamina propria.

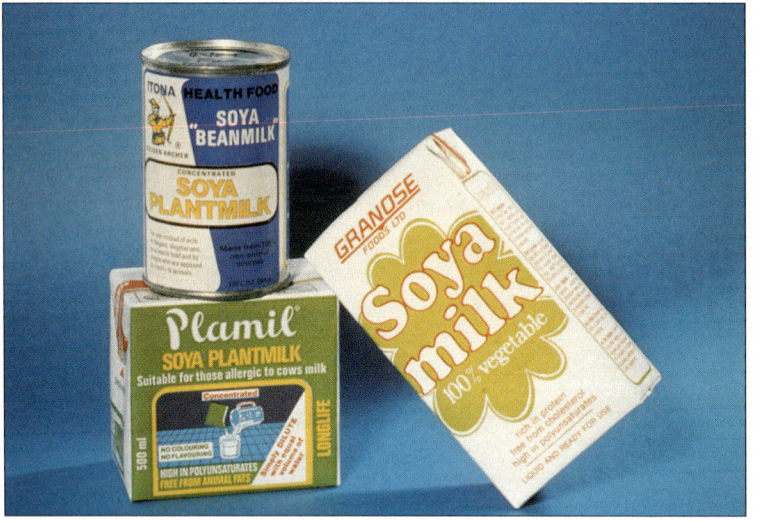

Fig. 4.18 Cows' milk protein intolerance: inappropriate infant feeds. The removal of cows' milk from the diet is central to the management of cows' milk protein intolerance. However, it is crucial that the replacement formula is nutritionally complete, and a number of potentially dangerous and nutritionally incomplete soya drinks are available in health-food stores. These should not be given to infants and children as a substitute for cows' milk formula.

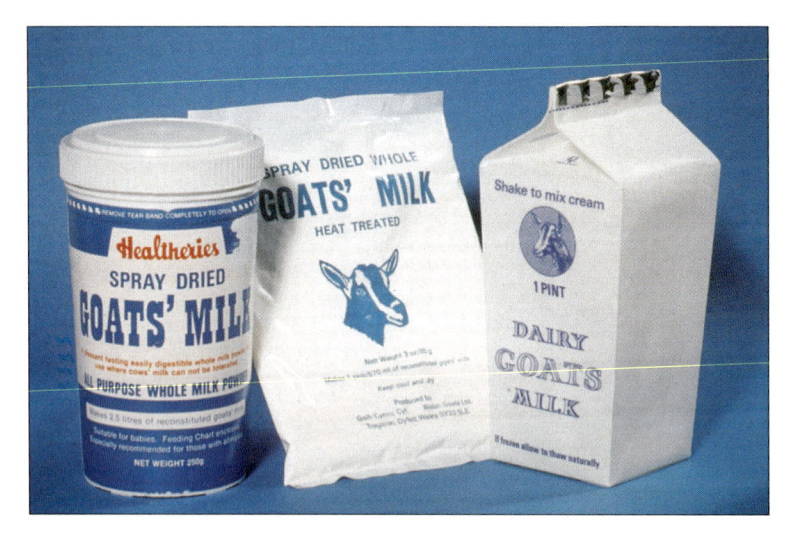

Fig. 4.19 Cows' milk protein intolerance: goats' milk. Goats' milk is an inappropriate replacement for cows' milk formula in patients with cows' milk protein intolerance. Its protein and electrolyte content are too high for infants and toddlers and it is deficient in folate. There is also considerable immunological cross-reactivity between goats' milk and cows' milk antigens.

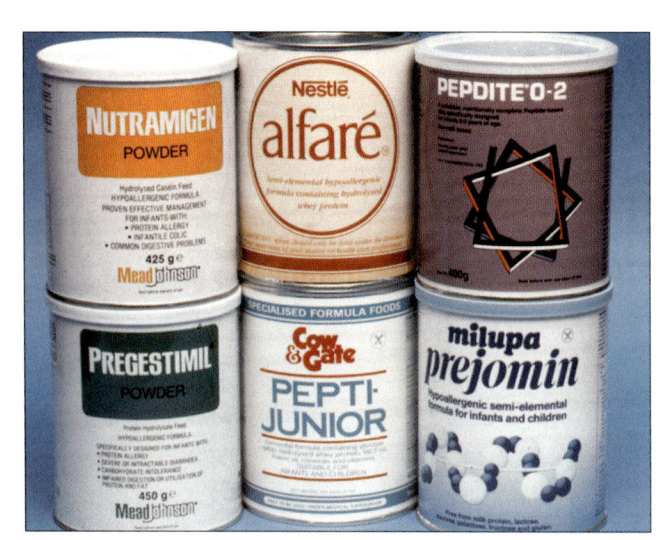

Fig. 4.20 Cows' milk protein intolerance: nutritionally complete replacement formulas. Soya formulas have the advantages of lower cost and greater palatability compared with protein hydrolysates (shown here) or feeds based on amino acids. However, perhaps 10–20% of patients intolerant to cow's milk are, or will become, intolerant to soya. The provision of a cows' milk substitute is nutritionally important, as cows' milk is normally a key source of energy and protein and the sole source of calcium for infants and young children. A supervised challenge with cows' milk is appropriate at about 2 years of age, by which time most children have outgrown their intolerance.

MICROVILLOUS INCLUSION DISEASE

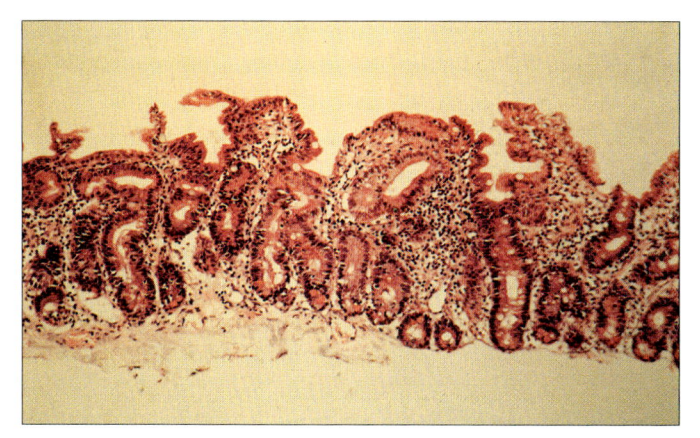

Fig. 4.21 Microvillous inclusion disease (microvillus atrophy). Microvillus inclusion disease presents with severe, protracted, watery diarrhoea within the first 2 weeks of life. It is invariably fatal, although long-term parenteral nutrition often prolongs life for several years. Inheritance is autosomal recessive. Jejunal biopsy reveals a hypoplastic villous atrophy (villous atrophy without crypt hypertrophy, producing a thin mucosa).

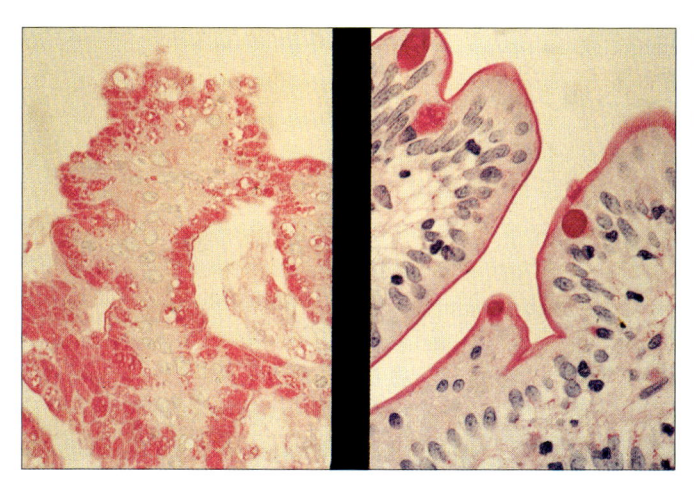

Fig. 4.22 Microvillus inclusion disease: PAS stain. Periodic acid–Schiff staining of jejunal biopsy sections shows a ragged brush-border membrane, with uptake of stain (left). A normal biopsy is on the right.

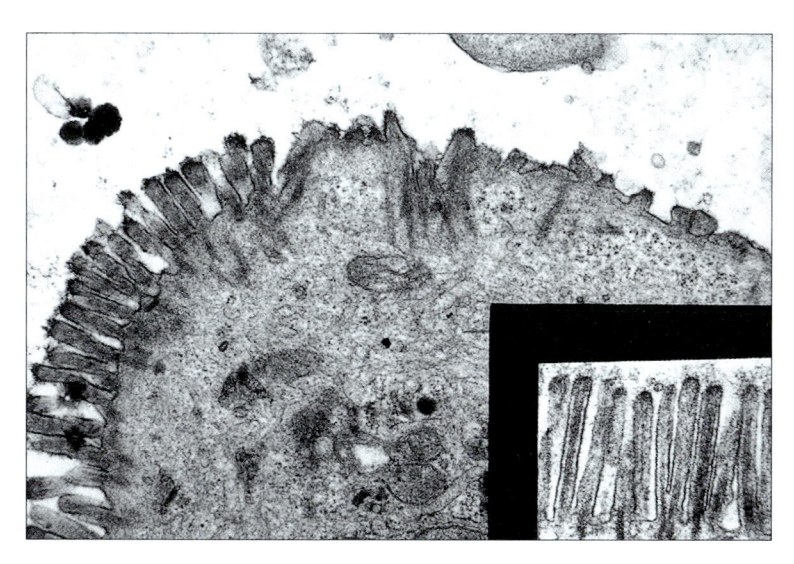

Fig. 4.23. Microvillous inclusion disease: electron microscopy. The diagnostic hallmarks are seen on electron microscopy of the jejunal mucosa. The microvilli are usually shortened or absent, although some microvilli appear normal. Lysosomal bodies are increased. Normal microvilli are shown in the inset.

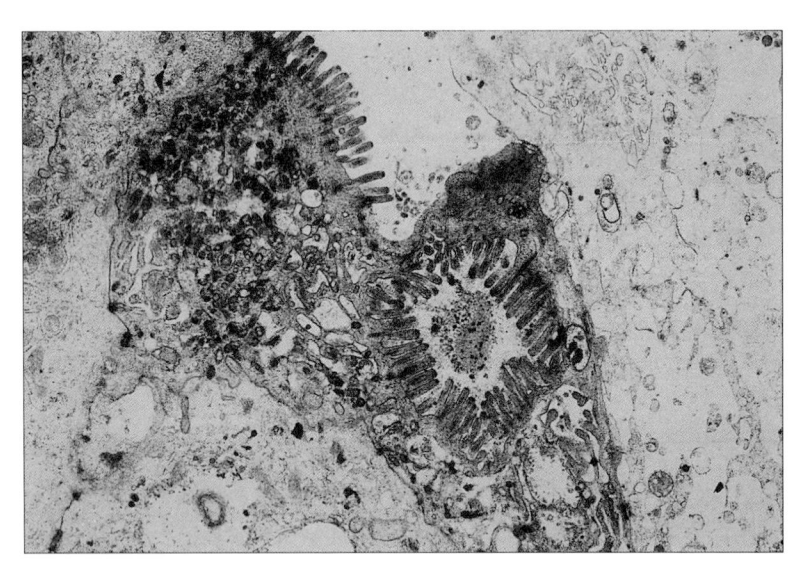

Fig. 4.24 Microvillous inclusion disease: inclusion bodies. Inclusion bodies below the apical membrane are the major diagnostic feature. The inclusions contain microvillus membrane. Similar lesions have been described in the colonic mucosa of affected patients.

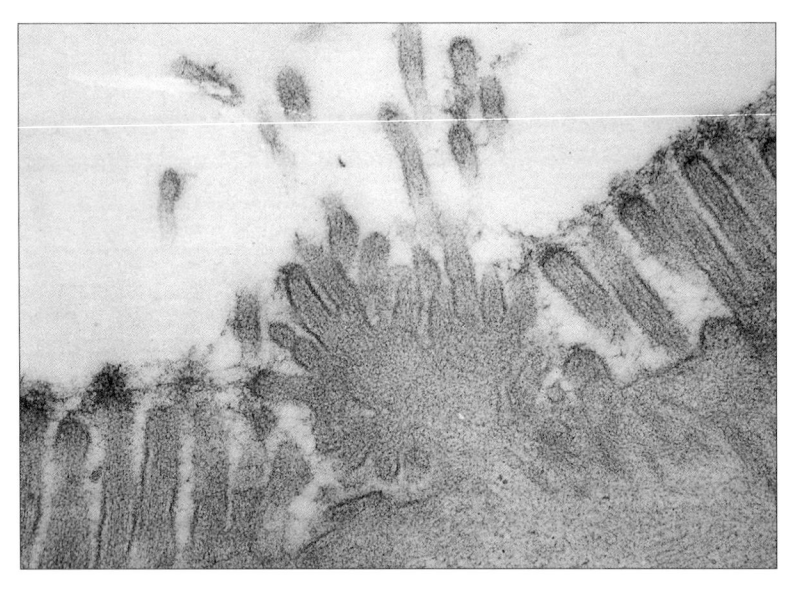

Fig. 4.25 Microvillous dystrophy. A less dramatic lesion has been described in which the microvillus inclusions are absent, but in which the microvilli are shortened or missing. Some microvilli appear tufted. The prognosis is similarly poor and inheritance is probably autosomal recessive.

Small Intestine Diseases

CONGENITAL SECRETORY DIARRHOEA

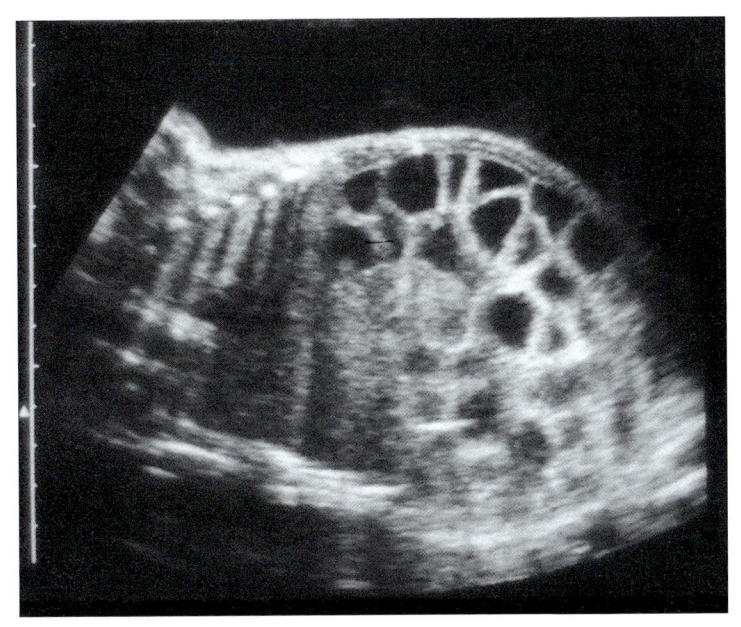

Fig. 4.26 Congenital sodium diarrhoea. A defect in the Na^+/H^+ exchanger in the jejunal brush-border membrane leads to congenital diarrhoea, in which stool Na^+ concentrations are high, often more than 100 mmol/litre. Patients present *in utero* with maternal polyhydramnios. Maternal ultrasound scanning reveals that the fetal abdomen is distended with fluid-filled loops of bowel. Abdominal distension is present at birth, meconium is absent, and profuse watery diarrhoea is present from birth. Provided fluid and electrolyte losses are replaced in the first few months of life, the prognosis is generally good.

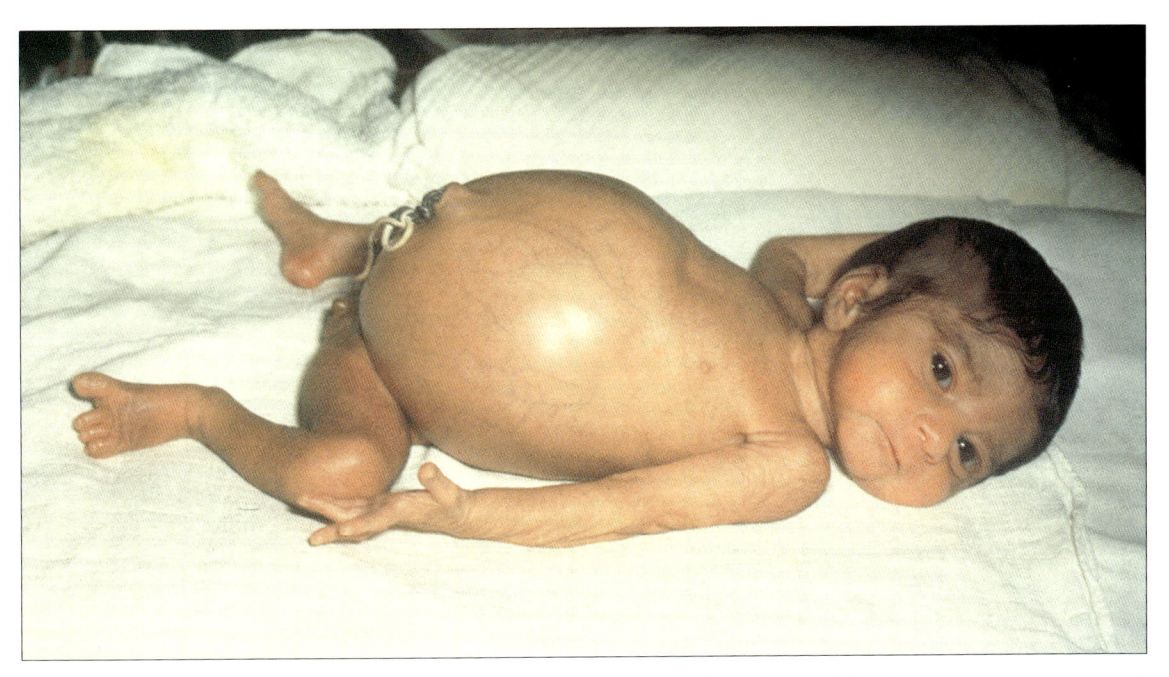

Fig. 4.27 Congenital chloride diarrhoea. Affected babies are clinically indistinguishable from patients with congenital sodium diarrhoea. Abdominal distension at birth may be marked in each disorder, and can lead to a diagnosis of suspected intestinal obstruction. Stool may be so profuse and watery that it is mistaken for urine. Congenital chloride diarrhoea may be distinguished from congenital sodium diarrhoea because the stool chloride concentrations are greater than the sum of sodium and potassium. It is also the only diarrhoeal disorder with a persistent mild metabolic alkalosis. The prognosis is good. Inheritance is autosomal recessive.

ABETALIPOPROTEINAEMIA

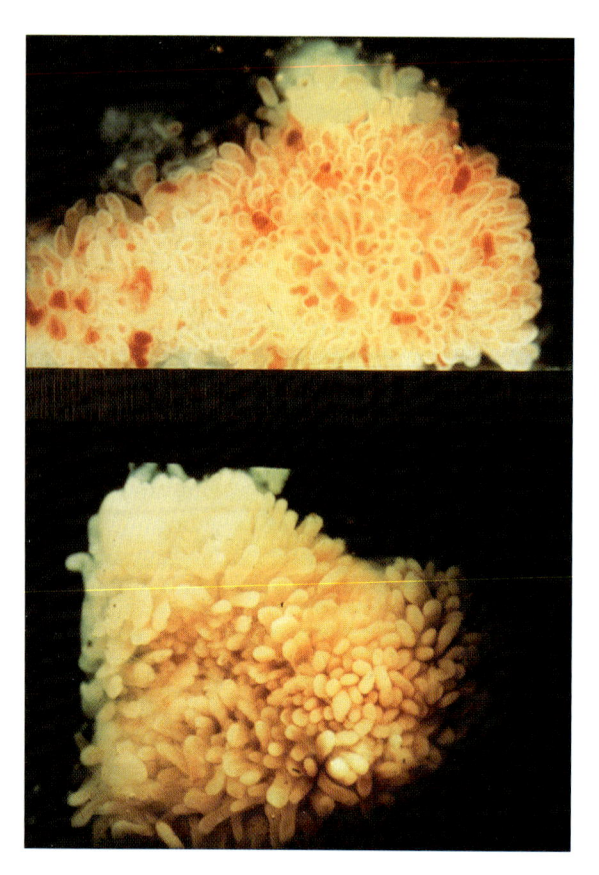

Fig. 4.28 Abetalipoproteinaemia.
Abetalipoproteinaemia (ABL) is an autosomal recessively inherited defect in the synthesis of apolipoprotein (apo B), or in the intracellular assembling of apo B with lipid. Apo B, low density lipoprotein (LDL), very low density lipoprotein (VLDL), and chylomicrons are absent from plasma. Dietary triglyceride cannot be re-packaged into chylomicrons and accumulates in small intestinal enterocytes. Steatorrhoea and fat-soluble vitamin malabsorption, particularly of vitamin E, result. Acanthocytosis of red cells is seen on a wet film. Under the dissecting microscope, the jejunal biopsy has a characteristic chalky white, 'sea anemone' appearance due to accumulation of lipid within enterocytes.
Normal (top); ABL (bottom).

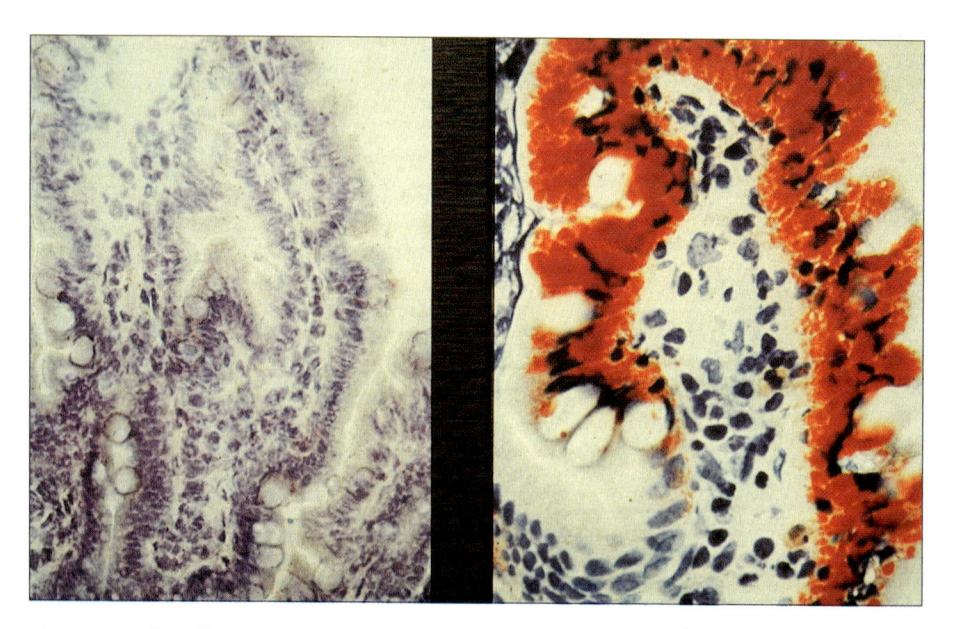

Fig. 4.29 Abetalipoproteinaemia: jejunal biopsy. Shown here is the appearance of the jejunal biopsy following fat staining with Oil Red-O. In contrast to the normal biopsy on the left, the enterocytes in abetalipoproteinaemia (right) are stuffed with lipid, particularly at the villus tips.

Small Intestine Diseases

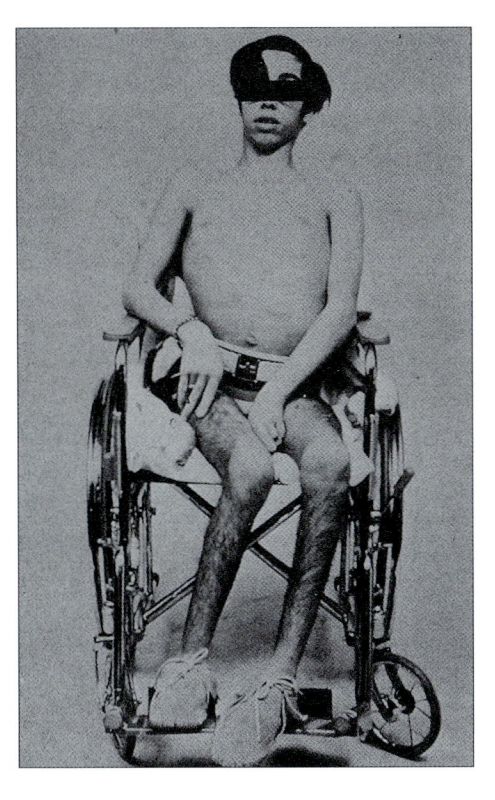

Fig. 4.30 End-stage untreated abetalipoproteinaemia (Bassen–Kornsweig syndrome). Untreated abetalipoproteinaemia leads to progressive, disabling neurological deterioration with some similarities to Friedreich's ataxia. However, early treatment with large oral doses of vitamin E prevents the neurological sequelae completely. This, along with other observations, led to the recognition that vitamin E is important for normal neurological function.

IMMUNOLOGICAL DISORDERS

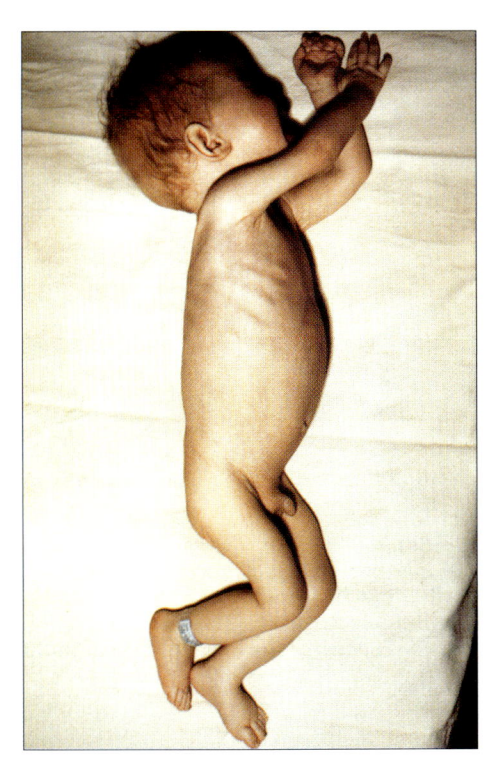

Fig. 4.31 Autoimmune enteropathy. This patient presented with severe protracted diarrhoea at 2 months of age. He had a severe enteropathy caused by circulating anti-enterocyte antibodies, which failed to respond to corticosteroids and cyclosporin. A family history of autoimmune disease is common in this disorder, and affected infants may develop other autoimmune phenomena, including thyroid disease, pernicious anaemia, and diabetes. The severity of autoimmune enteropathy is highly variable. Some patients respond to dietary manipulation, but most require immunosuppression, to which not all respond. In these, the outcome is often fatal, as it was in the infant shown.

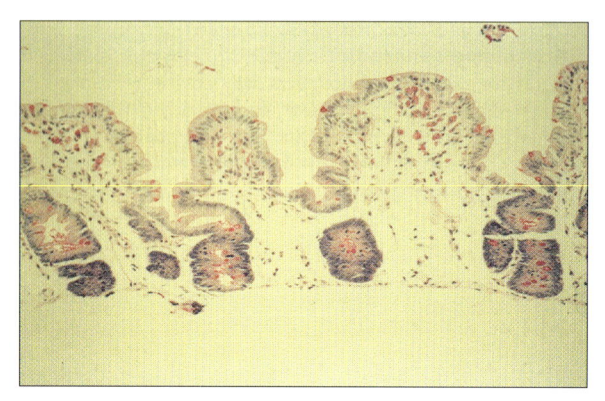

Fig. 4.32 Severe combined immunodeficiency: enteropathy. In addition to multiple severe infections, infants with severe combined immunodeficiency frequently present with protracted diarrhoea and marked failure to thrive. Persistent gastrointestinal infection, often with multiple organisms, explains the associated enteropathy only incompletely. PAS-positive macrophages at the tips of the villi are frequent. The enteropathy is usually intractable without bone marrow transplantation.

GRAFT VERSUS HOST DISEASE

In GVHD, donor lymphocytes (graft) survive in the recipient (host) and recognise and damage the host tissue. GVHD occurs most commonly after bone marrow transplantation or when viable lymphocytes are infused into an immunodeficient host. In acute GVHD, symptoms of nausea, vomiting, and profuse diarrhoea occur within 3–8 weeks of lymphocyte transfer. Confluent desquamative skin disease and cholestasis may occur. Chronic GVHD occurs between 3 and 12 months after transfer, and most intestinal symptoms relate to oesophageal inflammation and fibrosis.

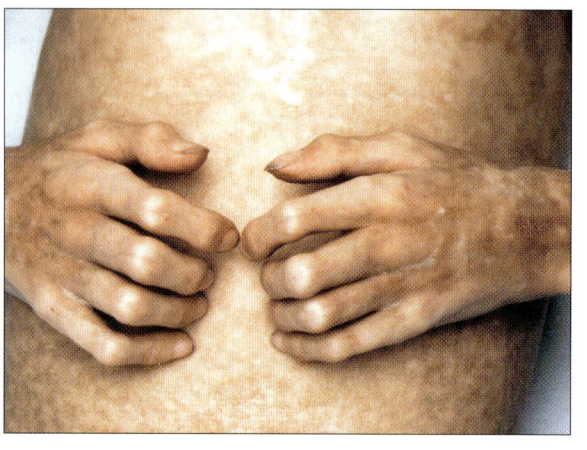

Fig. 4.33 Graft versus host disease. Chronic liver disease is common, and skin changes (seen here) are a major feature. This patient with chronic GVHD has increased pigmentation, contractures, and a scleroderma-like syndrome.

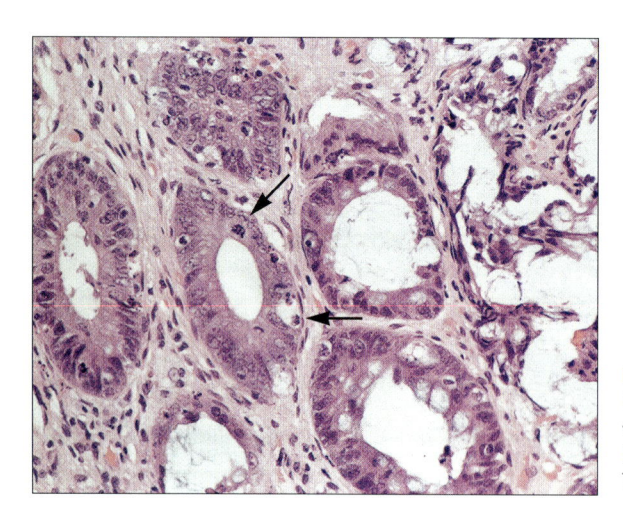

Fig. 4.34 Graft versus host disease. Children may have profuse diarrhoea due to involvement of the intestine with GVHD. The diagnosis is easily confirmed by a rectal biopsy, which demonstrates apoptotic bodies in the crypts. The liver may also be involved (*see* Chapter 16, **Fig. 16.25**).

Small Intestine Diseases

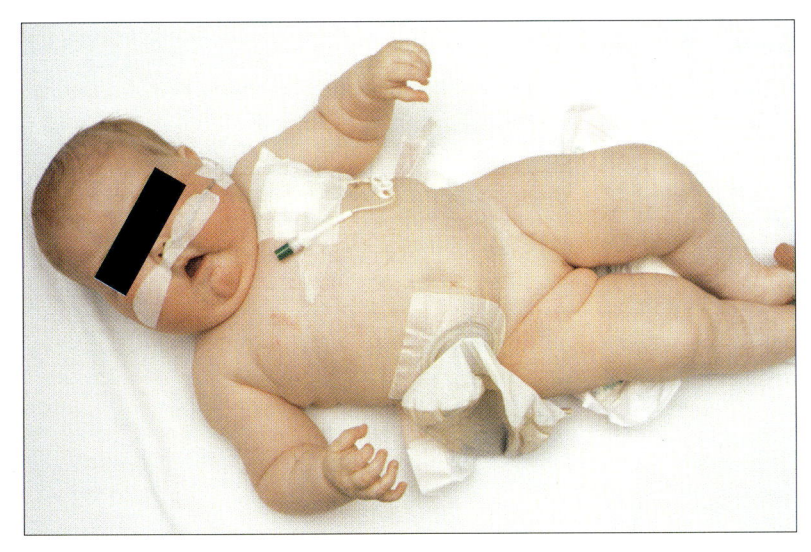

Fig. 4.35 Steroid-responsive enterocolitis. This patient developed a severe, panenteric inflammatory disorder at 1 month of age, affecting both the small and large intestines. The colitis was associated with stricturing and colectomy was required. However, the small intestinal inflammation responded to parenteral corticosteroids, which were required for 3 years before withdrawal was possible. As a result, the patient became markedly Cushingoid. The disorder is rare and of unknown cause.

SEQUELAE OF MASSIVE INTESTINAL RESECTION (SHORT BOWEL SYNDROME

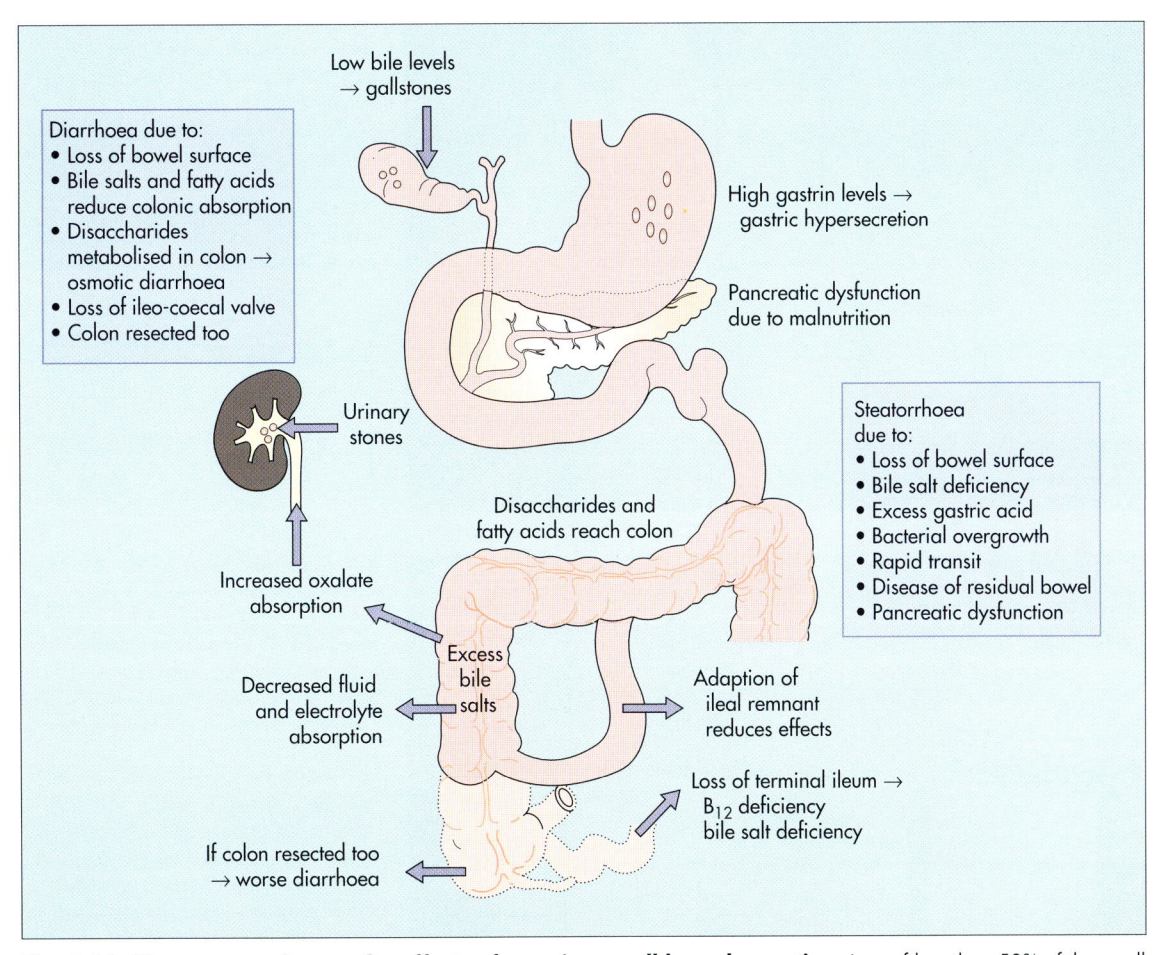

Fig. 4.36. Short gut syndrome: the effects of massive small bowel resection. Loss of less than 50% of the small intestine is unlikely to lead to major nutritional sequelae. Above 75% loss, nutritional support is almost invariable. Redrawn from *Clinical Nutrition in Gastroenterology*, RV Heatley et al. Courtesy of Churchill Livingstone.

45

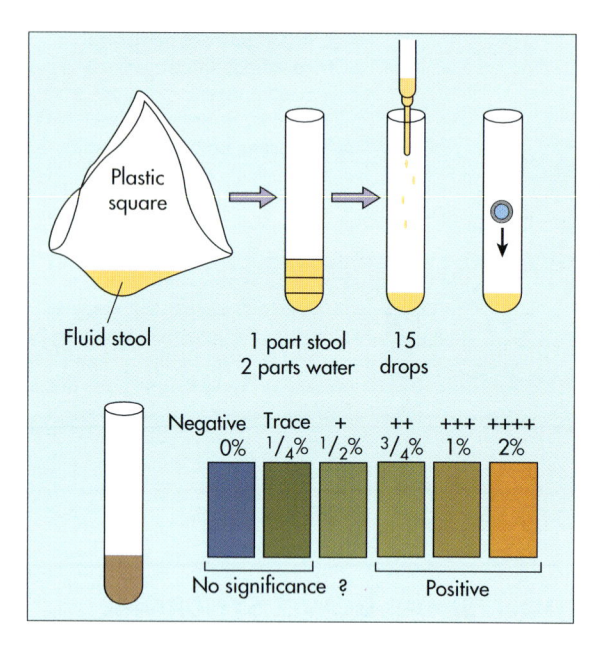

Fig. 4.37 Testing stool for reducing substances. The detection of carbohydrate intolerance is important in the investigation and management of patients with diarrhoea. Reducing sugars in the stool can be detected using a modified Clinitest procedure. Stool water must be collected (which is not always easy) and either tested immediately or frozen until testing is possible. Sucrose, which is not a reducing sugar, can be detected by prior hydrolysis, either by boiling the stool water or treating it with 6N HCl.

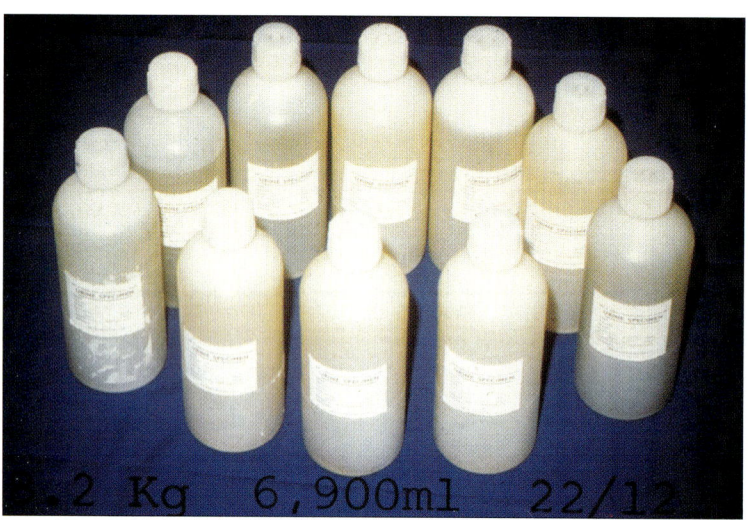

Fig. 4.38 Secretory diarrhoea: 24-hour stool output. Stool output from patients with secretory diarrhoea can be profuse. This patient's stool output was cholera-like in volume and continued on fasting. Stool sodium concentrations were high (>70 mmol/l). Despite extensive investigation, a diagnosis could not be made. The disorder was fatal, despite parenteral nutrition.

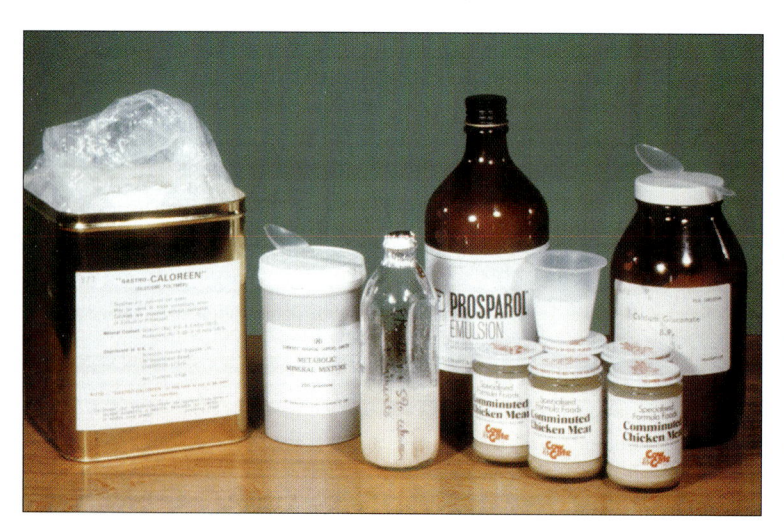

Fig. 4.39 Modular feeds. Modular feeds are frequently useful in the management of patients with protracted diarrhoea who have failed to respond to commercially available formulas based on peptides or amino acids. The concentration of the individual nutrients can be varied independently and the feed tailored to an individual patient's tolerances. Chicken meat is frequently used as the nitrogen source because of its low osmolality and allergenicity. The feeds are complex to prepare and should only be used under the supervision of an experienced paediatric dietician.

Small Intestine Diseases

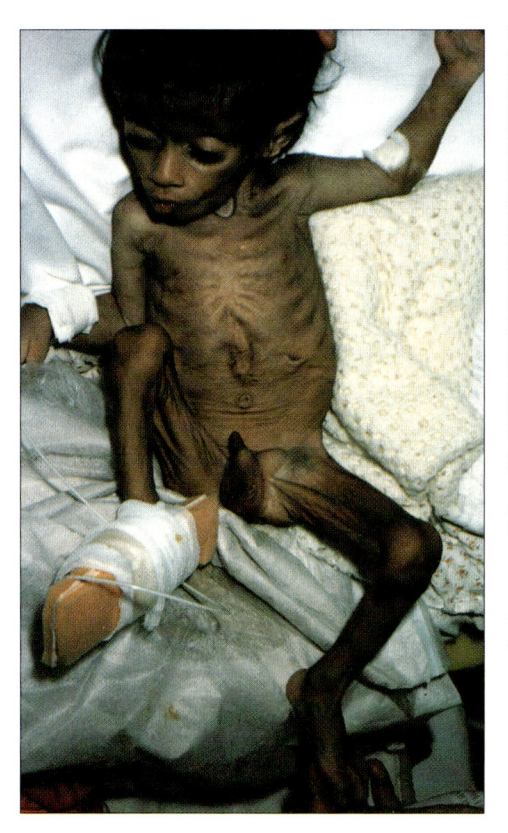

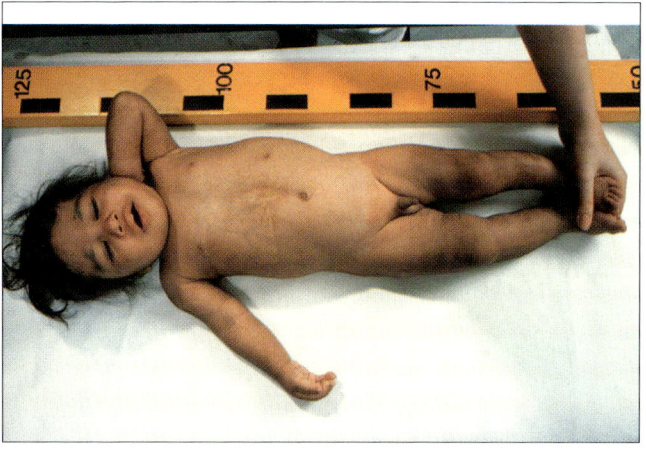

Figs 4.40, 4.41 Protracted diarrhoea: parenteral nutrition.
The effects of severe, protracted diarrhoea can be devastating, and patients develop severe protein energy malnutrition. This patient (**4.40**, left) had severe protracted diarrhoea for 5 weeks, following acute gastroenteritis. Under such circumstances, parenteral nutrition can be life-saving. In **4.41** (above) the same patient is shown after 2 months of parenteral nutrition.

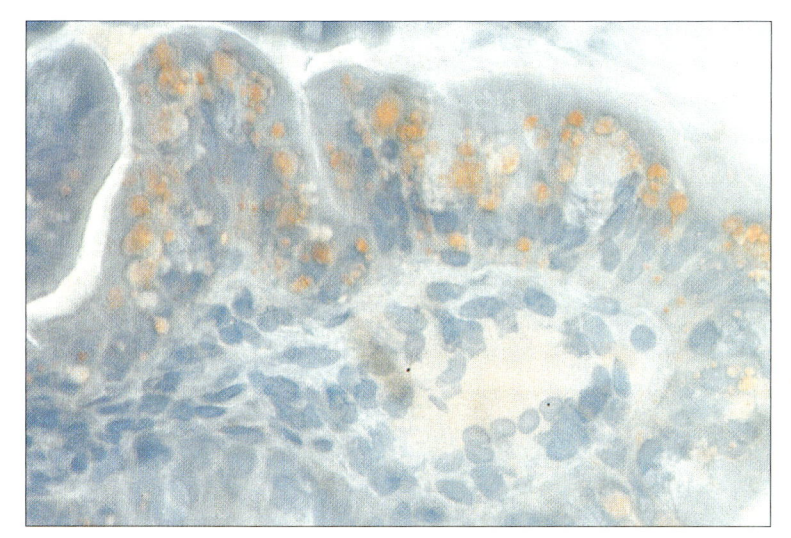

Fig. 4.42 Chylomicron retention disease (Anderson's disease).
This small intestinal biopsy has been stained with a fat stain (Oil Red-O) and shows marked accumulation of dietary triglyceride within the enterocytes. The disease is rare and is characterised by an inability to export dietary fat as chylomicrons. The precise cause is uncertain, but it appears to be due to a defect in chylomicron assembly or exocytosis. The disorder presents with steatorrhoea and failure to thrive. In contrast to abetalipoproteinaemia, betalipoproteins are present in the plasma, although in reduced quantities.

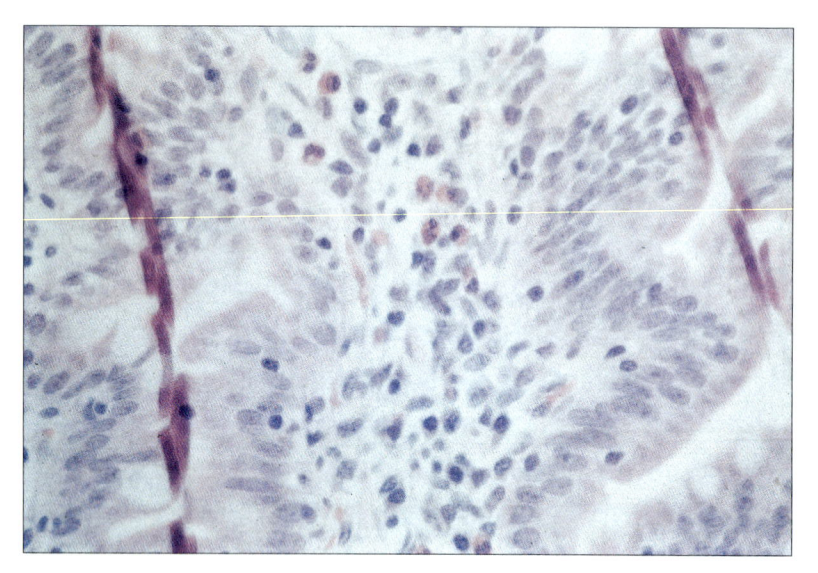

Fig. 4.43. Eosinophilic gastroenteritis. Eosinophilic gastroenteritis is an uncommon disorder that affects any part of the gut from the oesophagus to the rectum. The cause is unknown, but the disorder is characterised by eosinophilic infiltration of one or more areas of the gastrointestinal tract, usually the stomach and small intestine (as shown here). Diarrhoea, failure to thrive, protein-losing enteropathy, iron deficiency, and a strong family history of atopy are characteristic clinical features. Management is by dietary exclusion and/or steroids and immunosuppression.

5. Gastrointestinal Infections

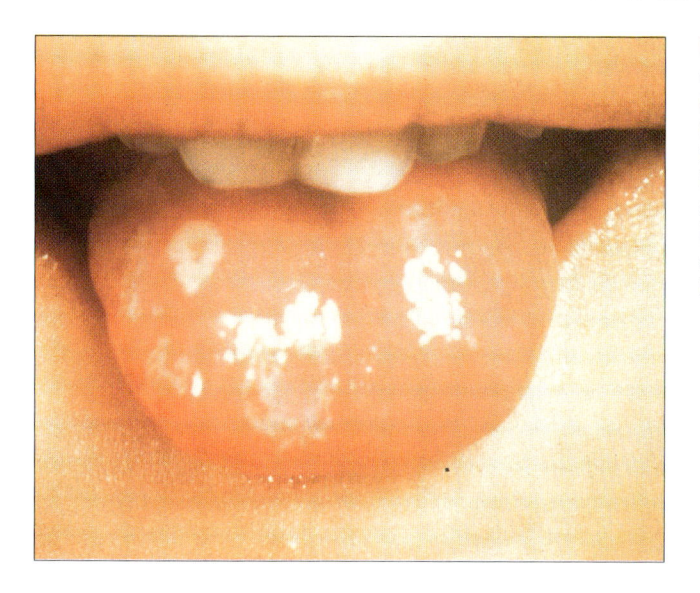

Figs 5.1, 5.2 Candidiasis. Candidiasis is a common cause of oral mucous membrane infection (thrush) (**5.1**, above) and perineal skin infections (**5.2**, below) in newborn infants. *Candida albicans* is the most common candidal species to cause infection in the newborn. Most infections are diagnosed clinically, but scrapings of the skin lesions demonstrate hyphae or yeast forms. Invasive candidiasis is rare in newborns, but is common in immunosuppressed patients.

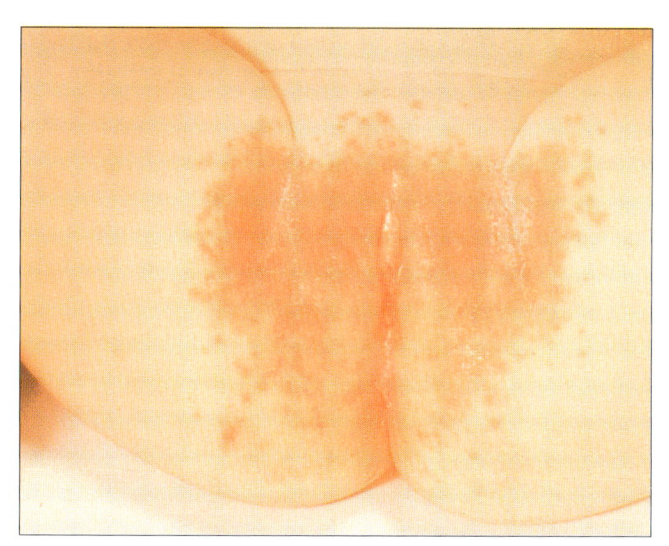

Pediatric Gastroenterology and Hepatology

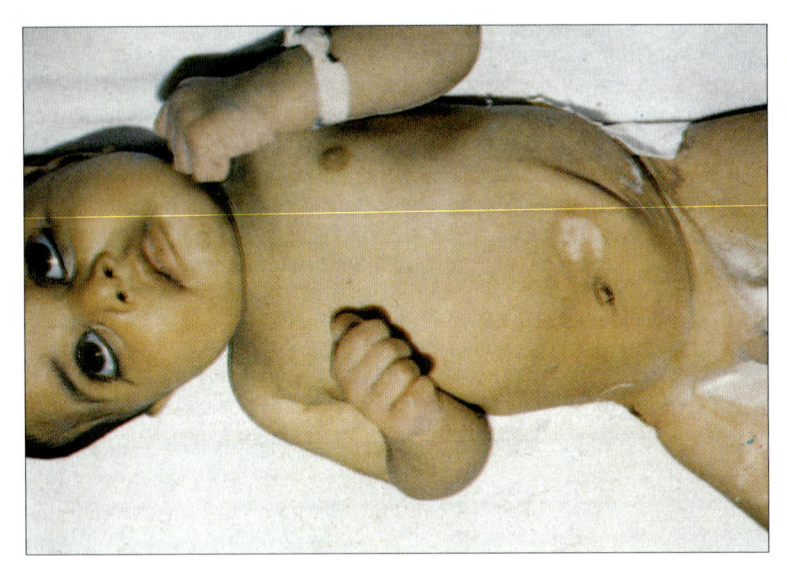

Fig. 5.3 Acute gastroenteritis: dehydration. This patient is severely dehydrated, and has lost 10% of body weight as a result of rotavirus diarrhoea. Tissue turgor is markedly reduced, and on the anterior abdominal wall a lifted skin-fold does not spring back into place. The eyes are also sunken and the baby is markedly apathetic.

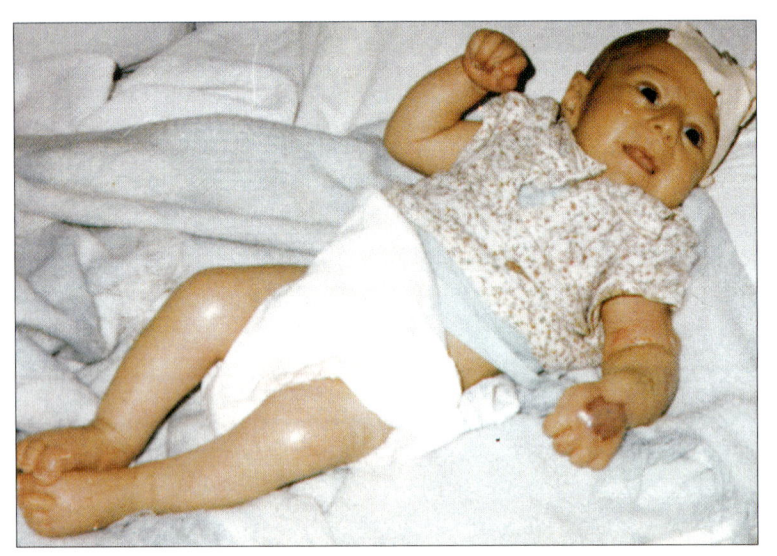

Figs 5.4, 5.5 Acute gastroenteritis: dehydration. This baby (**5.4**, middle) has severe hypernatraemic dehydration (serum sodium = 170 mmol/litre). The peripheral signs of dehydration, such as reduced tissue turgor, are not present, the skin on the legs is shiny, and the muscles were doughy on palpation. The infant was extremely irritable and had already suffered two generalised convulsions. Tissue necrosis due to hyperviscosity is already present on the dorsum of the left hand; by the next day this had progressed (**5.5**, bottom) to involve most of the left arm.

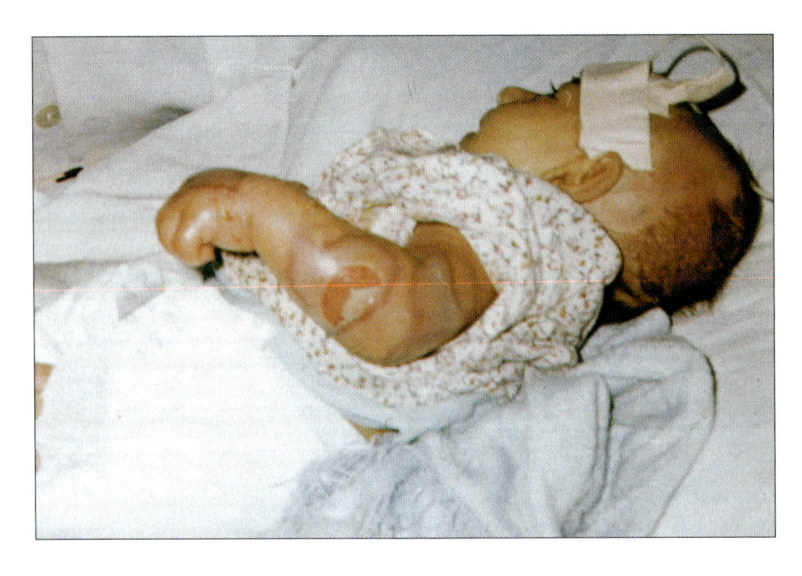

Gastrointestinal Infections

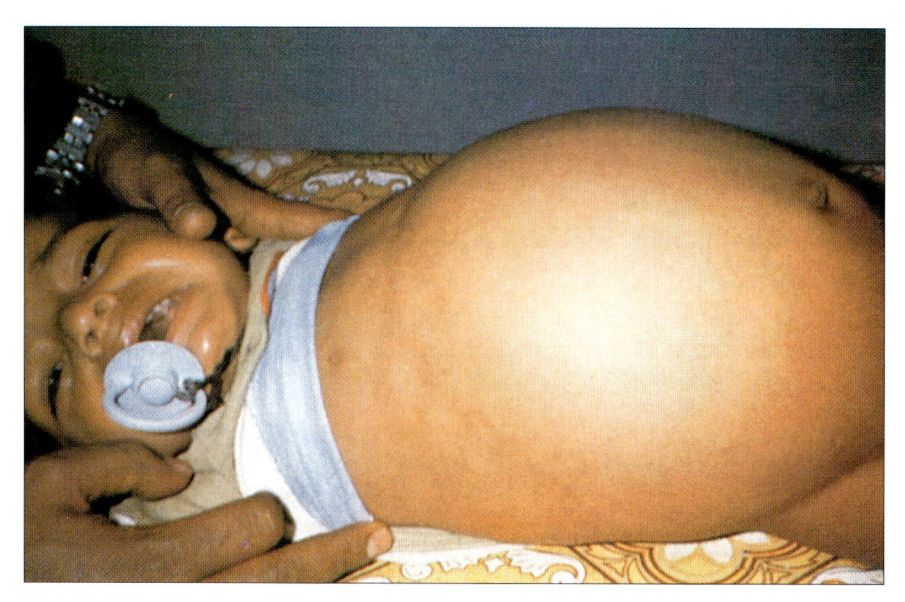

Fig. 5.6 Acute gastroenteritis complicated by ileus induced by opioids.
Antisymptomatic drugs are contraindicated in gastroenteritis. Agents that affect gut motility, such as diphenoxylate, codeine, or loperamide, may result in severe ileus, as shown here.

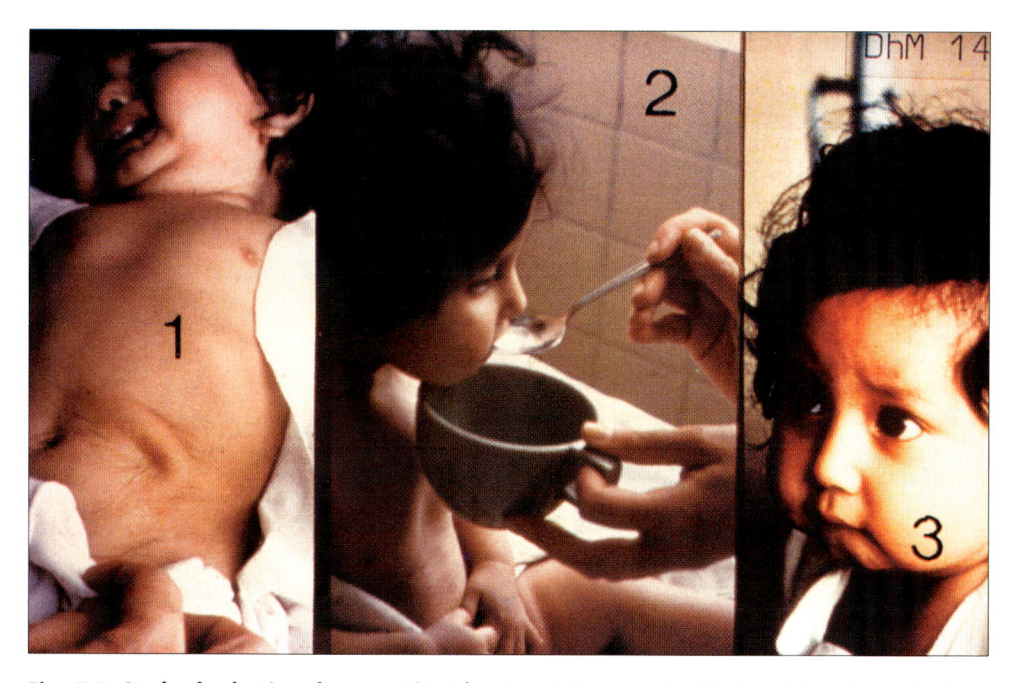

Fig. 5.7 Oral rehydration therapy. This infant (panel 1) is severely dehydrated (note the markedly reduced tissue turgor). Following treatment with WHO oral rehydration solution, given initially by cup and spoon because of vomiting (panel 2), dehydration was corrected successfully. The infant is shown in panel 3, 10 hours after the start of treatment.

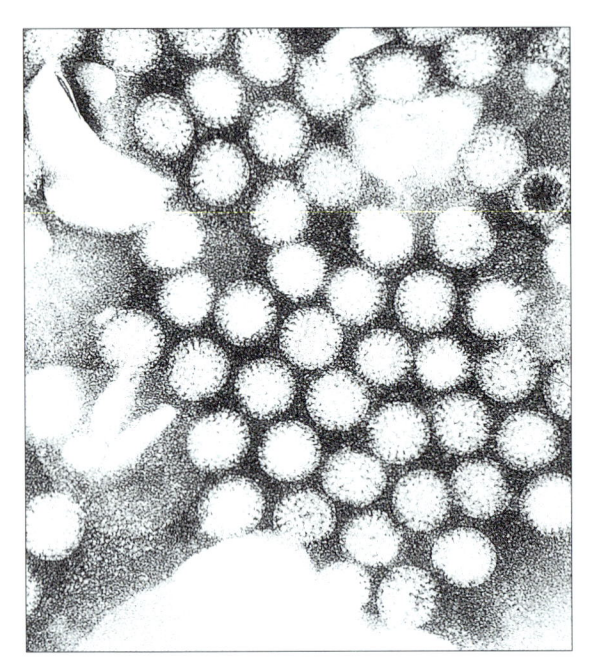

Fig. 5.8 Rotavirus. Electron microscopy (EM) of a Rotavirus which belong to the Reoviridae family and have a wheel-like 70 nm double-stranded RNA structure. They are the most common cause of infantile diarrhoea throughout the world, being responsible for more than a million deaths worldwide. There are seven groups which are distinguished by different antigenic and RNA patterns. The infection is commonest in winter and in infants less than 2 years of age. (EM ×120,000.)

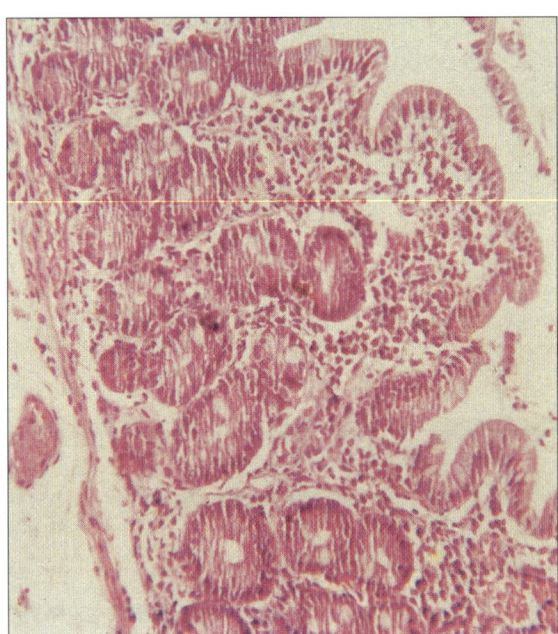

Fig. 5.9 Rotavirus. Rotavirus replicate in the differentiated columnar epithelial cells of the small intestinal villi. Characteristically, there is fever, vomiting, and profuse watery diarrhoea. Rotavirus infection is usually a self-limited disease, although dehydration may lead to hospitalisation or death. Secondary disaccharidase deficiency may result. The diagnosis is made by identifying the virus in the stool or by enzyme-linked immunosorbent assay (ELISA) (Haematoxylin and Eosin, ×20.).

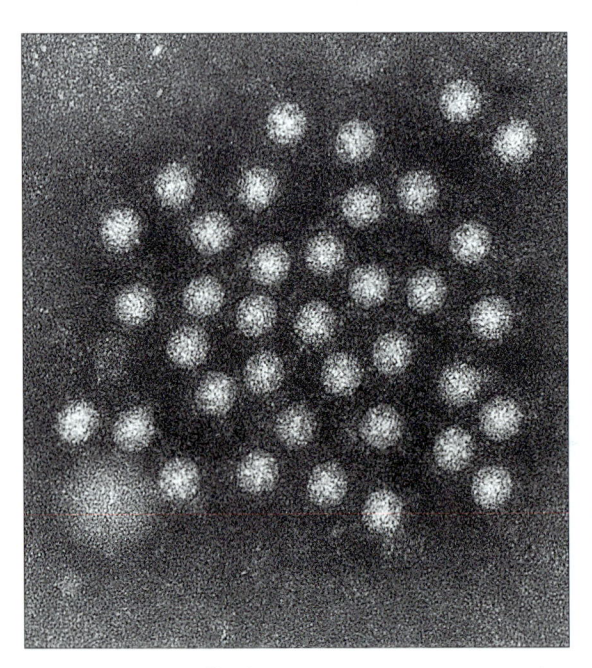

Fig. 5.10 Norwalk virus. Acute gastroenteritis may also be due to small round viruses or Norwalk virus (30–35 nm). The clinical presentation is similar to rotavirus. The identification of the virus is by EM of the stool (EM ×120,000.)

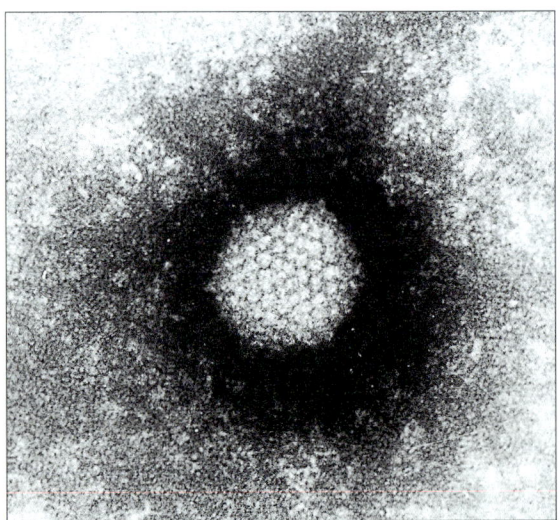

Fig. 5.11 Adenoviruses. Adenoviruses are DNA viruses (70–80 nm) primarily responsible for acute respiratory infections in infants, but may also cause conjuctivitis, haemorrhagic cystitis, acute diarrhoea, encephalomyelitis, and acute liver failure. The laboratory diagnosis is made either serologically, by a rise in adenovirus antibodies, or by growing the virus in culture from respiratory secretions or stool (EM ×160,000.)

Gastrointestinal Infections

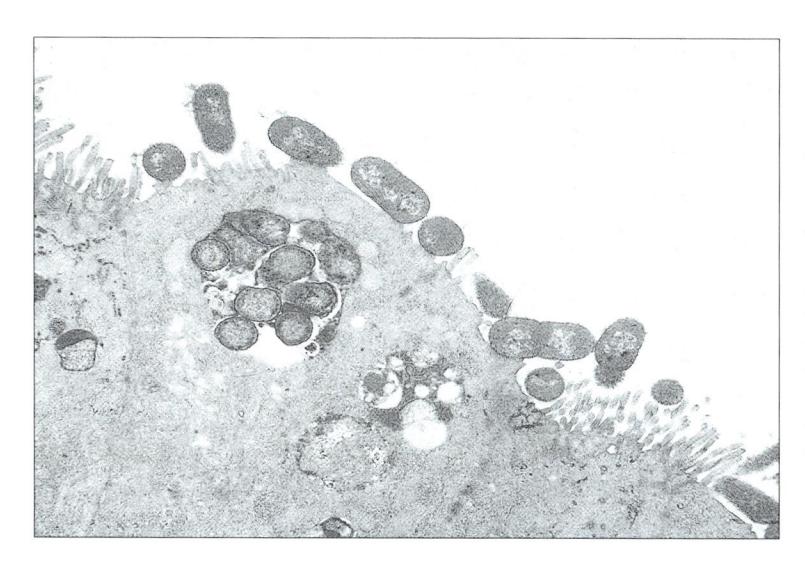

Fig. 5.12 Bacterial infections.
Bacterial infections of the small intestine include *Escherichia coli* (*E. coli*), *Salmonella*, and *Shigella*, but *E. coli* is the most common. *E. coli* may be enterotoxogenic (which produces a heat-labile enterotoxin resulting in watery stools), enteroinvasive (which produces a bloody diarrhoea), or enteropathogenic (which is associated with infantile gastroenteritis). This electron microscopy view demonstrates an enteropathogenic *E. coli* that is blunting microvilli in the small intestine. Management involves the treatment of dehydration and of fluid and electrolyte imbalance. Antimicrobial therapy is usually inappropriate. (EM ×5000.)

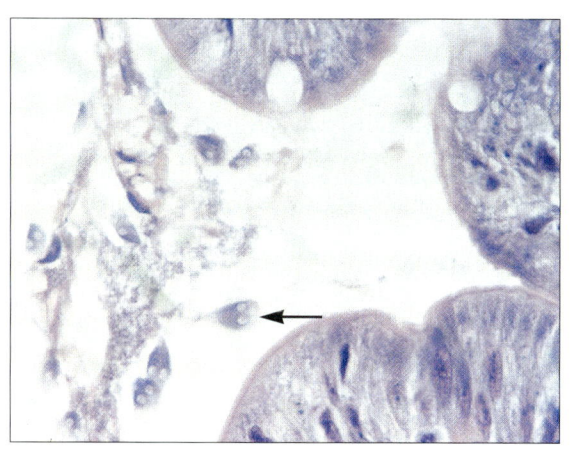

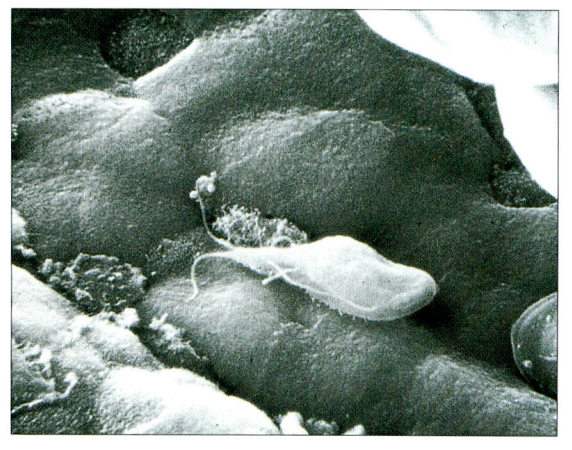

Figs 5.13, 5.14 *Giardia lamblia*. *G. lamblia* is a flagellate protozoan and a common cause of infective diarrhoea worldwide. Infection is by the ingestion of water-borne cysts. Once the cysts reach the upper small intestine they divide into four trophozoites, which colonise the lumen of the duodenum and jejunum (**5.13**, Giemsa ×33, left, **5.14**, EM, right, 10–20 μm). The most common clinical presentation is with diarrhoea, weight loss, crampy abdominal pain, steatorrhoea, malabsorption, and failure to thrive. The diagnosis can be made on identifying the protozoa in a jejunal aspirate or biopsy, or by identifying the cysts in stools. Treatment with metronidazole is usually necessary.

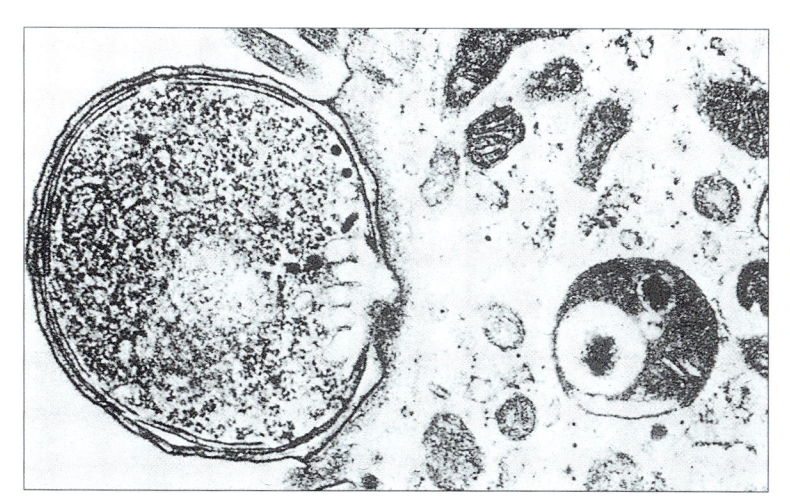

Fig. 5.15 Cryptosporidiosis.
Cryptosporidiosis is an intestinal infection by the protozoan *Cryptosporidium* which causes a self-limiting watery diarrhoea in normal children, but may produce protracted diarrhoea in immunosuppressed patients. Infection occurs by ingesting the cysts from infected faeces. The trophozoite divides in the jejunal mucosa and attaches to the mucosa. (EM, 2–5 μm, ×10,000.).

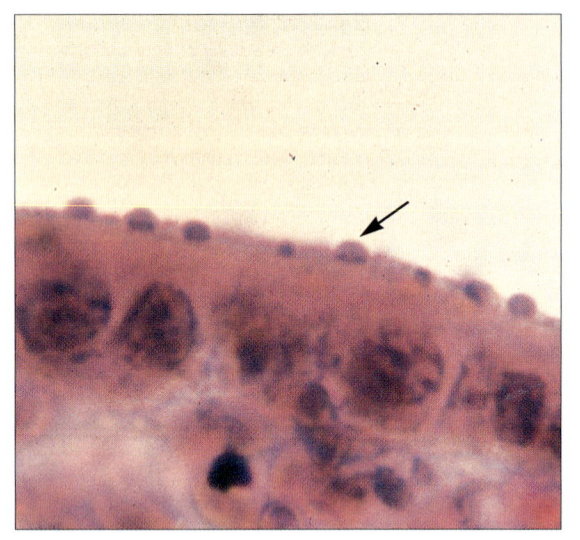

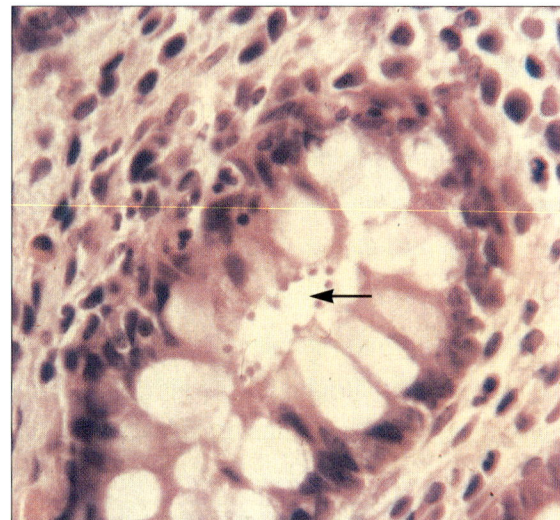

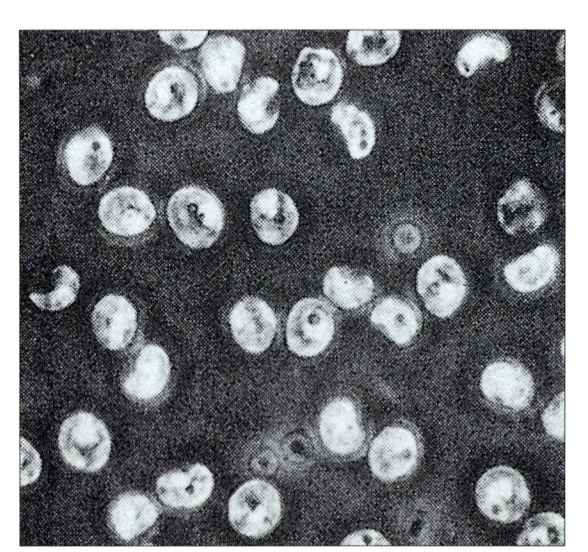

Figs 5.16–5.18 Cryptosporidiosis. The majority of infections take place in the small intestine, as in **5.16** (top left, Haematoxylin and Eosin, ×25), but in immunocompromised patients there may be an associated colitis with crypt abscesses (**5.17**, top right, Haematoxylin and Eosin, ×25). Infection is usually self-limiting, lasting 10–14 days. Diagnosis is difficult and is based upon identifying cysts in the stool (**5.18**, middle left, EM ×4000). Treatment is non-specific, except in immunosuppressed patients.

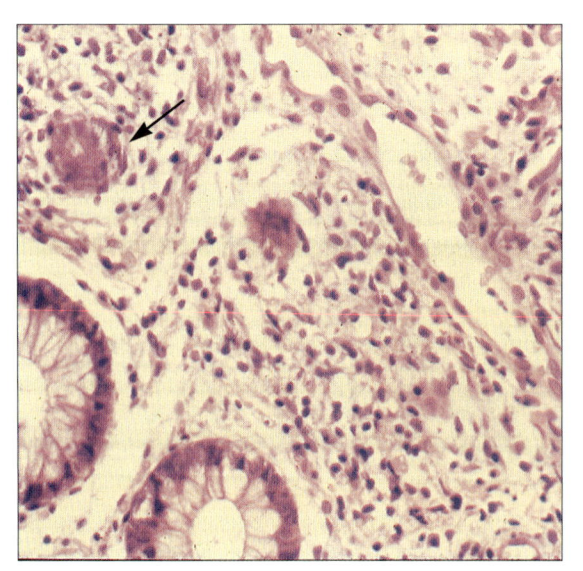

Fig. 5.19 Campylobacter gastroenteritis.
Campylobacter gastroenteritis is usually associated with *Campylobacter jejuni*. Symptoms include fever, malaise, myalgias, diarrhoea, and bloody stools. Over 90% of older children may have associated abdominal pain. The majority of patients have a self-limiting illness, but there may be a prolonged course in 20%. Persistent infection may mimic inflammatory bowel disease, as in this patient with a granuloma containing the organisms seen on rectal biopsy. The diagnosis is confirmed by stool culture. Uncomplicated campylobacter enteritis requires supportive therapy, but oral erythromycin may reduce the spread of disease (Haematoxylin and Eosin, ×25).

Gastrointestinal Infections

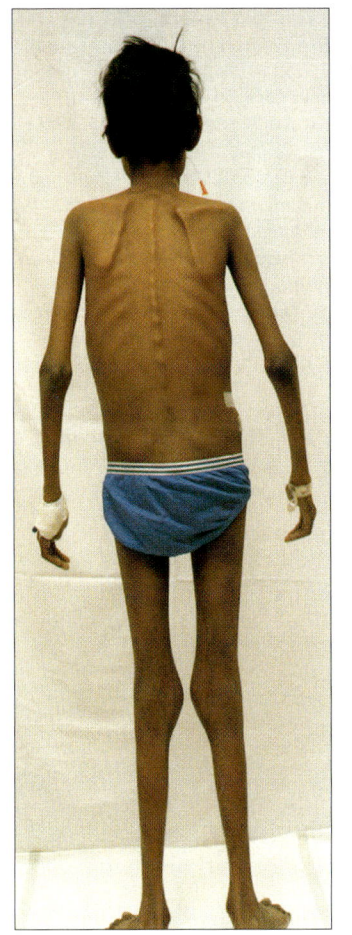

Fig. 5.20 Intestinal tuberculosis. Intestinal tuberculosis is uncommon in developed countries. In the UK it tends to occur in children whose families originated in the Indian sub-continent. Presentation is with recurrent abdominal pain and weight loss, and a right ileac fossa mass, as in this patient. The initial diagnosis was Crohn's disease. The Mantoux test was strongly positive. More recently, *Mycobacterium tuberculosis* and atypical species have been recognised as important opportunistic infections in acquired immunodeficiency syndrome.

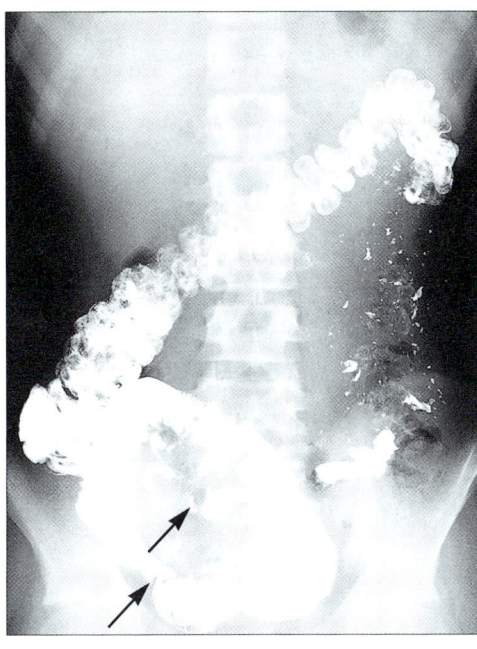

Fig. 5.21 Intestinal tuberculosis (barium follow-through). The distal ileum and caecum, the most commonly affected sites, are grossly abnormal. The wall of the gut is grossly thickened and there are areas of irregular narrowing and dilatation. The differential diagnosis is Crohn's disease.

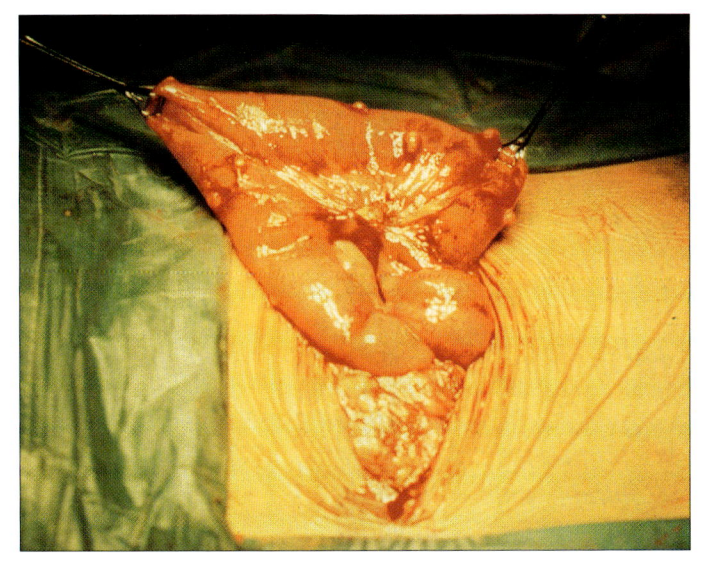

Fig. 5.22 Intestinal tuberculosis. At laporotomy the wall of the distal ileum is grossly thickened and the lumen narrowed. The serosal surface is studded with tubercles. Histological sections revealed transmural inflammation with non-caseating giant cell granulomas. Acid-fast bacilli were shown to be present with Ziehl–Neelsen's stain. Intestinal obstruction and caecal perforation leading to peritonitis have been reported.

55

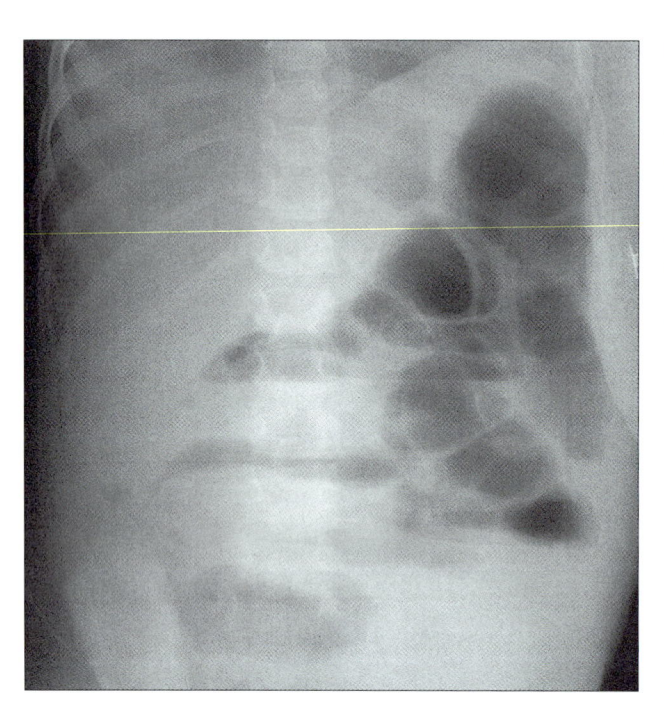

Figs 5.23, 5.24 Yersinia enterocolitica.
Yersinia enterocolitica is associated with diarrhoea, mesenteric adenitis, and terminal ileitis. Septicaemia may develop in children with diabetes, cirrhosis, or iron overload. This 4-year-old girl with thalassaemia intermedia and serum ferritin of 3690 mmol/litre developed a severe enterocolitis and peritonitis and septicaemia following an appendicectomy (**5.23**, top, note fluid levels and dilated bowel loops). *Yersinia enterocolitica* was isolated from blood and peritoneal fluid, and identified using a methylene-blue stain (**5.24**, bottom). She made a good recovery following a laparotomy, jejunostomy, and broad-spectrum antibiotics.

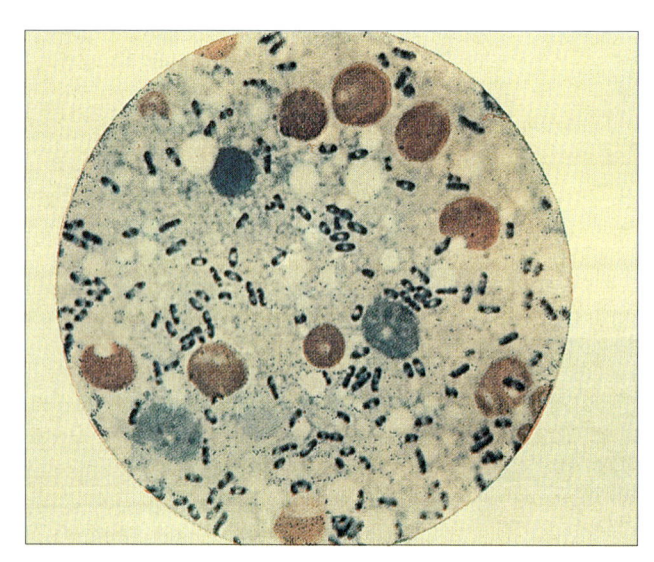

6. Inflammatory Bowel Disease

CROHN'S DISEASE

Crohn's disease is a transmural, focal, subacute or chronic inflammatory disorder, affecting any part of the gastrointestinal tract from mouth to anus, but most commonly the distal ileum, colon, and anorectal areas.

There are two peaks of incidence, in early and late adult life, but between one-quarter to one-third of patients present before the age of 20 years. In the past 40 years there has been an increase in the incidence of Crohn's disease in all age groups, ranging from 100 to 400%.

The cause is not known, but familial and racial clustering support a racial predisposition. Intestinal inflammation may be the result of an appropriate response to an as yet unidentified infection, antigen or toxin Alternatively, the disease may result from an inappropriate response to normal laminal factors consequent upon a defective mucosal barrier or immune regulation.

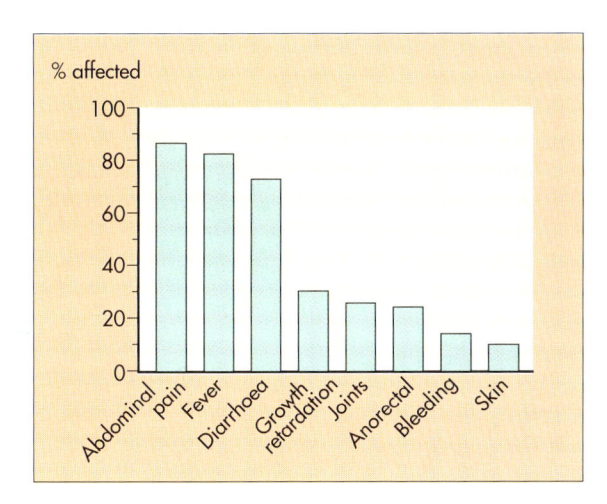

Fig. 6.1 Initial symptoms of Crohn's disease.
Abdominal pain (often colicky, periumbilical, and worse after meals), diarrhoea, and growth failure are the classic triad. However, the disease is frequently insidious in onset, so the diagnosis is often delayed, especially in those patients who present with extra-intestinal symptoms or whose disease is confined to the terminal ileum and right colon.

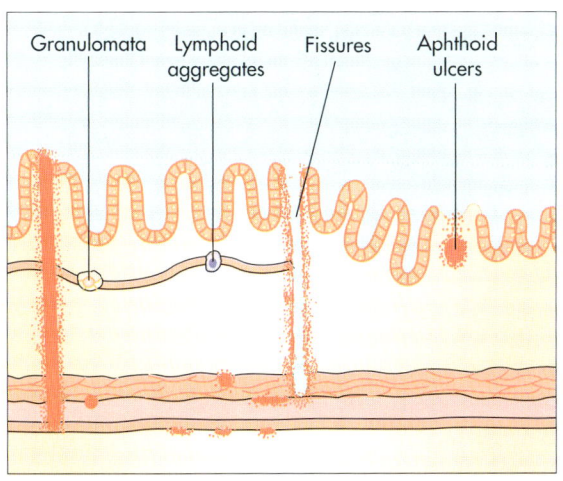

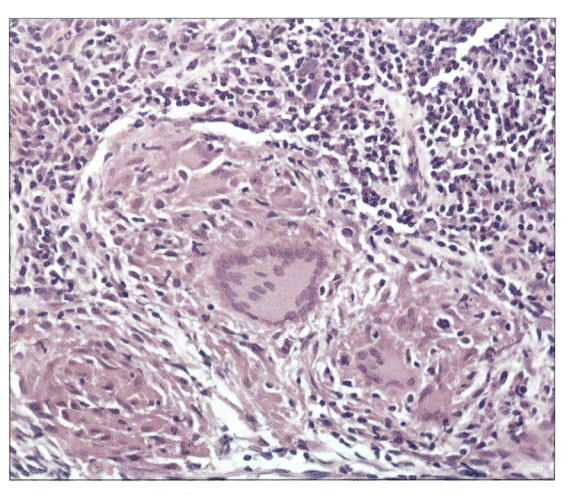

Figs 6.2, 6.3 Pathology of Crohn's disease. Characteristically, transmural inflammation involving intestinal fat and serosa is present, together with mucosal ulceration and fissuring (**6.2**, left). The diagnostic hallmark is the presence of non-caseating epithelioid cell granulomata, found in at least 50% of cases (**6.3**, right).

Pediatric Gastroenterology and Hepatology

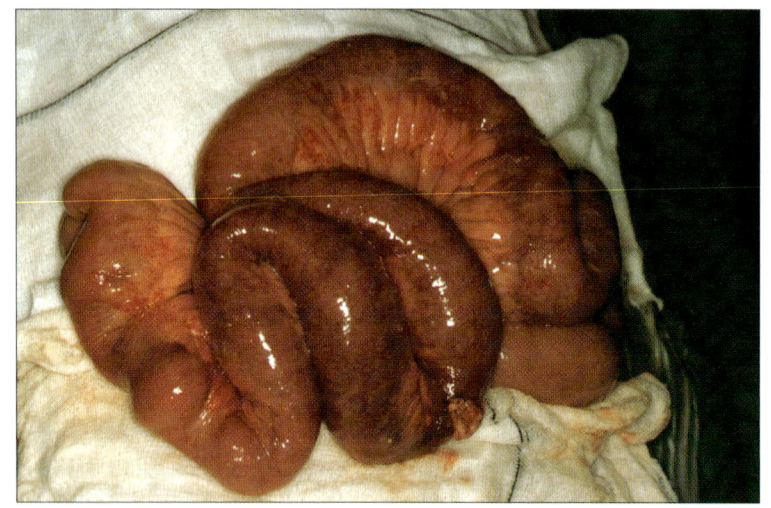

Fig 6.4. Macroscopic appearance of Crohn's disease: small intestine. The affected small intestine is thickened and hosepipe-like. A variable degree of stenosis is found in the thickened segment, leading to subacute obstruction. Deep penetrating ulceration may lead to sinuses, fistulae, and abscesses, although these complications tend to be uncommon in childhood.

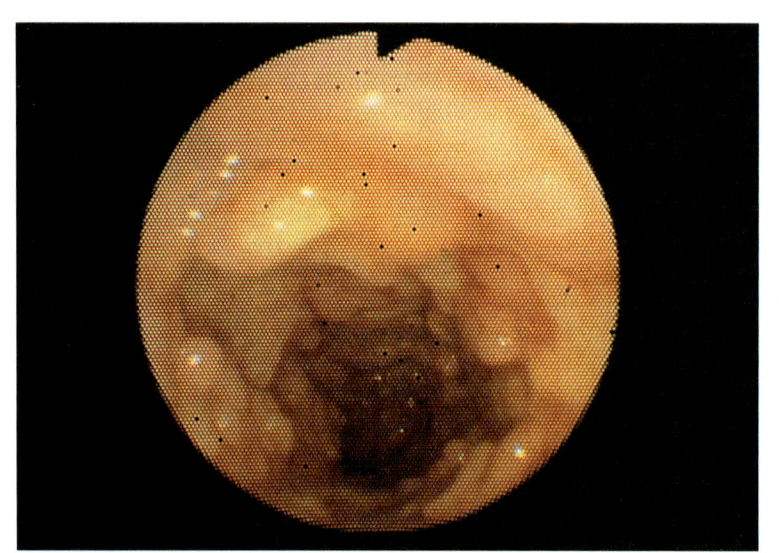

Fig. 6.5 Colonoscopic appearances of severe Crohn's colitis. The mucosa shows a cobblestone pattern. There are residual areas of oedematous mucosa between deep, linear ulcers. In less severe disease, the inflammation is often asymmetric and discontinuous. Aphthous ulceration and serpiginous linear ulceration are characteristic. The rectum is often spared.

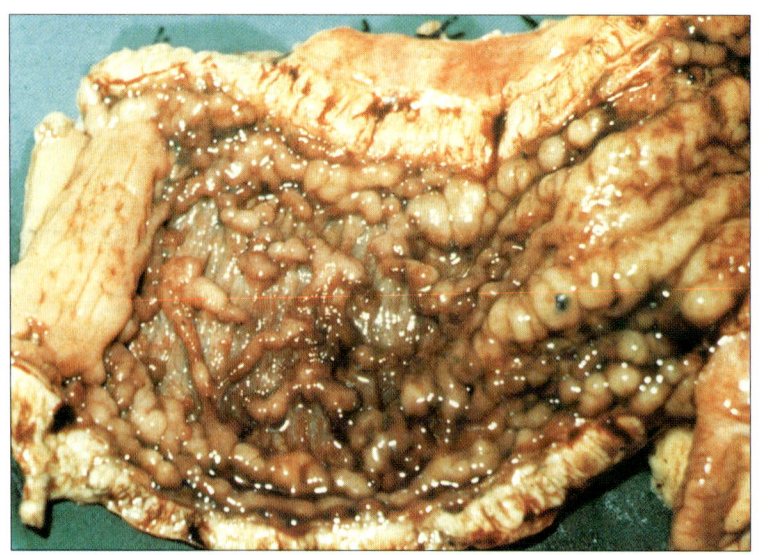

Fig. 6.6 Toxic megacolon complicating severe Crohn's colitis. Toxic megacolon may complicate Crohn's colitis, but is a less common cause of this disorder than ulcerative colitis. In this case, the mucosa has disappeared over wide areas and the underlying smooth muscle is clearly visible. Not surprisingly, the colon had perforated in several places.

Inflammatory Bowel Disease

Diagnostic features in Crohn's disease

Barium follow-through

- Segmental involvement, mural thickening, stenotic loops
- Abnormal terminal ileum: rigid, constricted, nodular
- Partial obstruction
- Abdominal mass

Colonoscopy

- Patchy inflammation
- Aphthous ulcers

Histology

- Lymphoid hyperplasia
- Nodular granulomata
- Submucosal oedema

Fig. 6.7 Diagnostic features in Crohn's disease.

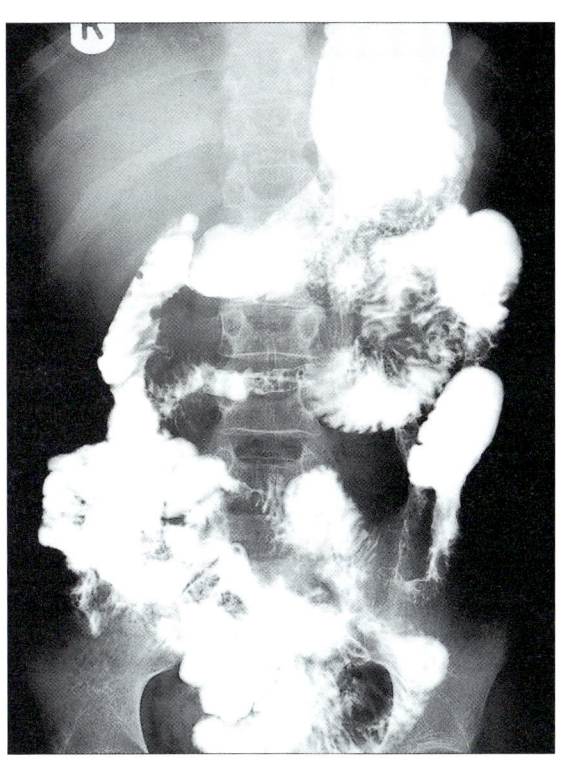

Fig. 6.8 Barium meal and follow-through in induced small intestinal Crohn's disease. Extensive jejunal Crohn's disease is present. The wall of the jejunum is thickened, which has led to marked separation of the column of barium, together with areas of extreme narrowing (string sign), deep penetrative (rose thorn) ulcers and areas of dilatation.

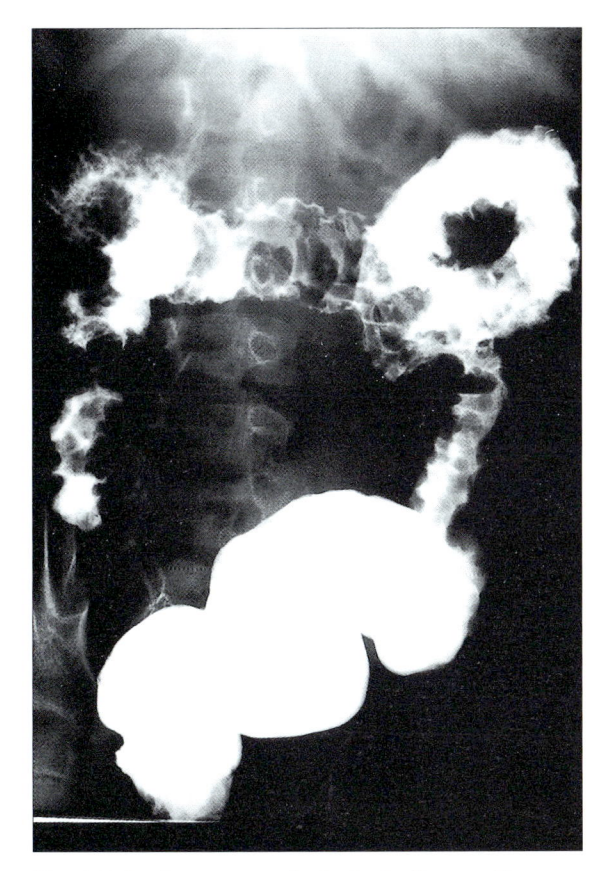

Fig. 6.9 Barium enema in Crohn's disease. The rectum is spared, but the remaining colon is severely affected with deep penetrating ulcers, asymmetric involvement of the bowel wall, and 'cobblestoning'.

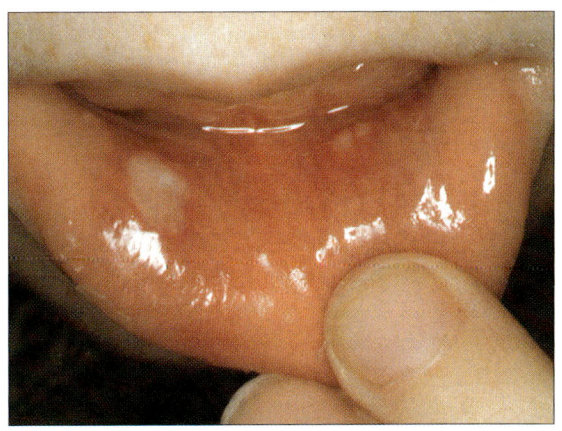

Fig. 6.10 Oral ulceration. About 10% of patients will experience oral ulceration at some stage during their disease; this causes pain and soreness of the mouth or tongue and interferes with eating and drinking. Occasionally, ulcers may be asymptomatic and missed unless the mouth is inspected carefully. Angular cheilitis (cracking and fissuring at the corners of the mouth) is also common.

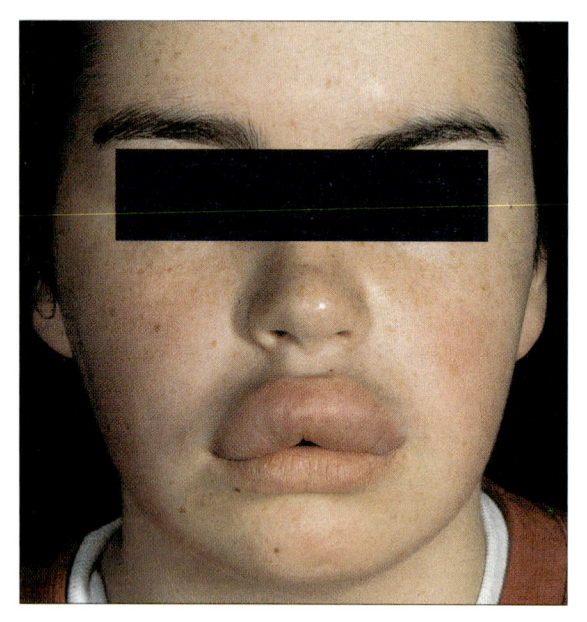

Fig. 6.11 Oral Crohn's disease (orofacial granulomatosis). More extensive involvement of the mouth leads to swelling of the lips and cheeks, often with considerable disfigurement. The buccal mucosa usually reveals a fissured, cobblestone appearance, with or without aphthous ulceration. Biopsy of the mucosa almost always reveals non-caseating granulomata. In some patients this may be the only clinical manifestation of Crohn's disease, although there may be radiological or endoscopic evidence of disease. When there is no other evidence of disease, the disorder is often called orofacial granulomatosis, although many patients go on to develop typical Crohn's disease.

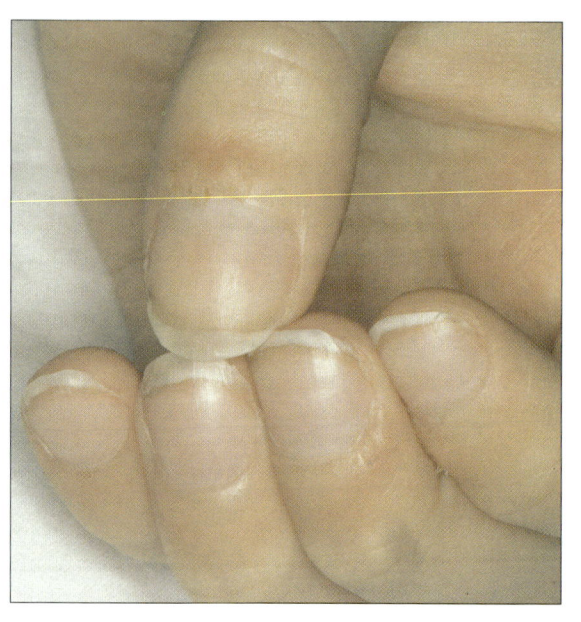

Fig. 6.12 Extra-intestinal manifestations: finger clubbing. About 10% of children with Crohn's disease have clubbing. It is rarely gross and more likely in patients with small-intestinal disease. It usually regresses after surgery and correlates well with disease activity and the degree of fibrosis in the surgical specimen.

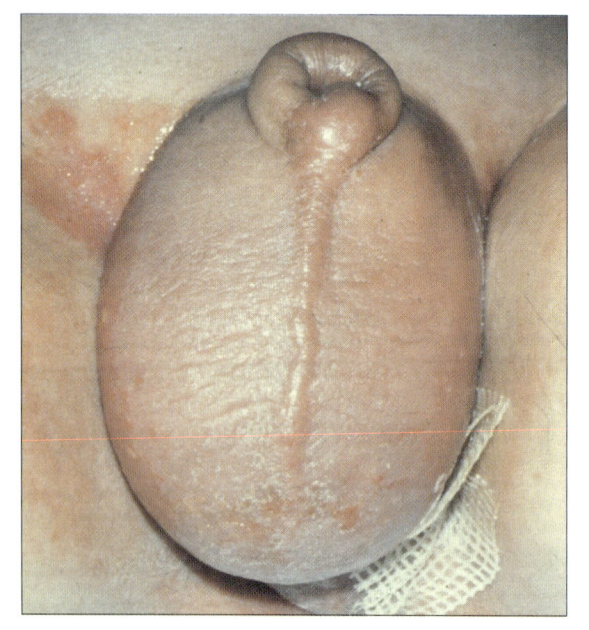

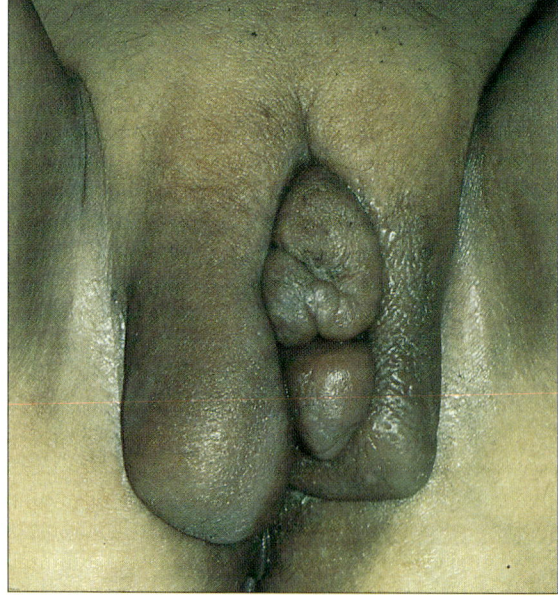

Figs 6.13, 6.14 Genital Crohn's disease. Rarely, Crohn's disease may involve the genitalia, sometimes in association with perianal disease.

Inflammatory Bowel Disease

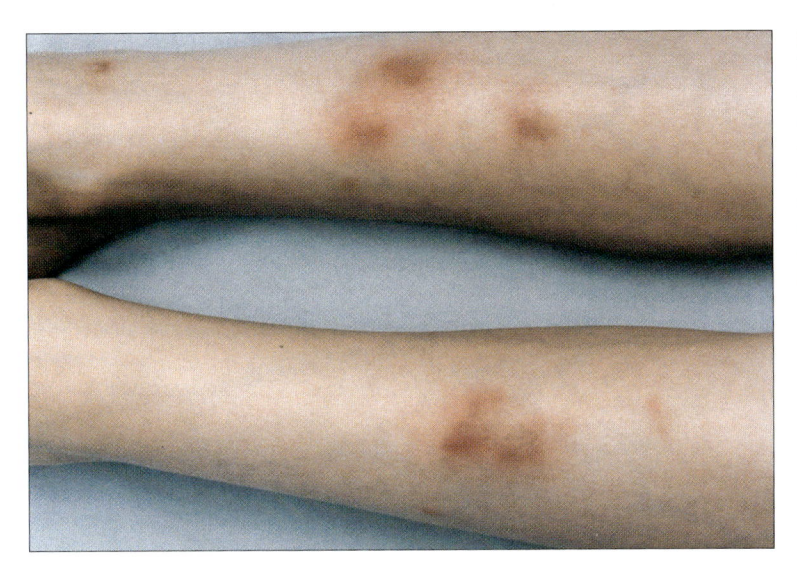

Fig. 6.15 Erythema nodosum. The lesions are sited characteristically on the shins and are raised, red, tender nodules. They occur in 5–10% of children with Crohn's disease, particularly those with Crohn's colitis, and indicate that the underlying disease is active. The lesions subside in a few days, leaving a transient brownish discoloration of the skin.

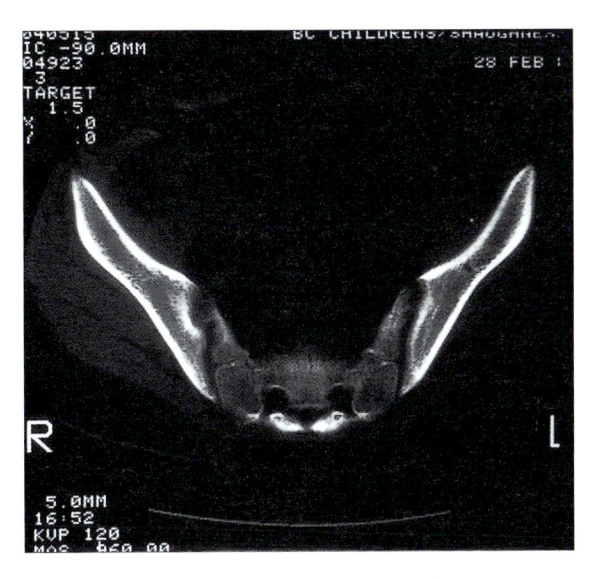

Fig. 6.16 Sacroiliitis. Sacroiliitis and ankylosing spondylitis, in which most patients are HLA-B27 positive, are uncommon complications of inflammatory bowel disease in children. A CT scan of this patient shows right-sided sacroiliac erosion with lateral border sclerosis.

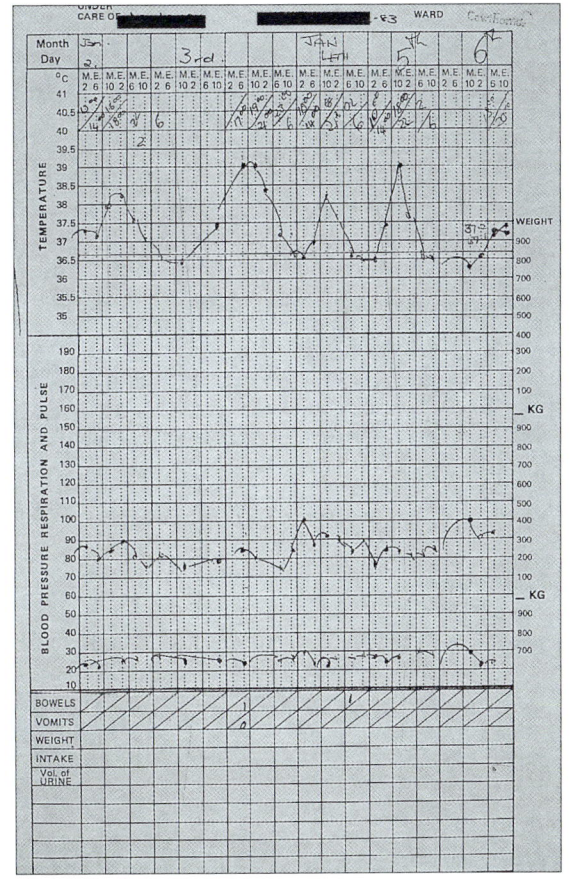

Fig. 6.17 Pyrexia. A swinging pyrexia occurs in about a quarter of patients at diagnosis and is usually low grade and intermittent. It settles as the disease enters remission. Occasionally, a more dramatic swinging fever may be present; if this occurs with weight loss, but in the absence of gastrointestinal symptoms, a provisional diagnosis of malignancy or connective tissue disease may be given.

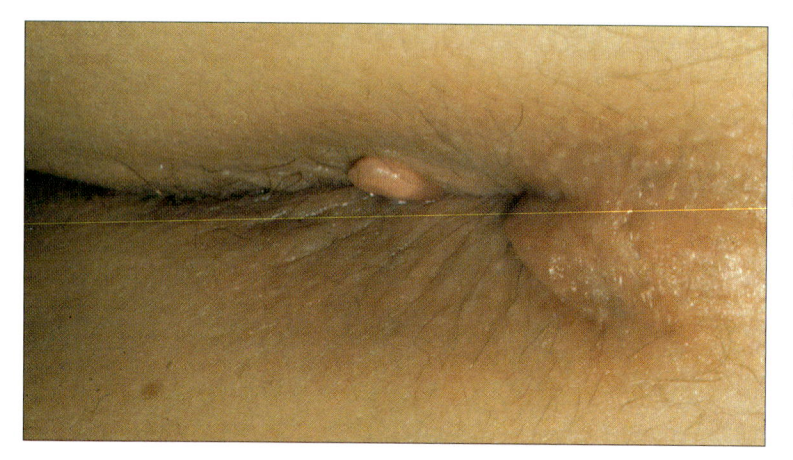

Fig. 6.18 Perianal abnormality. In the child shown here, this perianal abnormality, virtually diagnostic of Crohn's disease, had been missed. He presented with anorexia and weight loss and had diffuse small intestinal disease.

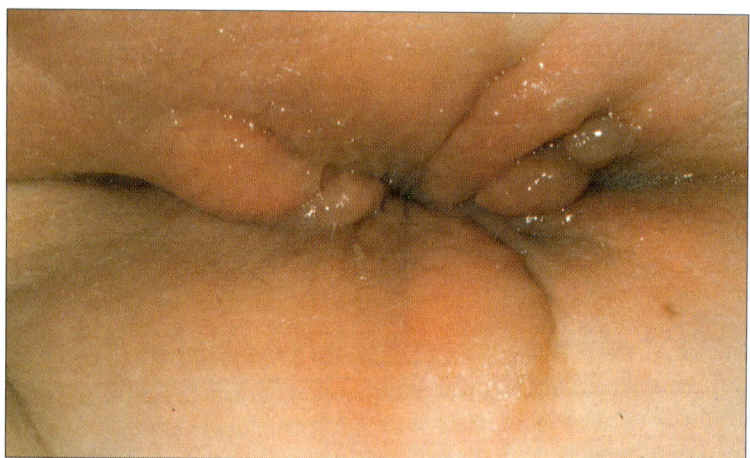

Fig. 6.19 Perianal disease: fissures and skin tags. Nearly 50% of children have a perianal abnormality. Skin tags are uncommon in children, so they are an important diagnostic clue. There is a broad spectrum of severity, ranging from oedematous skin tags, through anal fissures (both seen here), to anal fistulas, erosive perianal ulceration, and deep abscesses. In the absence of abscesses, the lesions are usually remarkably painless, despite their florid appearance. The abnormality reflects overall disease activity, tending to be progressive when proximal bowel disease is active.

Fig. 6.20 Cutaneous Crohn's disease. Rarely, Crohn's granulomata may be found in organs remote from the gut, so-called metastatic Crohn's disease. This 5-year-old girl had extensive colonic Crohn's disease and at presentation was noted to have a generalised erythematous papular rash, which histologically showed typical non-caseating granulomata.

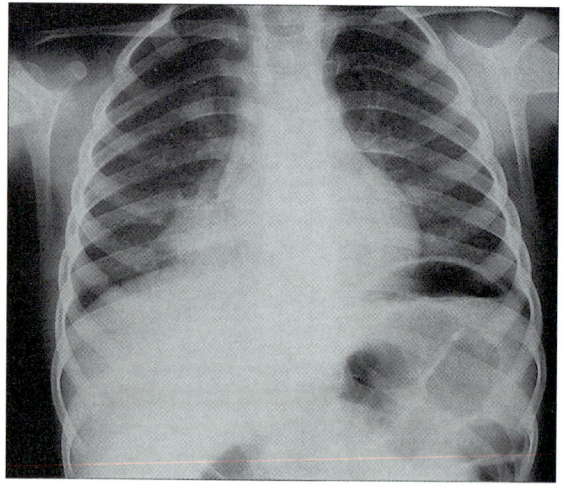

Fig. 6.21 Pulmonary Crohn's disease. Crohn's disease in the lung is rare. This 3-year-old presented with swollen gums and a persistent abnormality on his chest radiograph. Lung biopsy showed multiple non-caseating epithelioid granulomas, and granulomatous inflammation was also found in the buccal mucosa; an anal skin tag and a microscopic colitis were also present. Sarcoidosis is the main differential diagnosis.

Inflammatory Bowel Disease

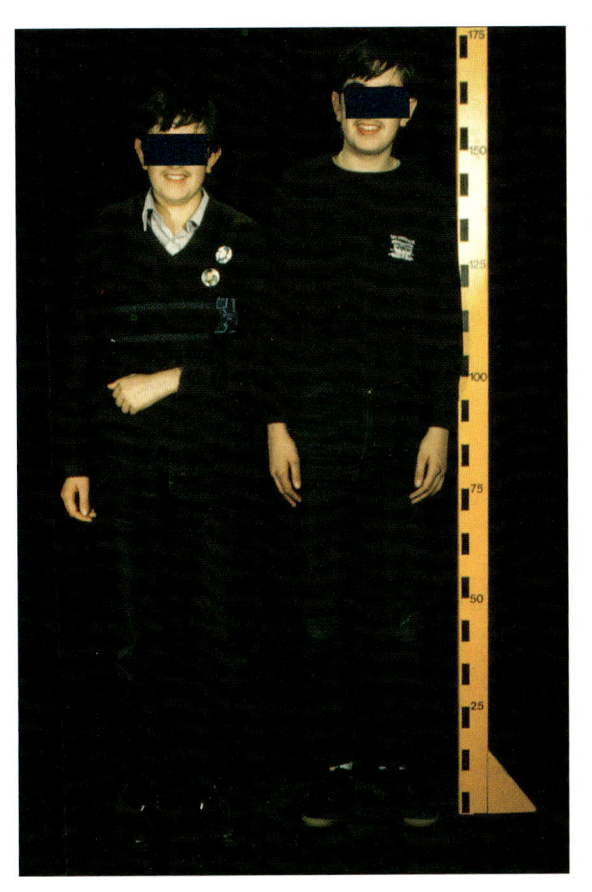

Fig. 6.22 Growth failure. Growth failure affects approximately one-third of patients with Crohn's disease and is associated with pubertal delay and a retarded bone age. Of these identical twins, the child on the left was referred to a growth clinic as his height was falling further behind that of his normal twin. Gastrointestinal symptoms were absent and growth hormone secretion was normal. A barium follow-through showed diffuse small bowel Crohn's disease.

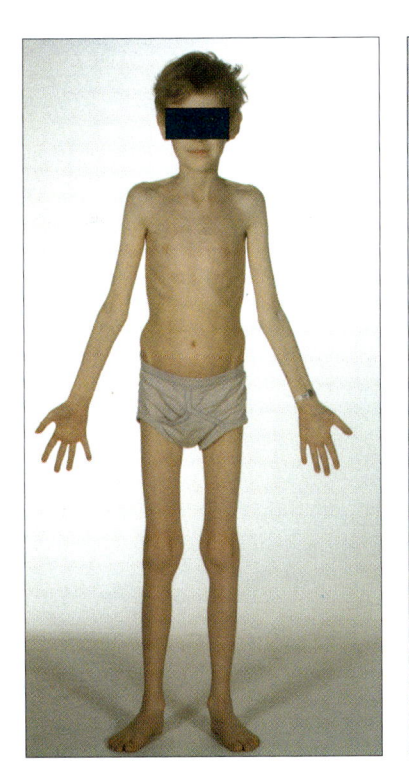

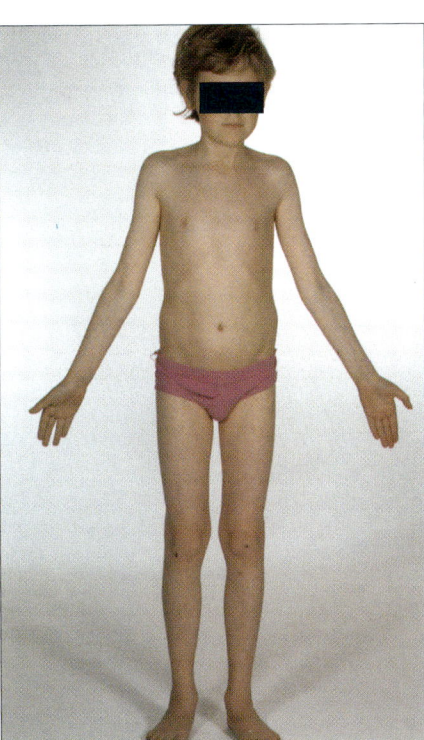

Figs 6.23, 6.24 Response to an elemental diet. This patient presented at the age of 11 years with a 2-year history of diarrhoea, weight loss, abdominal pain, and oral ulceration. He was severely malnourished and a barium follow-through showed Crohn's disease of the distal ileum (**6.23**, left). He was treated with a chemically defined diet, with amino acids providing the nitrogen source, and 6 months later was still in remission, his weight had increased, and he had started to show some acceleration in linear growth (**6.24**, right). An elemental diet is now the treatment of choice, rather than corticosteroids, in children with small intestinal Crohn's disease.

ULCERATIVE COLITIS

Ulcerative colitis is a recurrent, inflammatory, and ulcerative disease that involves only the mucosa of the colon. The entire large bowel is usually affected. In contrast to Crohn's disease, the incidence of ulcerative colitis has not changed recently; the overall incidence of Crohn's disease and ulcerative colitis now appears to be similar. As in the case of Crohn's disease, the aetiology is unknown.

Ulcerative colitis presents most commonly with bloody diarrhoea, although this is not invariable, and blood may be absent from the stools (**6.25**). It is important to note that while 60% of children present with mild diarrhoea of somewhat insidious onset, with or without bleeding, 10% present with a fulminating colitis, possibly with toxic megacolon, and require emergency treatment when first seen.

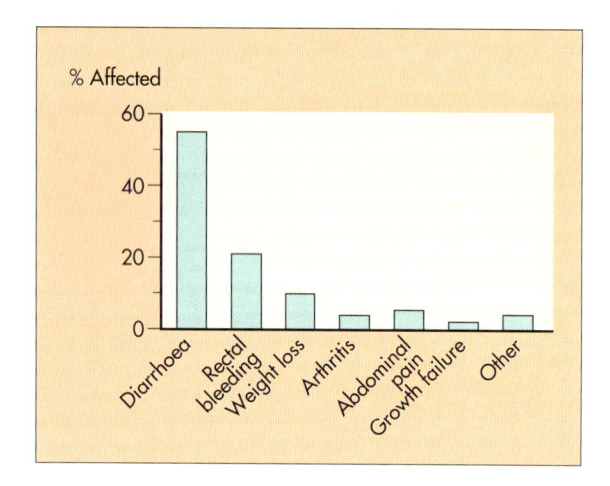

Fig. 6.25 Initial symptoms of ulcerative colitis.

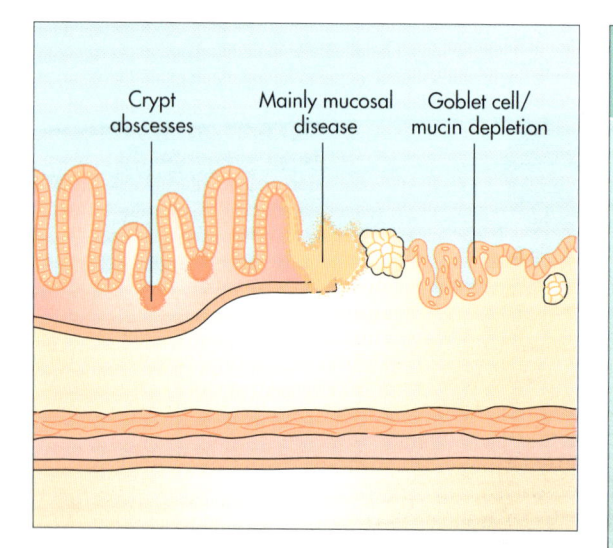

Fig. 6.26 Histology. Microscopically, the inflammatory process is confined initially to the mucosa, but may spread to the submucosa if the overlying epithelium is destroyed. Vascular congestion, crypt abscesses, loss of goblet cells, crypt branching, and the appearance of Paneth cells within the crypts are all commonly seen but none are pathognomic. Fibrosis is minimal, even in chronic disease. In fulminating disease, extensive mucosal ulceration is accompanied by severe destruction of the submucosa to expose the colonic musculature, which may be covered by a thin layer of granulation tissue only.

Patterns of clinical presentation of ulcerative colitis

Mild disease

Diarrhoea (intermittently with blood);
No fever, no weight loss;
Normal physical examination;
Colonoscopy: mild distal disease;
No hypoalbuminaemia.

Moderate disease

Bloody diarrhoea (less than six stools per day);
Abdominal pain (cramps preceding defaecation);
Intermittent fever: weight loss;
Possible tenderness on abdominal palpation;
Colonoscopy: friability and loss of vascular pattern.

Severe disease

Severe bloody diarrhoea (more than six stools per day);
Significant weight loss;
Systemic manifestations: fever; tachycardia;
Abdominal diffuse tenderness on palpation;
Limited sigmoidoscopy: findings of fulminant colitis (diffuse ulceration, pseudopolyps);
Hypoalbuminaemia.

Fig. 6.27 Patterns of clinical presentation of ulcerative colitis.

Diagnostic features in ulcerative colitis

Radiology

- Continuous involvement
- Foreshortening; loss of haustra
- Irregularity of mucosal margins
- Normal terminal ileum

Colonoscopy

- Friability
- Lack of vascular pattern
- Diffuse rectosigmoid ulceration
- Crypt abscesses
- Pseudopolyps

Histology

- Acute inflammation infiltrate
- Crypt distortion
- Goblet cell depletion

Fig. 6.28 Diagnostic features in ulcerative colitis.

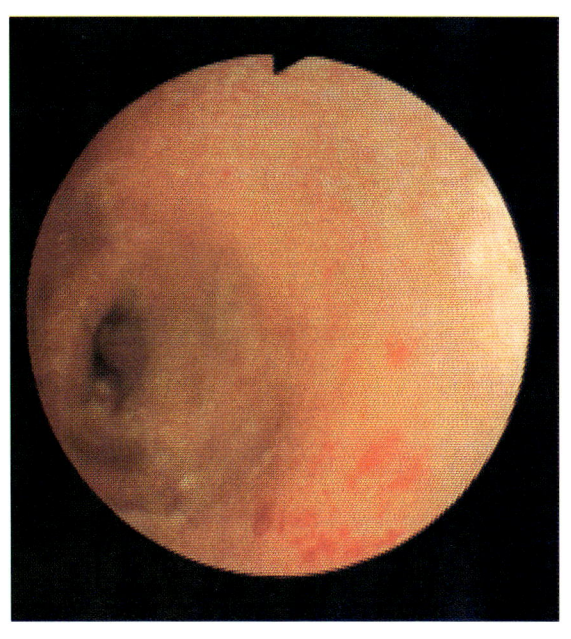

Fig. 6.29 Colonoscopic appearances. Colonoscopy is now the diagnostic method of choice, having superseded barium enema. Loss of the normal vascular pattern is the initial abnormality, followed by hyperaemia, granularity, and contact bleeding. As seen here, the haemorrhagic mucosa subsequently becomes patchily and superficially ulcerated, but without fissuring. Inflammatory polyposis, as distinct from the cobblestones seen in Crohn's disease, is commonly seen in the colon. In contrast to Crohn's colitis, the disease is continuous and predominantly left-sided.

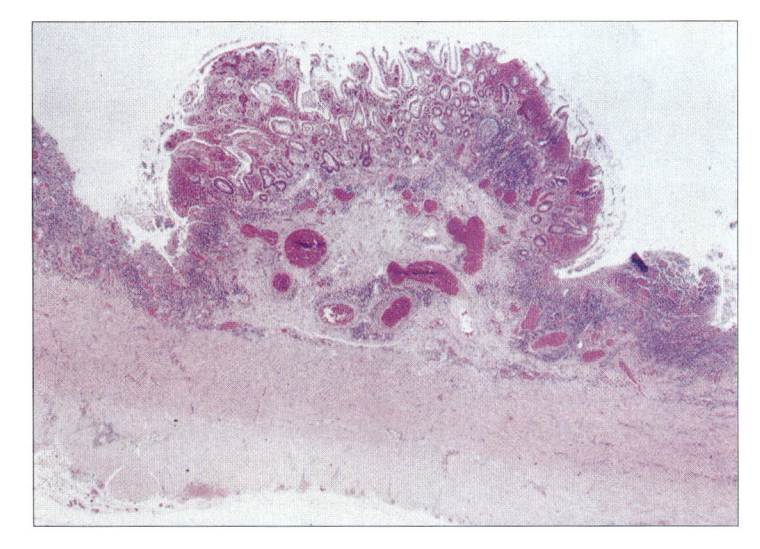

Fig. 6.30 Inflammatory polyp (pseudopolyp). Inflammatory polyps result from exuberant regeneration of the affected epithelium. They are found in the colon, but not in the rectum, and are a sign of long-standing disease.

Pediatric Gastroenterology and Hepatology

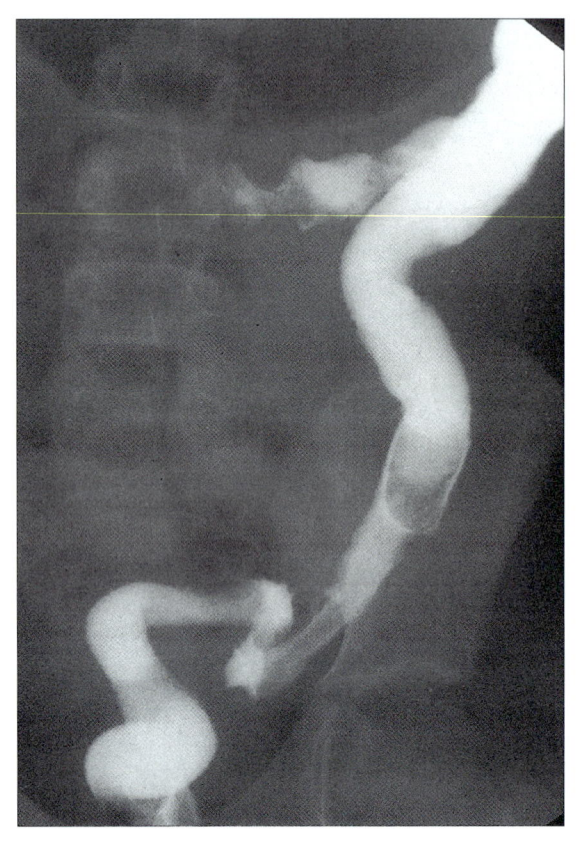

Fig. 6.31 Barium enema. This 10-year-old girl had moderately severe disease. There is loss of haustra leading to a somewhat tubular appearance. Mucosal ulceration is present and is best seen in the sigmoid colon. Marked mucosal oedema is seen in the transverse colon. In long-standing disease the colon becomes short, and in patients with pan-colitis the last few centimetres of ileum may appear dilated and featureless, indicating a 'backwash' ileitis.

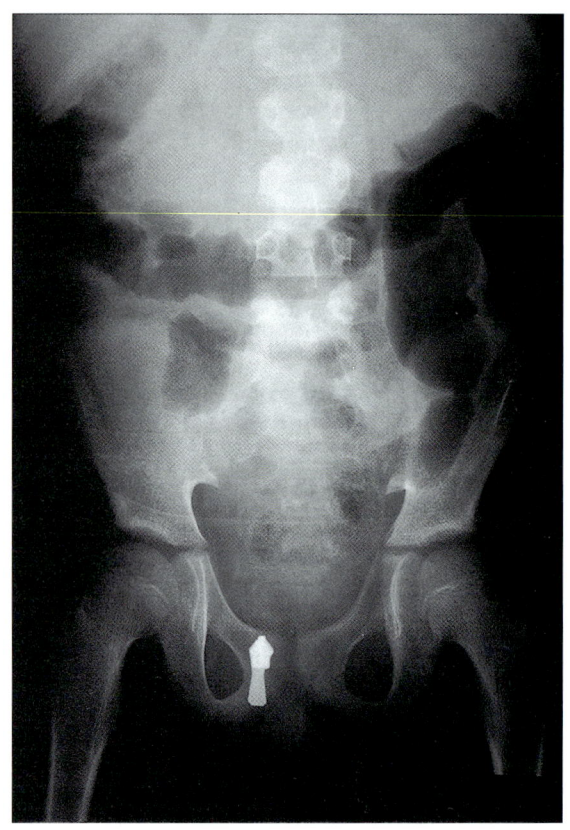

Figs 6.32, 6.33 Toxic megacolon. This patient had severe fulminating colitis and was febrile, had a tachycardia, hypoalbuminaemia, and anaemia. Her abdomen was slightly distended and tender, and bowel sounds were absent. The plain abdominal film shows marked colonic dilatation with obvious mucosal oedema in the transverse colon (**6.32**, top right). She failed to respond to 48 hours of intensive medical treatment, but a sub-total colectomy was life-saving. The colectomy specimen shows the haemorrhagic mucosa and there is widespread ulceration (**6.33**, bottom).

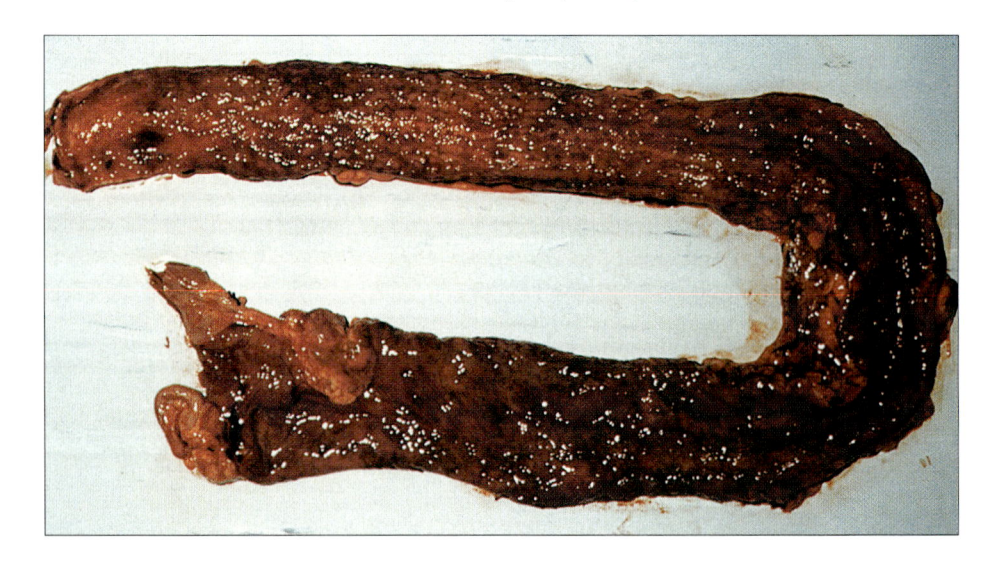

Inflammatory Bowel Disease

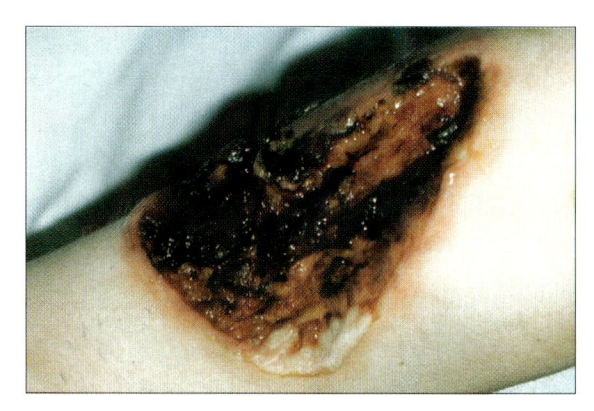

Fig. 6.34 Pyoderma gangrenosum. Pyoderma gangrenosum is rare and occurs in only 1% of patients with ulcerative colitis. It produces a deep, painful ulcer with undermined purple edges. The patient presents with sudden skin necrosis, sometimes with blistering, followed by ulceration, including both fat and muscle. The cause is unknown, but it usually occurs in association with active colonic inflammation.

Proctocolectomy with ileal reservoir and anal anastomosis

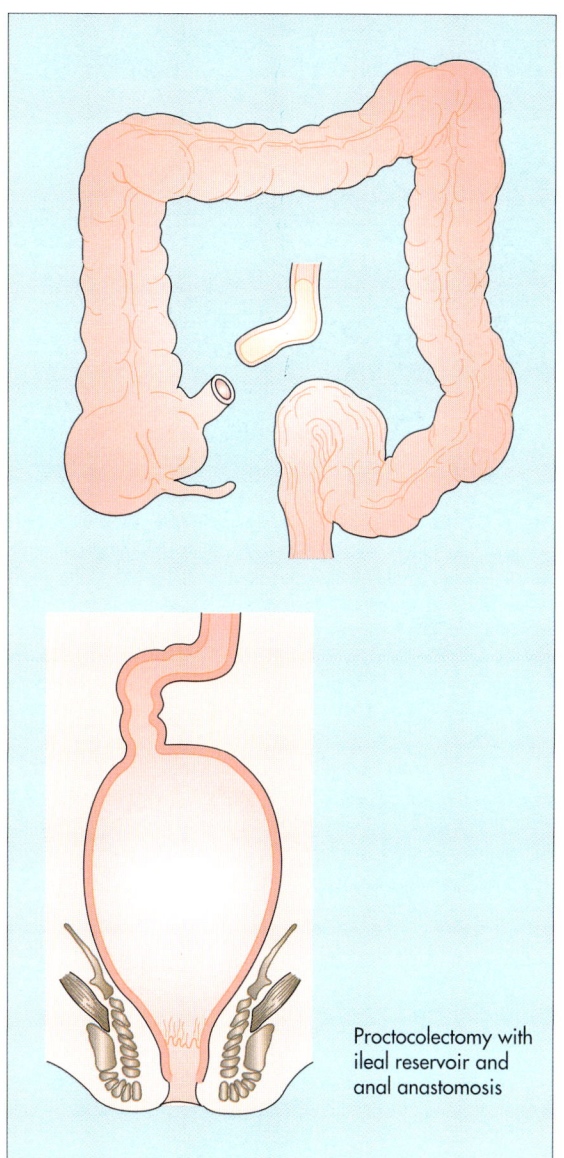

Fig. 6.36 Proctocolectomy with ileal reservoir and anal anastomosis. Total colectomy, mucosal proctectomy, with ileal pouch–anal anastomosis has become a popular option for patients who require colectomy. All mucosal disease is removed, the normal route for defaecation is maintained, and the anal sphincter is undisturbed. The procedure involves abdominal colectomy, excision of the distal rectal mucosa from the underlying upper internal anal sphincter and lower rectal muscular cuff, the fashioning of an ileal pouch, and anastomosis of the ileal mucosa to the anoderm.

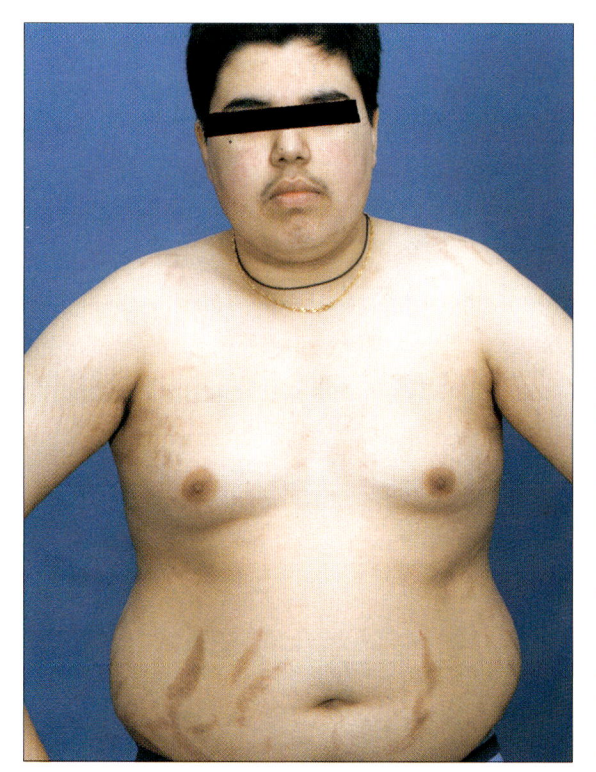

Fig. 6.35 Cushingoid appearance secondary to steroid administration. This patient had chronic ulcerative colitis and had refused a colectomy. He had been on oral steroids for 2 years and developed these characteristic facial appearances, together with obesity, striae, and hirsutism. His linear growth had become poor, but he showed good catch-up following colectomy.

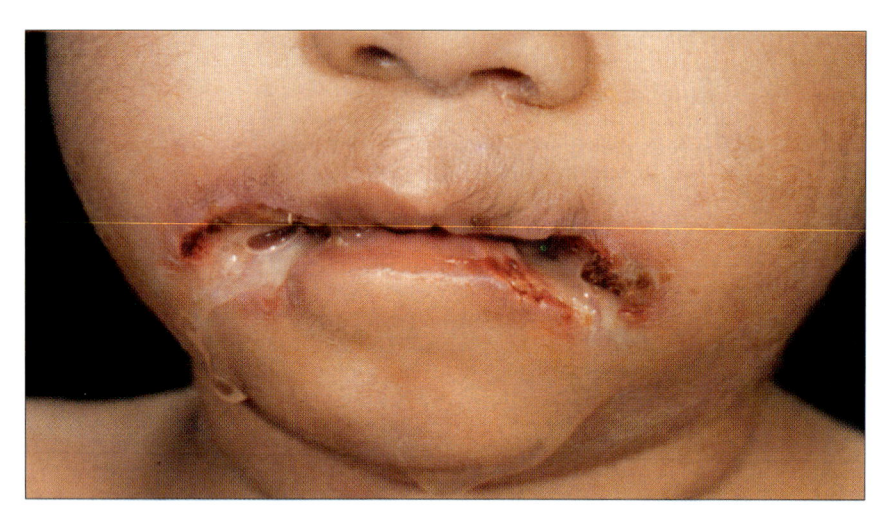

Fig. 6.37 Behçet's disease. Behçet's disease is a multisystem vasculitic disorder of unknown aetiology. Major symptoms comprise recurrent, painful oral ulceration, recurrent genital ulcers, uveitis, cutaneous vasculitis, synovitis, meningo-encephalitis, and cutaneous hyper-reactivity to minor trauma. The frequency of gastrointestinal involvement is highly variable, but has been reported in up to 15% of cases. Clinically and radiologically, Behçet's mimics Crohn's disease. In contrast to Crohn's, there is less inflammation in the area surrounding ulcers (which occur most commonly in the ileocaecal region) and granulomas are not seen. Treatment is with corticosteroids or other immunosuppressants.

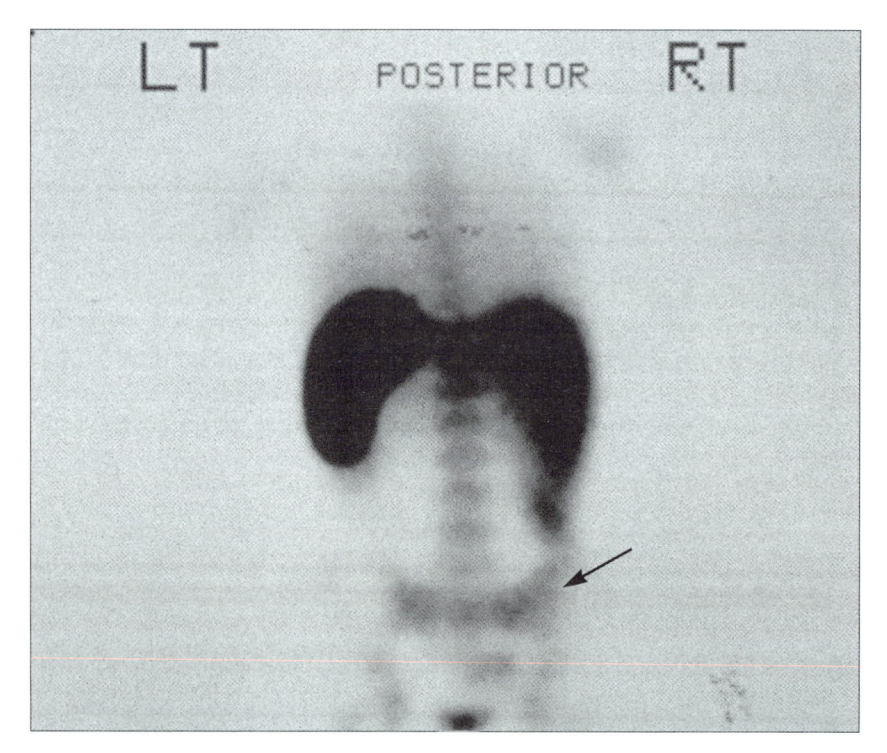

Fig. 6.38 Technetium HMPAO-labelled white cell scan. The technitium white cell scan is a sensitive test for alimentary bowel disease in the small bowel and colon. White blood cells, separated from the patient and labelled with technitium, are injected intravenously and migrate to areas of inflammation. In this study, the 3.5-hour scan shows increased activity in the ascending and transverse colon. High activity in the upper abdomen is in the liver and spleen; high activity in the pelvis is in the bladder.

7. Motility and Constipation

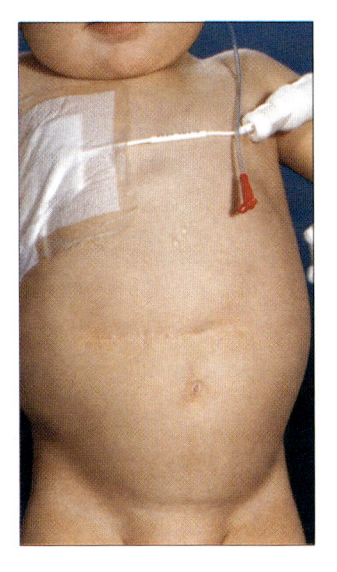

Fig. 7.1 Intestinal pseudo-obstruction. Intestinal pseudo-obstruction in children (vomiting and constipation, usually with abdominal distension, but without a mechanical cause) usually presents in the first few months of life. In some children it is due to a neuropathy of the myenteric plexus, whereas in others it results from a smooth muscle myopathy. Sometimes there is an associated lesion of the urinary tract (hollow visceral myopathy). Long-term parenteral nutrition is often necessary.

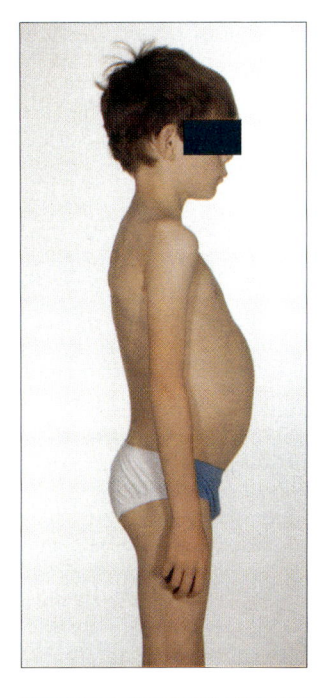

Fig. 7.2 Intestinal pseudo-obstruction. This patient has intestinal pseudo-obstruction and has been maintained on home parenteral nutrition since early childhood. While the very long-term prognosis for such patients is uncertain, most enjoy a good quality of life at home.

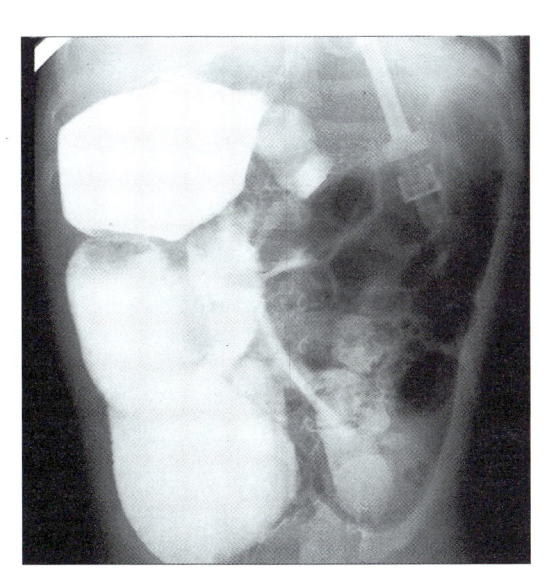

Fig. 7.3 Barium study in pseudo-obstruction complicating neonatal short gut syndrome. The most frequently encountered form of intestinal pseudo-obstruction is that which may complicate massive small intestinal loss in the neonate. This patient has a short, dilated, dysmotile small intestine (following resection for a gangrenous gastroschisis) which required parenteral nutrition for several months before spontaneous resolution.

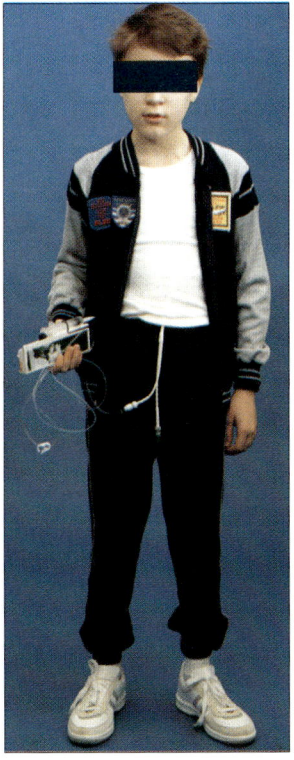

Fig. 7.4 Pseudo-obstruction and malrotation. Intestinal malrotation may be complicated by intestinal pseudo-obstruction. This boy has a malrotation and at 8 years of age presented with recurrent episodes of pain and profuse bile-stained vomiting, leading to two laparotomies, each of which failed to reveal a mechanical obstruction. His symptoms subsequently became persistent, with abdominal pain so severe that he required a morphine infusion (shown here). He also required parenteral nutrition, but his symptoms resolved on treatment with cisapride.

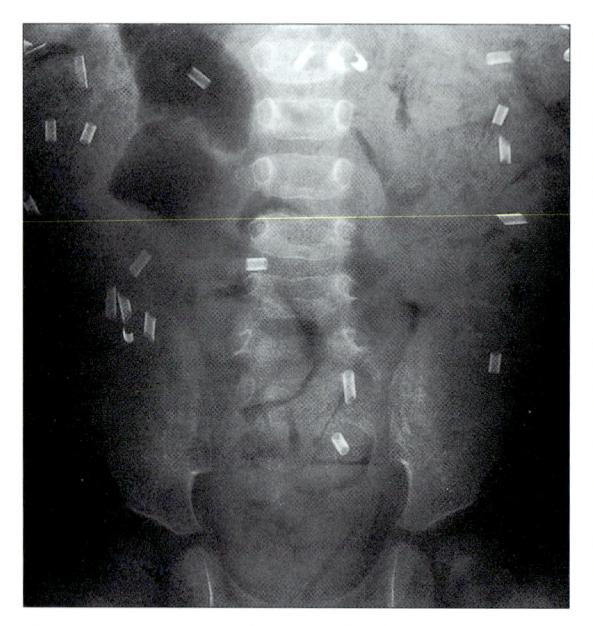

Fig. 7.5 Severe constipation. The diagnosis and assessment of the severity of constipation may be difficult, especially in children who present with spurious diarrhoea. This child presented with a history of several years of 'diarrhoea' associated with soiling. Although there may be obvious faecal retention on a plain abdominal film, parents and children have difficulty in understanding radiographs. In severely constipated children, the fact that most of the radio-opaque markers administered orally are retained, even after several days, is helpful in convincing parents of the diagnosis. The degree of marker retention also predicts the likely duration and difficulty of treatment.

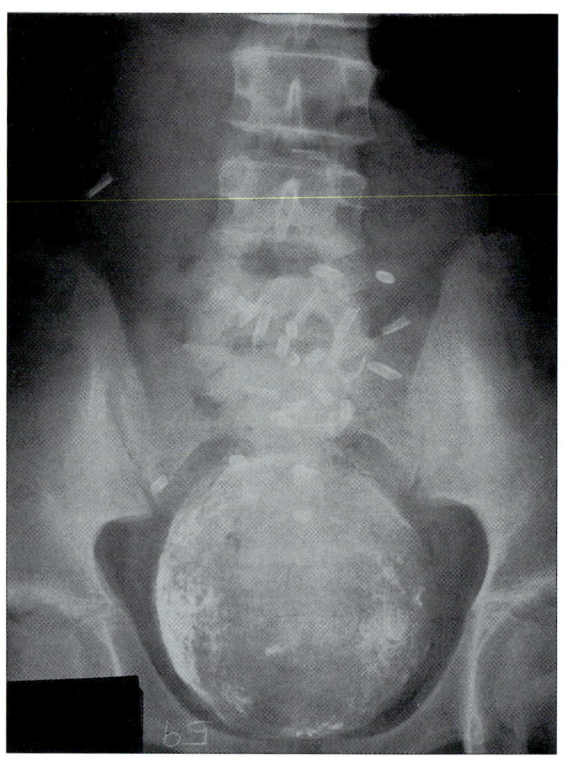

Fig. 7.6 Severe faecal impaction in a megarectum. This abdominal film, taken after the administration of radio-opaque markers, shows a large impacted faecal mass in a patient who presented with several years' soiling. Manual evacuation of such masses may be necessary.

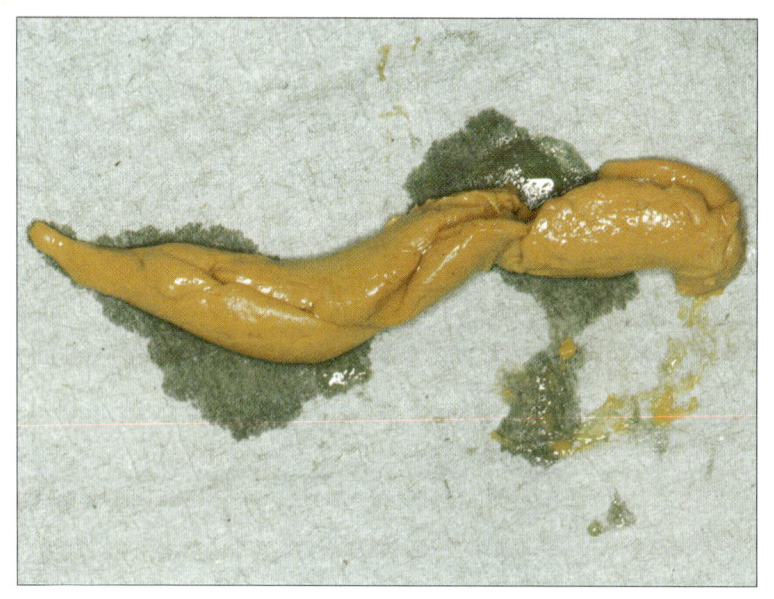

Fig. 7.7 Constipation: ribbon stool. Constipation is common in children living in developed countries. Nearly 1 in 40 of 7-year-old boys are affected, but only 1 in 140 of 7-year-old girls. In most children a structural basis is absent, but the 6-month-old child who produced this ribbon stool had experienced difficult, infrequent defaecation from early infancy. Mild anal stenosis was present, which resolved with repeated anal dilatation using metal dilators. Hirschsprung's disease (Chapter 1) is an important differential diagnosis, which can usually be excluded on clinical grounds. Other disorders which may more rarely present with constipation include coeliac disease, cows' milk protein intolerance, hypothyroidism, and hypercalcaemia.

8. General and Abdominal Pain

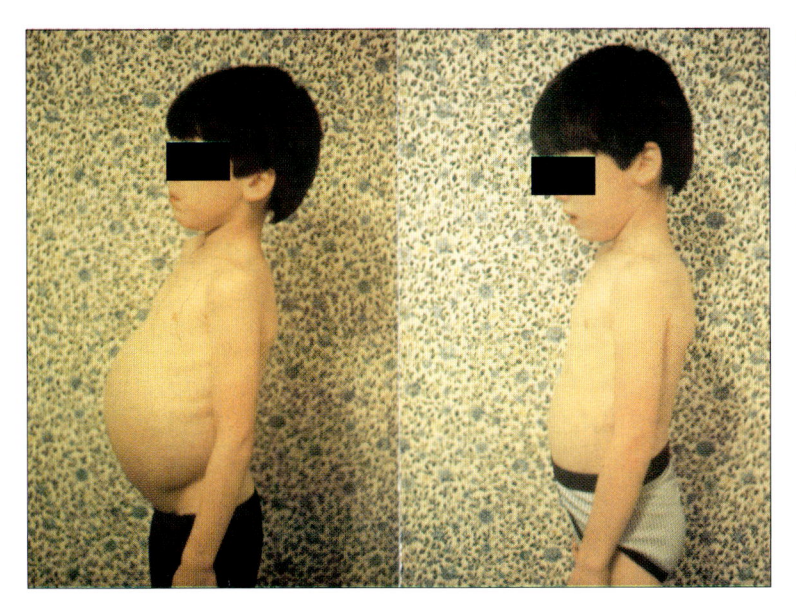

Fig. 8.1 Air swallowing. This child has a markedly distended abdomen during the day (the left-hand panel shows him at bedtime), but the distension is not present on waking (right-hand panel). This is due to air swallowing, not intestinal disease, and is particularly common in toddlers.

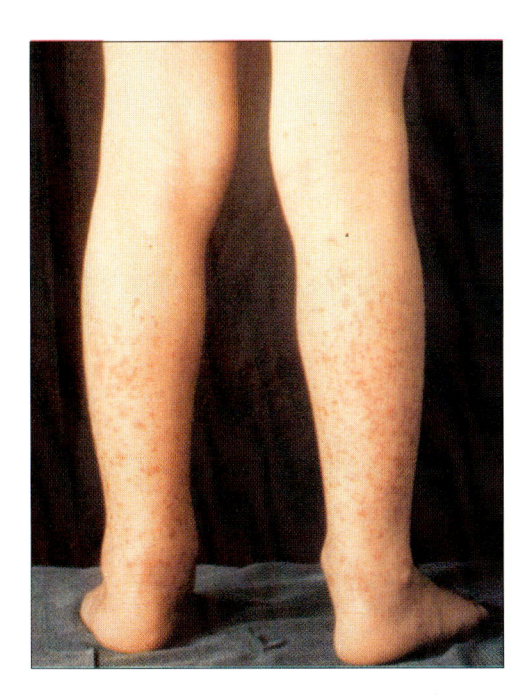

Fig. 8.2 Henoch–Schönlein purpura. There is a purpuric rash affecting the lower limbs. This begins as an urticarial rash which becomes purpuric and affects mainly the limbs and buttocks. There may be involvement of the gastrointestinal and renal tracts and of the joints.

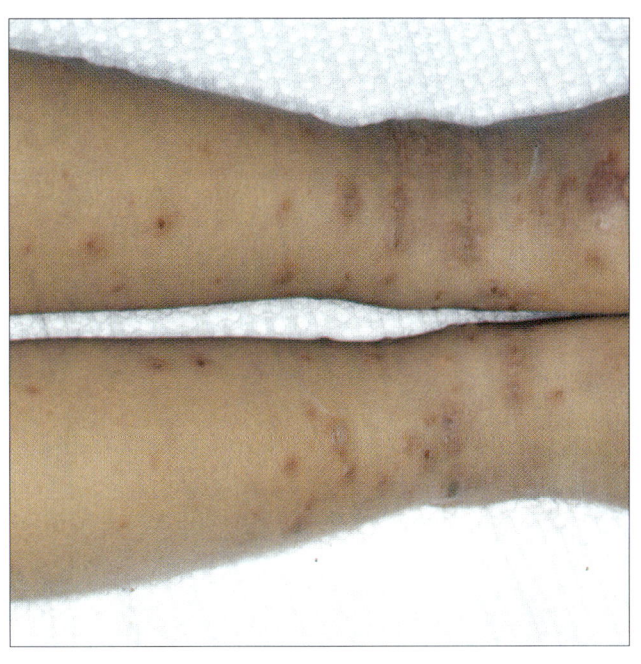

Fig. 8.3 Henoch–Schönlein purpura. The purpuric rash is again shown, but appears more blotchy and urticarial on the extensor surfaces near the ankle joints. The dorsal surfaces of both feet are swollen. Similar swelling may be seen on the hands and face.

Pediatric Gastroenterology and Hepatology

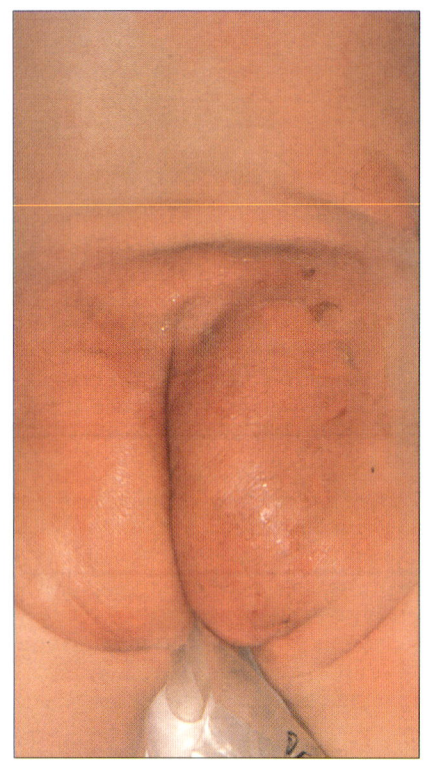

Fig. 8.4 Munchausen syndrome by proxy. This infant presented with severe buttock excoriation due to severe, protracted diarrhoea. Initial investigations failed to reveal a cause for the diarrhoea, but a laxative derivative (senna) was present in the urine. The diarrhoea stopped abruptly once the infant's mother had been separated from the patient.

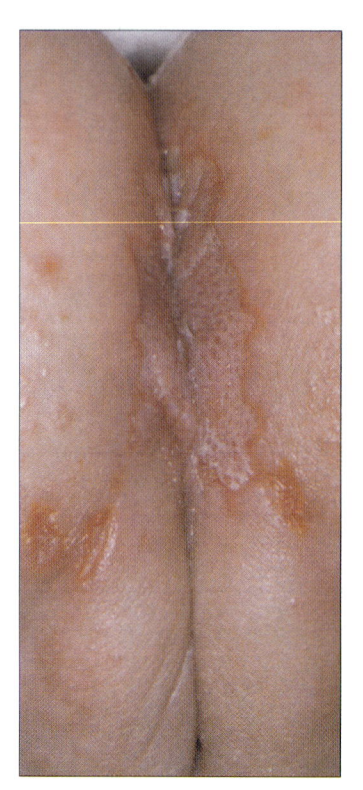

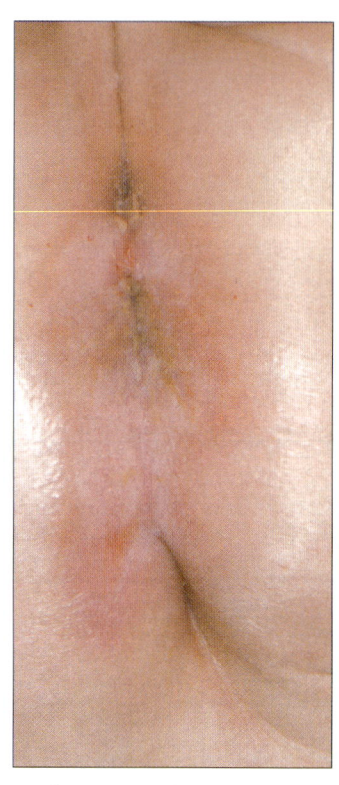

Figs 8.5, 8.6 Munchausen syndrome by proxy. The patient's mother complained that this curious excoriation (**8.5**, left) around the anus had been present for several weeks. Extensive investigation failed to reveal a cause, until the appearance of excoriated lesions around the nostril suggested Munchausen syndrome by proxy. Removal of the mother from the child took place one week before the appearance in **8.6** (right).

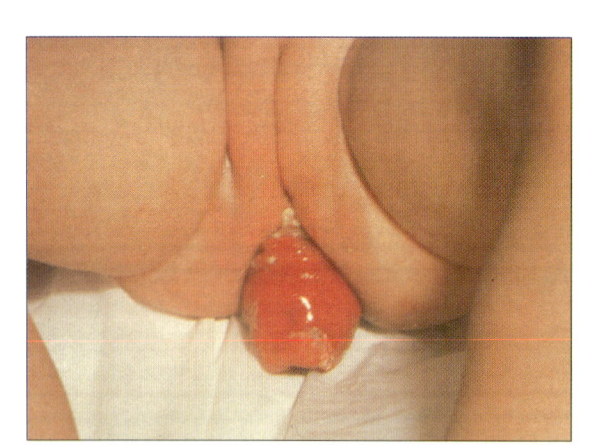

Fig. 8.7 Rectal prolapse. This may be associated with cystic fibrosis, malnutrition, or paralysis of the muscles of the pelvic floor (e.g., in spina bifida). Repeated recurrence following manual reduction may require submucosal injection of sclerosant.

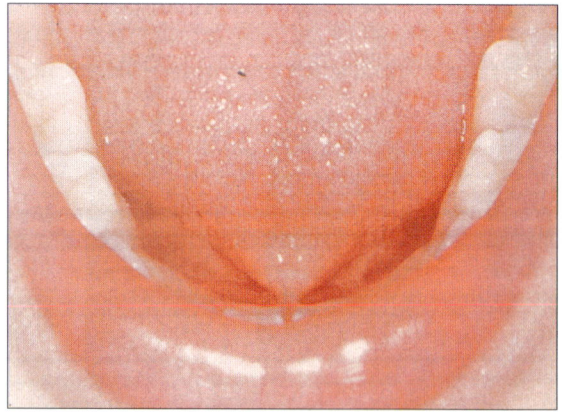

Fig. 8.8 Tongue tie (ankyloglossia). A short lingual frenum is present which extends to the tip of the tongue, and prevents tongue protrusion. Surgical intervention is seldom necessary as this anomaly is rarely responsible for difficulties in sucking or speech.

General and Abdominal Pain

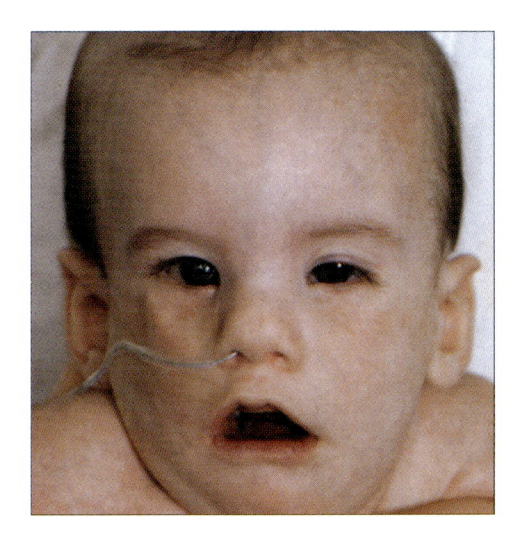

Fig. 8.9 Bulbar palsy (Möbius syndrome). This infant has dysphagia and chokes on liquid feeds. He has a flaccid (lower motor neurone) bulbar palsy and a facial diplegia. He presented with a poor suck, and nasal regurgitation of feeds. The nasogastric tube is used for enteral feeding.

RECURRENT ABDOMINAL PAIN

Recurrent abdominal pain (RAP) is common in childhood, and affects 10% of children at some stage. Most children (95%) do not have organic pathology, but it is important to recognise those that do, on the basis of the history (e.g., growth failure, other gastrointestinal symptoms, nocturnal pain) and a detailed examination.

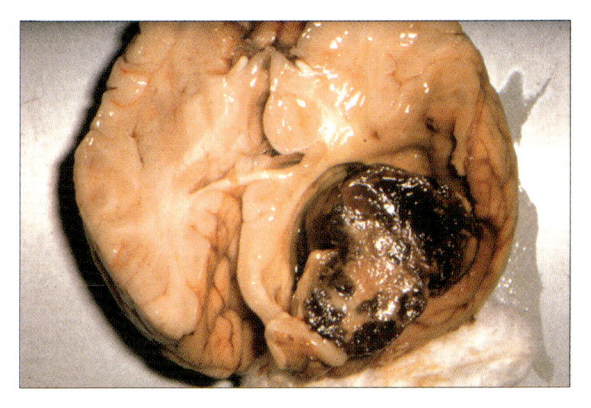

Fig. 8.10 Cerebral tumour. Extra-intestinal causes of RAP are important. The child with this large tumour presented with abdominal pain and papilloedema. Careful fundoscopy is therefore a crucial part of the clinical examination of every child with RAP.

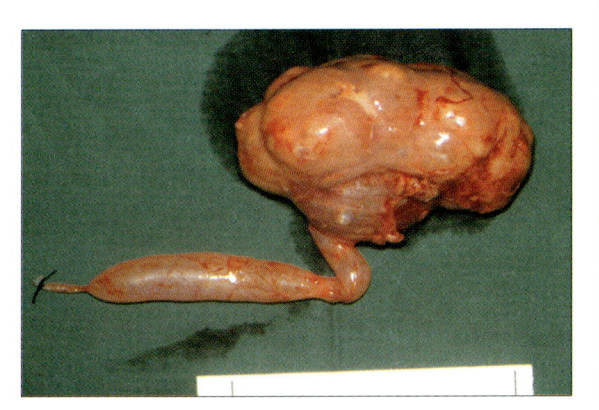

Fig. 8.11 Hydronephrosis. Urinary tract disease may present with RAP, with few or no urinary symptoms. The patient whose resected kidney is shown here had several years' RAP before a mass in the loin was found on examination. Urine microscopy and culture should be performed on every child with RAP, and there should be a low threshold for ultrasound examination of the abdomen.

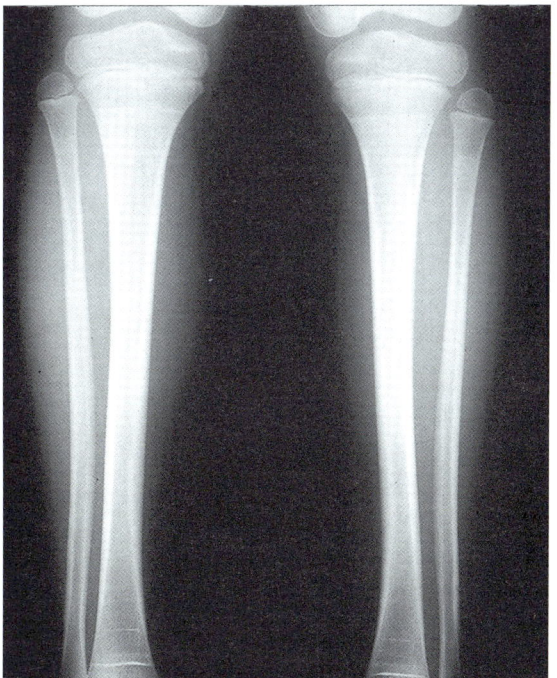

Fig. 8.12 Lead poisoning. Lead poisoning is now a rare cause of RAP in developed countries. This patient presented with colicky pain and anaemia, and the blood film showed basophil stippling. The radiograph shows dense 'lead lines' at the distal ends of each tibia. The patient, who was psychologically disturbed, had been gnawing painted surfaces in an old house.

Pediatric Gastroenterology and Hepatology

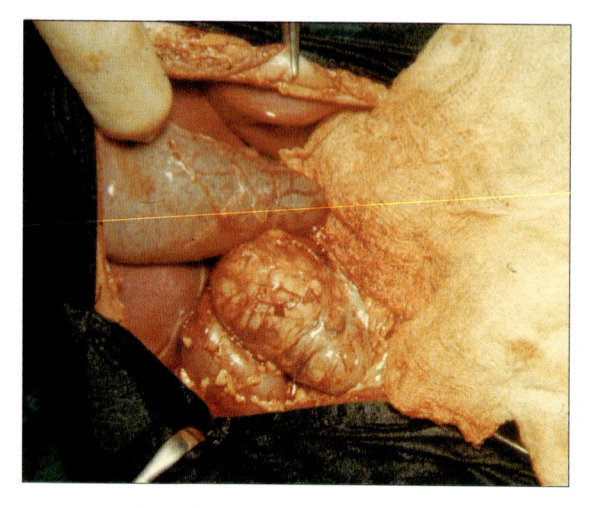

Fig. 8.13 Ganglioneuroblastoma. Right-sided pain in this patient was accompanied by hypertension. Abdominal ultrasound examination revealed a right-sided adrenal ganglioneuroblastoma, shown here between the gall bladder and right kidney at laparotomy. Although there are often some less-differentiated cells on histology, most tumours behave in a benign fashion, and local resection is usually curative (*see* VIP-secreting tumour, Chapter 9).

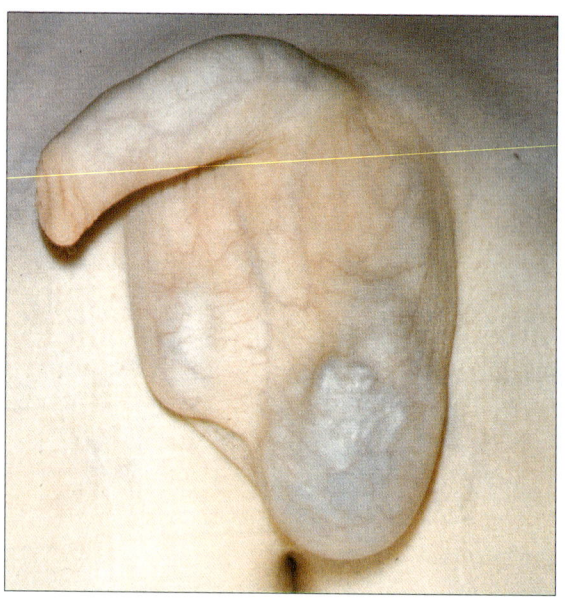

Fig. 8.14 Seminoma. Examination of the genitalia in this boy with RAP revealed a seminoma of the left testis.

MISCELLANEOUS DISORDERS

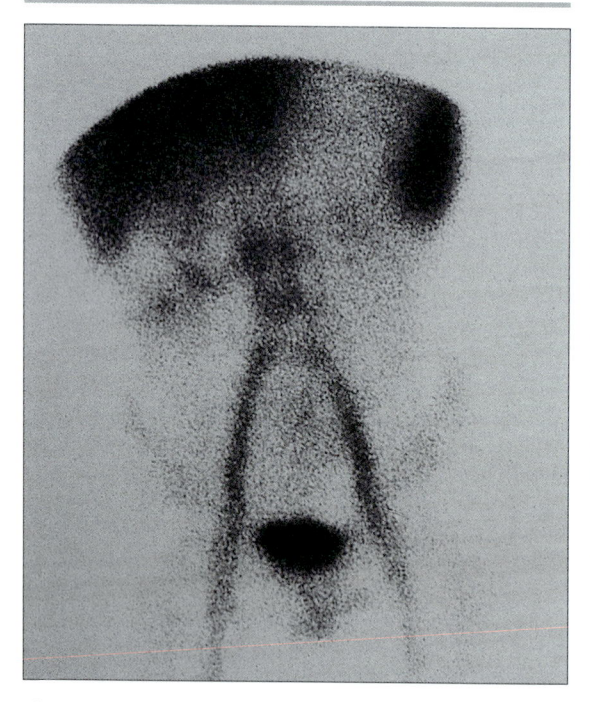

Fig. 8.15 Labelled red-cell scan. Some of the patient's own red cells are removed, labelled with technitium and re-injected. Extravasated red cells are detected on serial scanning. This patient had an angiodysplasia of the transverse colon. Initial scans showed extravasation at the hepatic flexure. On this later scan, extravasated blood has been carried into the transverse colon.

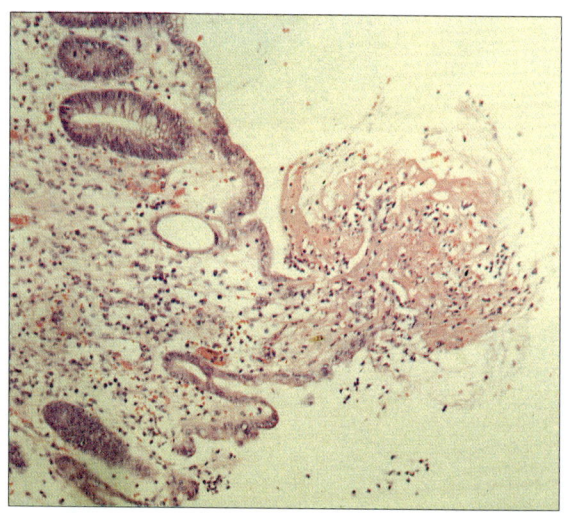

Fig. 8.16 Pseudomembranous colitis. Shown here is focal ulceration of the surface epithelium of the colon, with a volcano-like cap of inflammatory debris and cells. Endoscopically, these lesions appear flat and raised, varying in size from a few millimetres to nearly a centimetre. The intervening mucosa is hyperaemic. In most cases, infection with toxin-producing *Clostridium difficile* is responsible, usually following antibiotic exposure. In this case, the disease occurred secondary to Hirschsprung's disease.

9. Gastrointestinal Tumours

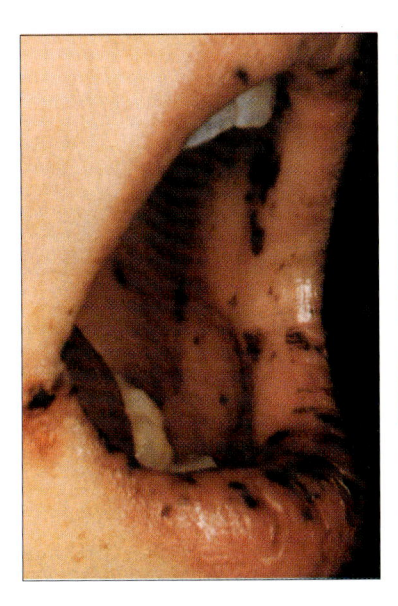

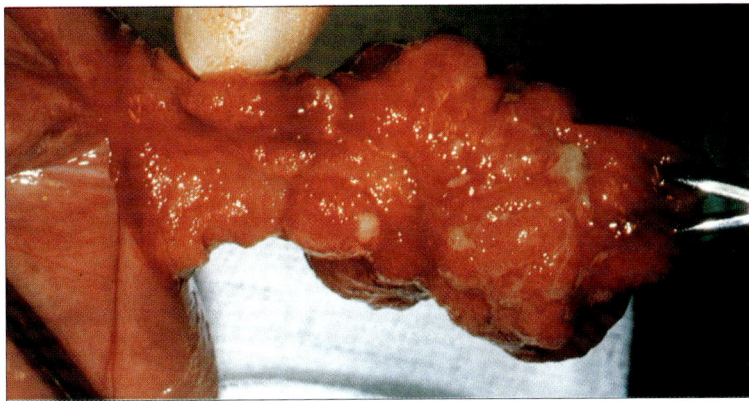

Figs 9.1, 9.2 Peutz–Jeghers syndrome. Mucocutaneous pigmentation around the nose, lips (**9.1**, top left), buccal mucosa, hands, and feet occurs in association with hamartomatous polyps in the stomach, small intestine (**9.2**, top right), and colon. Polyps occur most commonly in the small intestine and produce recurrent abdominal pain and intussusception. The syndrome is transmitted by autosomal dominant inheritance with variable penetrance. Without screening, 50% of patients develop either intestinal or extra-intestinal tumours (ovarian, breast, pancreas, cholangiocarcinoma, gall bladder, Sertoli cell), with a median age of 50 years at diagnosis. Screening of adults is required by colonoscopy, barium study, pelvic ultrasound (females), and gonadal examination (males).

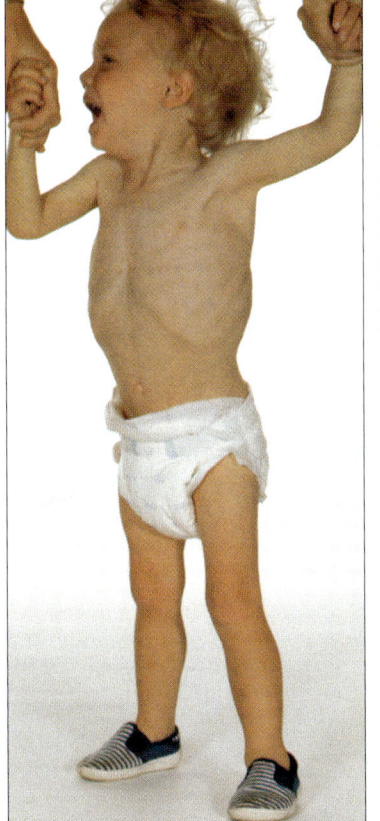

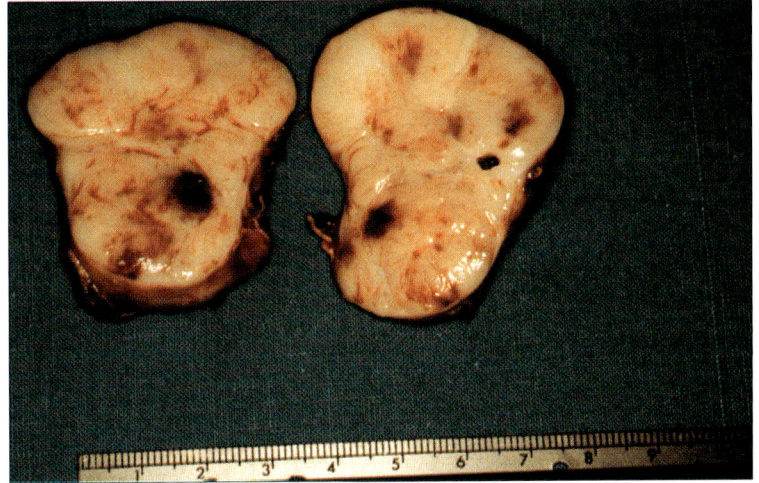

Figs 9.3, 9.4 Vasoactive intestinal peptide (VIP) secreting ganglioneuroblastoma. Watery diarrhoea, hypokalaemia, and a metabolic acidosis are the hallmarks of VIP-secreting tumours. Most are ganglioneuromas or ganglioneuroblastomas (which rarely metastasize) of the adrenals or, less commonly, of the sympathetic ganglia. This boy (**9.3**, bottom left) presented with a 6-month history of watery diarrhoea, and was found to have an adrenal ganglioneuroblastoma; a resected specimen from him is shown in **9.4** (lower right).

Pediatric Gastroenterology and Hepatology

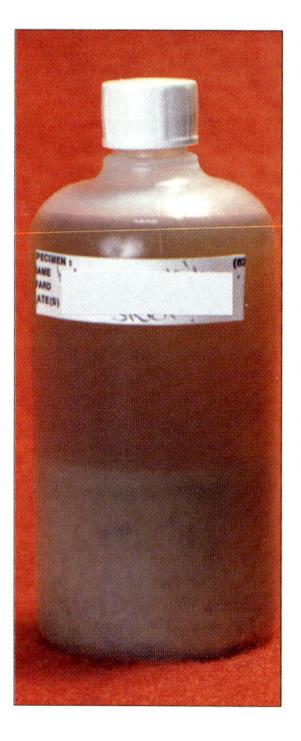

Fig. 9.5 VIP-secreting ganglioneuroblastoma. The onset of watery diarrhoea, particularly without a preceding infective episode, is an important symptom. Shown is the 24-hour stool collection from the patient shown in **Fig. 9.3**, which has the biochemical hallmark of a secretory diarrhoea: a low osmotic gap {290 −[(stool Na$^+$ + K$^+$) × 2] <50 mOsm/kg }. In an osmotic diarrhoea, the osmotic gap is usually more than 100 mOsm/kg.

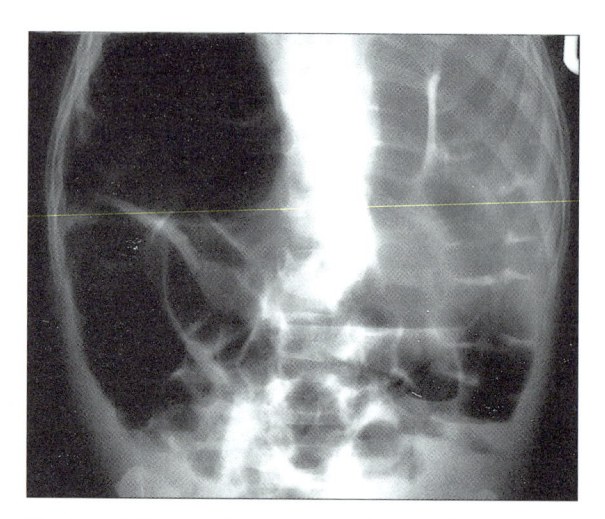

Fig. 9.6 VIP-secreting tumour. Abdominal distension is a common finding in patients with a VIP-secreting tumour. This radiograph shows considerable dilatation of both the small and large intestine, a variable diagnostic clue in children with persistent secretory diarrhoea. The dilatation persists despite correction of any hypokalaemia. About 50% of plain abdominal films show calcification in the adrenal tumour.

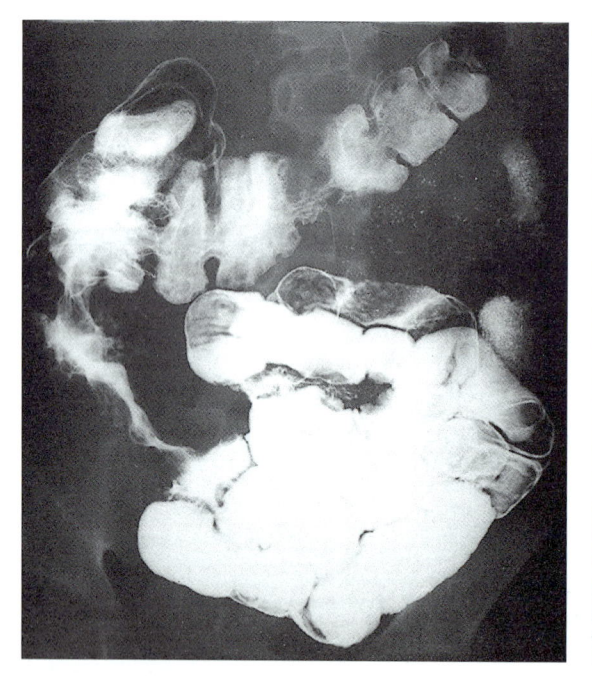

Fig. 9.7 Intestinal non-Hodgkin's lymphoma: barium radiograph. This patient presented with a 6-month history of recurrent abdominal pain and lethargy. Examination revealed a right iliac fossa mass, and Crohn's disease was considered as the most likely diagnosis. The barium meal and follow through shows stricturing of the terminal ileum and caecum, with ulceration and nodularity. At laparotomy, a partially necrotic ileo-caecal mass was resected which proved to be a B-cell non-Hodgkin's lymphoma.

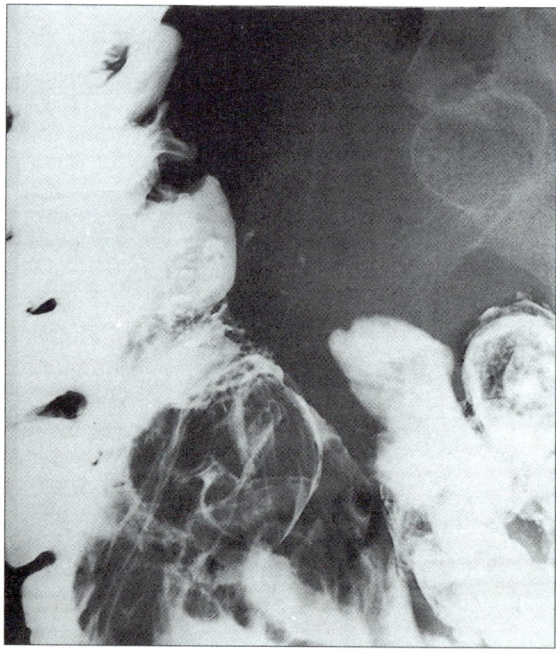

Fig. 9.8 Adenocarcinoma: radiograph. Adenocarcinoma of the small intestine is a rare tumour in childhood, and usually presents with obstruction from a circumferential tumour, or as a non-obstructing mass. This 14-year-old presented with anorexia, weight loss, and a severe iron-deficiency anaemia. A right iliac fossa mass was present which, on barium follow-through, was found to be related to a large filling defect in the caecum. At laparotomy, this proved to be a Duke's grade C adenocarcinoma, an extremely rare tumour at this age.

Gastrointestinal Tumours

FAMILIAL ADENOMATOUS POLYPOSIS

EARLY COLONIC DISEASE

Family adenomatous polyposis (FAP) is inherited as an autosomal dominant gene located on chromosome 5q. Adenomatous polyps develop in the colon (50% will have polyps at sigmoidoscopy by 15 years of age) and the number increases progressively until the colon becomes studded throughout its length. Without colectomy, colorectal cancer is inevitable and appears about 10 to 15 years after the appearance of polyposis.

In Gardner's syndrome, all the features of FAP occur in association with osteomas of the mandible, skull, and long bones, associated with a variety of benign soft tissue tumours.

HISTOLOGY

The polyps in FAP are adenomas, and therefore true neoplasms. Numerous microscopic adenomas of the colon are also present, which may involve a single colonic crypt. Polyps are also present in the upper gastrointestinal tract, which do not seem to progress to malignancy with the same rapidity as the colonic lesions.

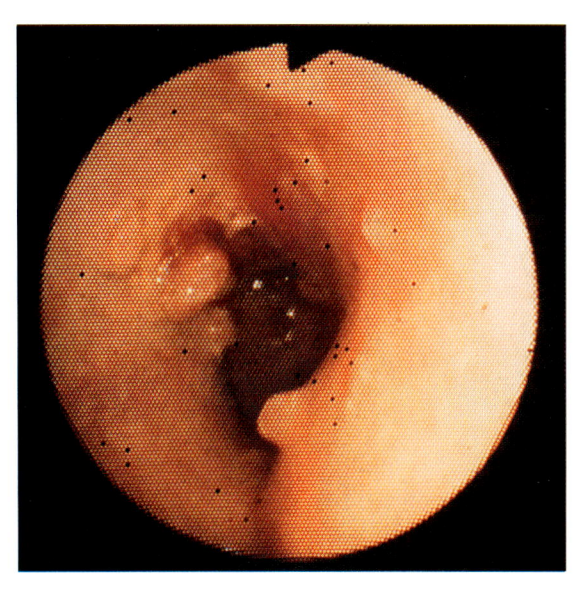

Fig. 9.9 Family adenomatous polyposis: early colonic disease. This patient already has several polyps at the age of 13. He had a positive family history, abnormal genetic markers, and congenital hypertrophy of retinal pigment epithelium. Colectomy is usually advisable as soon as polyps are identified, once puberty is complete.

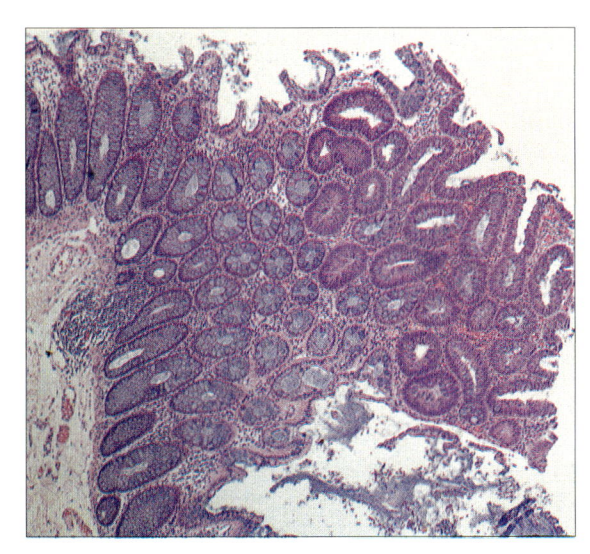

Fig. 9.10 Familial adenomatous polyposis. This polyp demonstrates the characteristic features of FAP – dense, closely packed glands with little stroma between the glands, which are lined with mucin-depleted cells. The premalignant changes may be compared to the normal mucosa beneath.

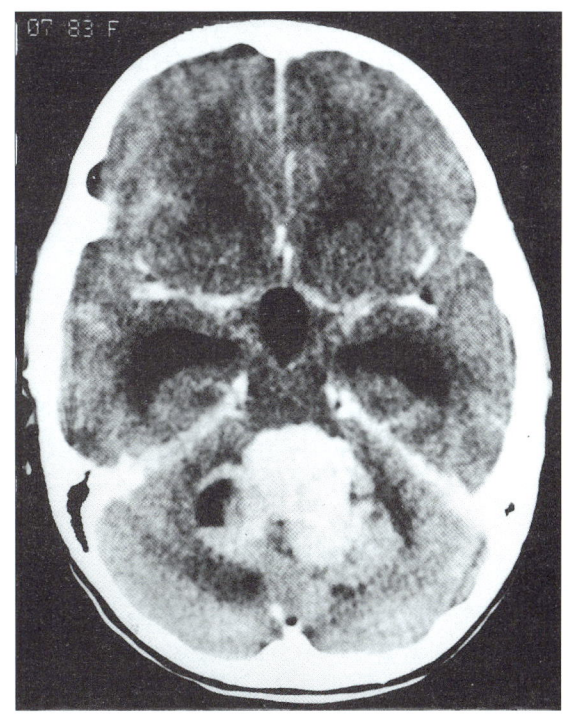

Fig. 9.11 Turcot's syndrome. In Turcot's syndrome, colonic adenomas, which are fewer than in classic familial adenomatous polyposis, occur in association with malignant brain tumours in childhood and adolescence (especially glioblastoma multiforme, a form of high-grade astrocytoma). Inheritance is autosomal recessive.

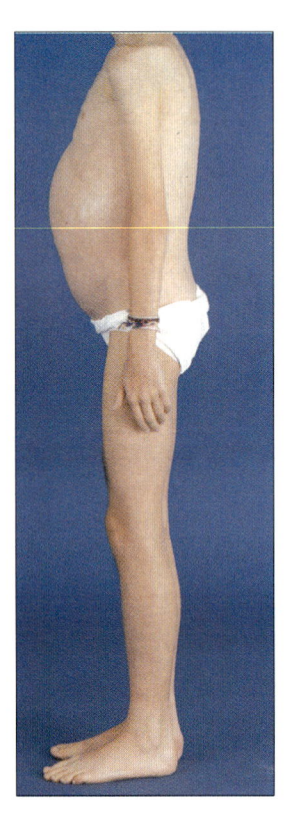

Fig. 9.12 Peritoneal mesothelioma. This 10-year-old girl presented with a 6-month history of marked abdominal distension, due to ascites. Cytology of the ascitic fluid demonstrated large numbers of abnormal mesothelial cells. The diagnosis of malignant peritoneal mesothelioma was confirmed at laparotomy, at which the peritoneum was found to be grossly abnormal, with thickening and oedema, and was studded throughout with white nodules. This is a rare tumour in childhood with a highly variable response to chemotherapy. Treatment is aimed primarily at disease control.

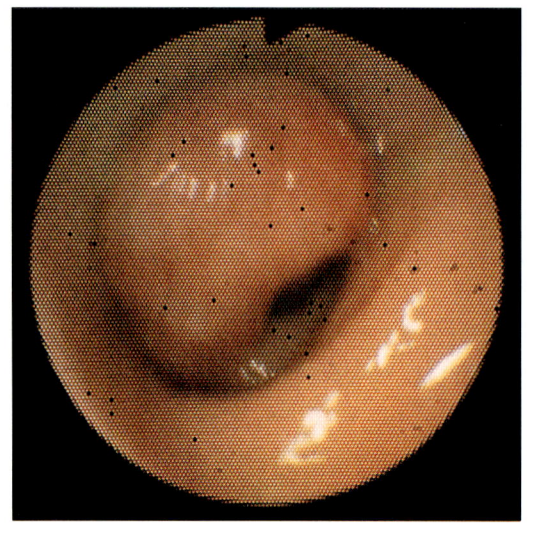

Fig. 9.13 Juvenile polyp: colonoscopic appearance. Here is shown the characteristic appearance of a juvenile polyp. Painless bleeding is the most common presentation, and is most often seen between the ages of 1 and 10 years. In children, 40% of those affected have more than one polyp, but usually not more than two or three. Three-quarters of these are located distal to the rectosigmoid colon. Following polypectomy, recurrence rate is about 5%.

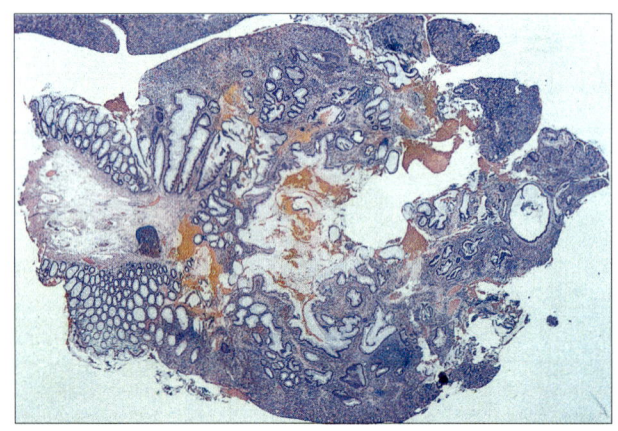

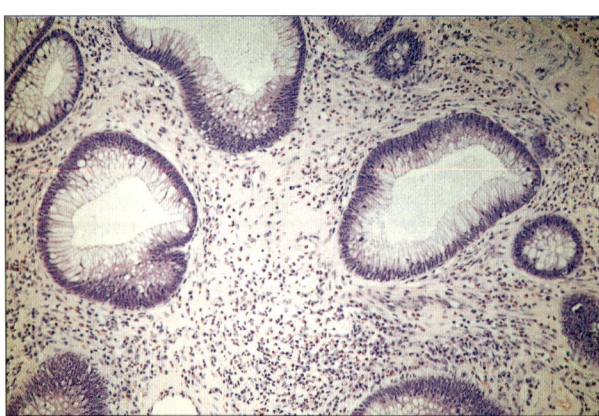

Figs 9.14, 9.15 Juvenile polyp: histology. The histology of juvenile polyp demonstrates marked cystic dilatation of glands with mucin retention (**9.14**, top), and an eosinophilic inflammatory infiltrate (**9.15**, bottom).

10. Pancreatic and Gallbladder Disease

GALLSTONE DISEASE

Gallstone formation may be secondary to liver disease, cystic fibrosis, ileal disease or resection, haemolytic disorders, or total parenteral nutrition. The majority of stones are found in the gallbladder and are asymptomatic. Less than 6% may occlude the cystic duct or common bile duct, leading to biliary obstruction, cholangitis, intrahepatic abscesses, and biliary fibrosis or pancreatitis.

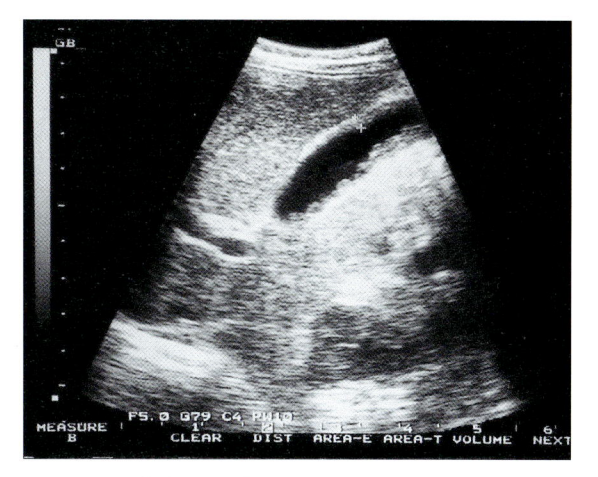

Fig. 10.1 Abdominal ultrasound. The easiest way to diagnose gallstones is by abdominal ultrasound, as in this boy (2 1/2 years old) with congenital spherocytosis, recurrent jaundice, abdominal pain, and abnormal liver function tests. He was successfully treated with a laparoscopic cholecystectomy.

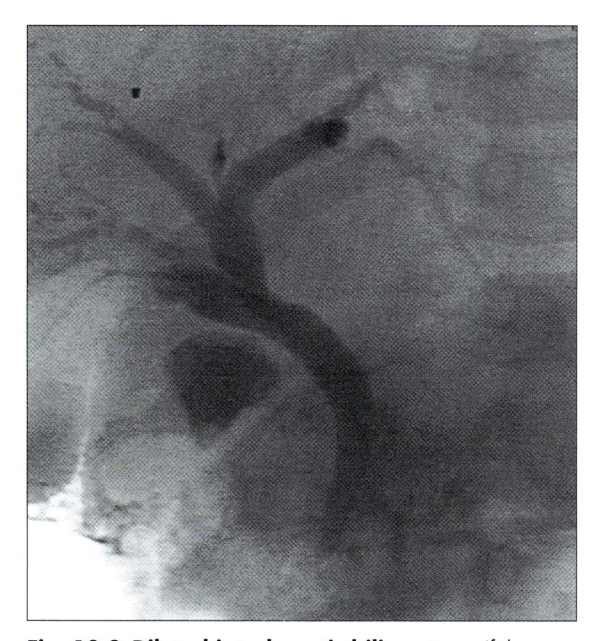

Fig. 10.2 Dilated intrahepatic biliary tree. If the abdominal ultrasound suggests a dilated intrahepatic biliary tree this should be confirmed with an endoscopic retrograde cholangiopancreatography (ERCP). This baby presented with recurrent obstructive jaundice following a traumatic delivery with extensive bruising. He was found to have stones in the gallbladder and common bile duct, and a dilated intrahepatic biliary tree was found on ERCP. He had a cholecystectomy with a spincterotomy of the ampulla of Vater.

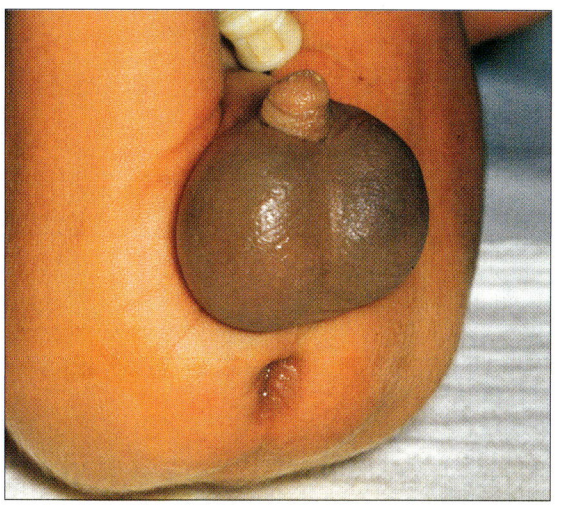

Fig. 10.3 Spontaneous perforation. Spontaneous perforation of the bile duct is a rare problem in the neonate. There is leakage of bile between the junction of the cystic duct and common duct. leading to biliary peritonitis and ascites, which may extend into the scrotum, as in this 5-day-old infant. The aetiology is unknown, but the condition may be secondary to gallstones or mucous plugs.

79

Pediatric Gastroenterology and Hepatology

ACUTE AND CHRONIC PANCREATITIS

Pancreatitis is rare in childhood. There are many causes, but abdominal trauma, infection, and congenital abnormalities are the most likely. Most children present with a long history of pain, which may or may not have been misdiagnosed as chronic recurrent abdominal pain.

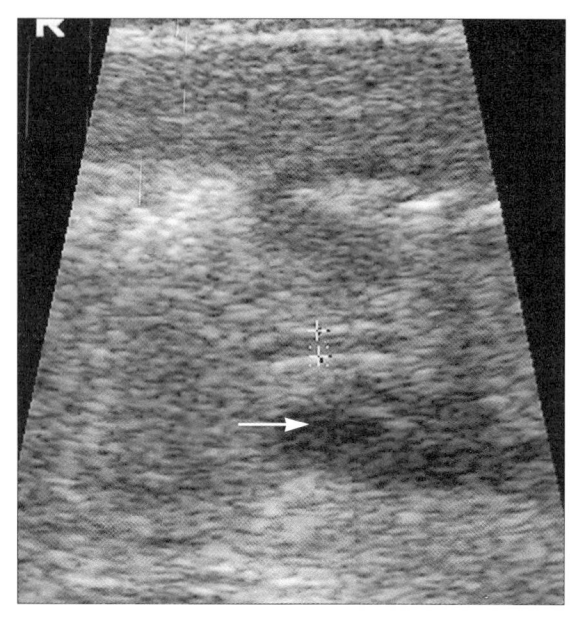

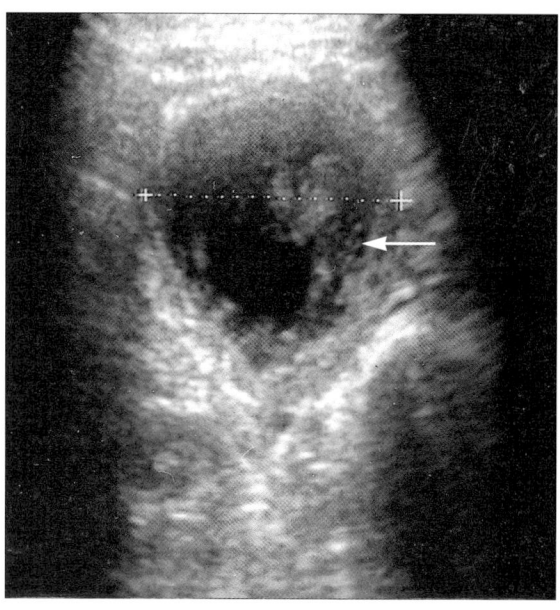

Figs 10.4, 10.5 Recurrent abdominal pain. Recurrent abdominal pain in association with an elevated serum or urine amylase is a common presenting symptom. Occasionally, abdominal ultrasound will demonstrate a dilated pancreatic duct (**10.4**, left) or a pseudocyst (**10.5**, right).

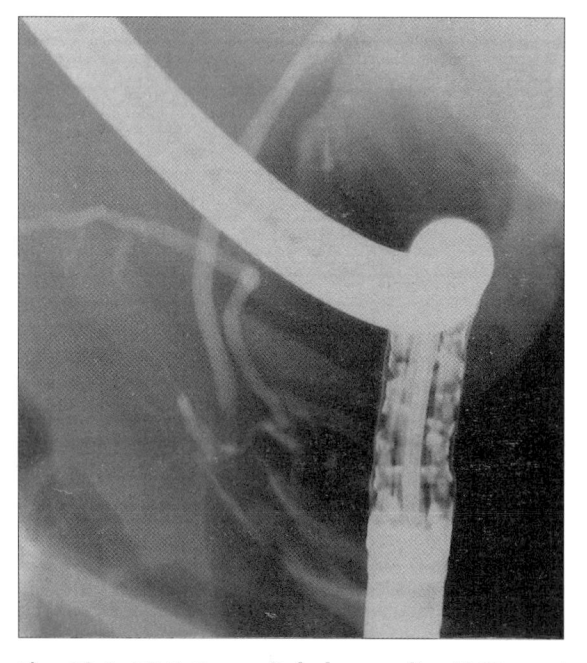

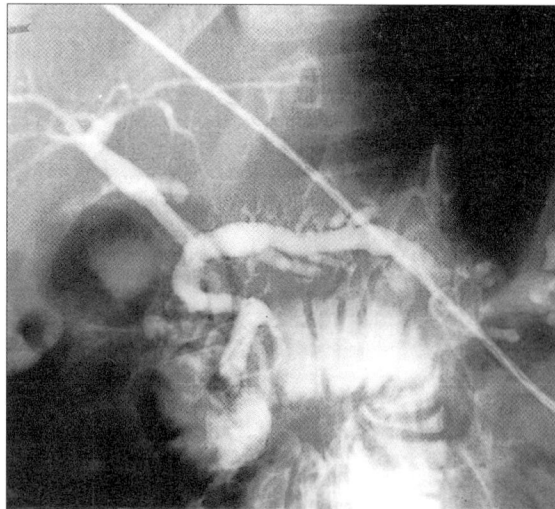

Figs 10.6, 10.7 Congenital abnormality. ERCP may demonstrate a congenital abnormality, e.g. reduplication of the pancreatic duct (**10.6**, left) or a dilated pancreatic duct with stunted side branches (**10.7**, right) secondary to chronic pancreatitis. Antioxidant therapy may reduce the incidence of recurrent pancreatitis, but partial or total pancreatectomy is usually necessary.

Pancreatic and Gallbladder Disease

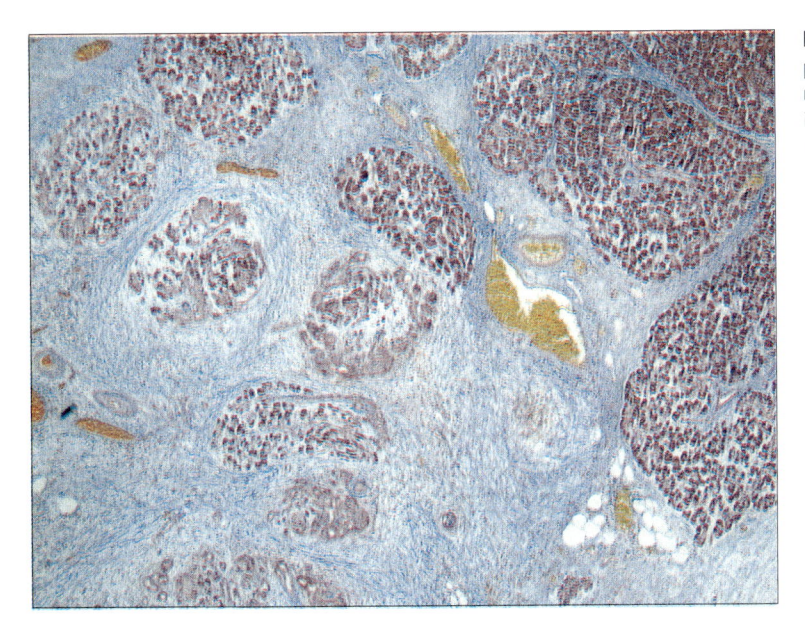

Fig. 10.8 Histology. In chronic pancreatitis, pancreatic histology reveals severe fibrosis with a little inflammation and atrophy of the acini (Haematoxylin and Eosin ×25).

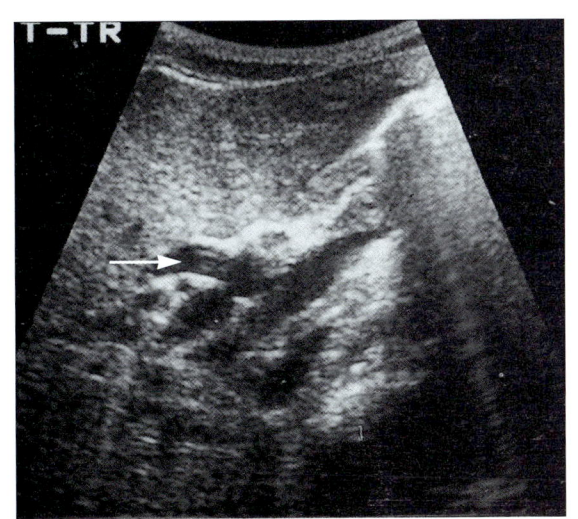

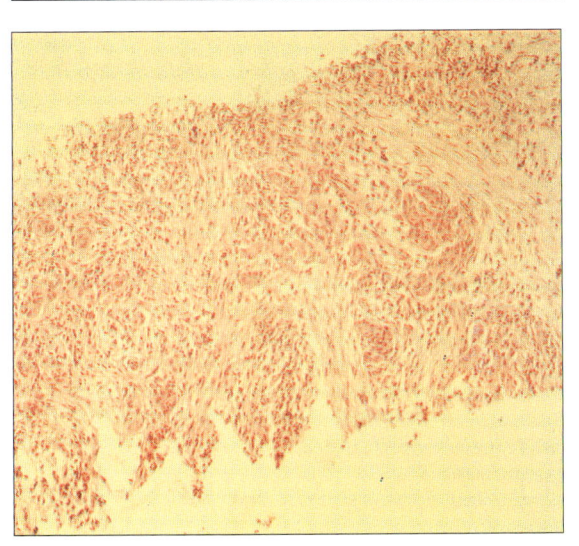

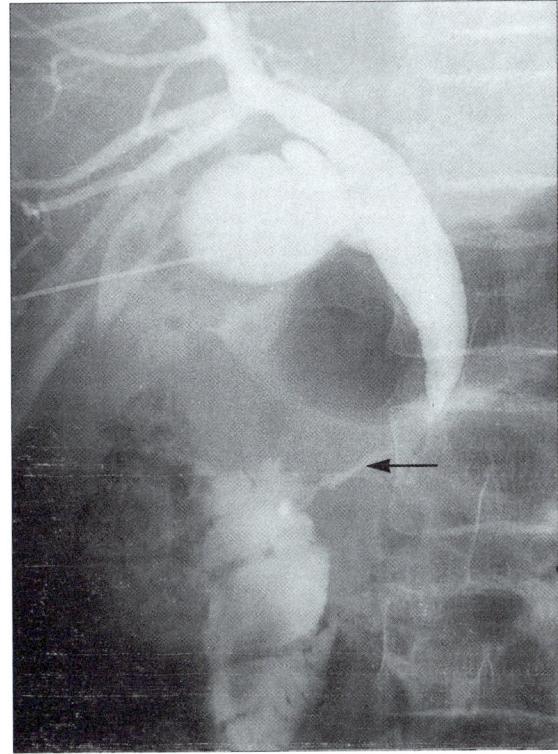

Figs 10.9–10.11 Chronic pancreatitis. This child with recurrent abdominal pain was noted to have dilated intrahepatic bile ducts on abdominal ultrasound (**10.9**, top left) secondary to a biliary stricture (**10.10**, top right), which was resected and a Roux-en-Y anastomosis created. He achieved complete remission from abdominal pain, but biopsy of his pancreas revealed severe fibrosis with chronic pancreatitis (**10.11**, Haematoxylin and Eosin ×10, bottom left) and he is now maintained on pancreatic supplements and daily insulin.

Pediatric Gastroenterology and Hepatology

CYSTIC FIBROSIS

Cystic fibrosis has an incidence of 1:2000 live births. Clinical features include chronic lung disease, pancreatic insufficiency, liver disease, and intestinal complications, such as meconium ileus and distal ileus obstruction syndrome.

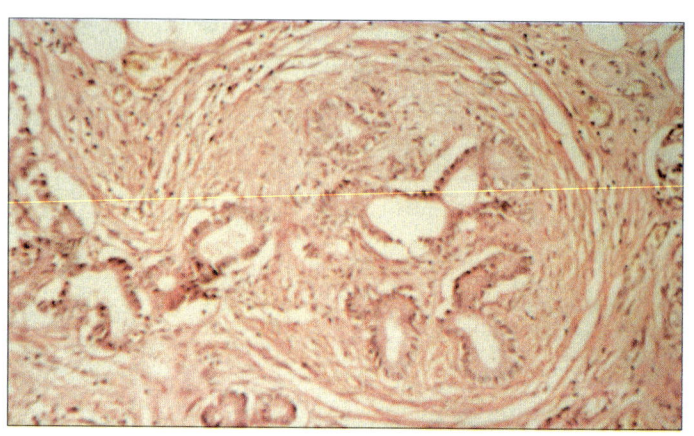

Fig. 10.12 Cystic fibrosis (CF). The primary abnormality in the pancreas is reduction of bicarbonate-dependent water secretion, leading to inspissated secretions which block the pancreatic ducts. This causes dilatation, with obstruction to the flow of digestive enzymes, subsequent degeneration of the acinar cells, and pancreatic fibrosis.

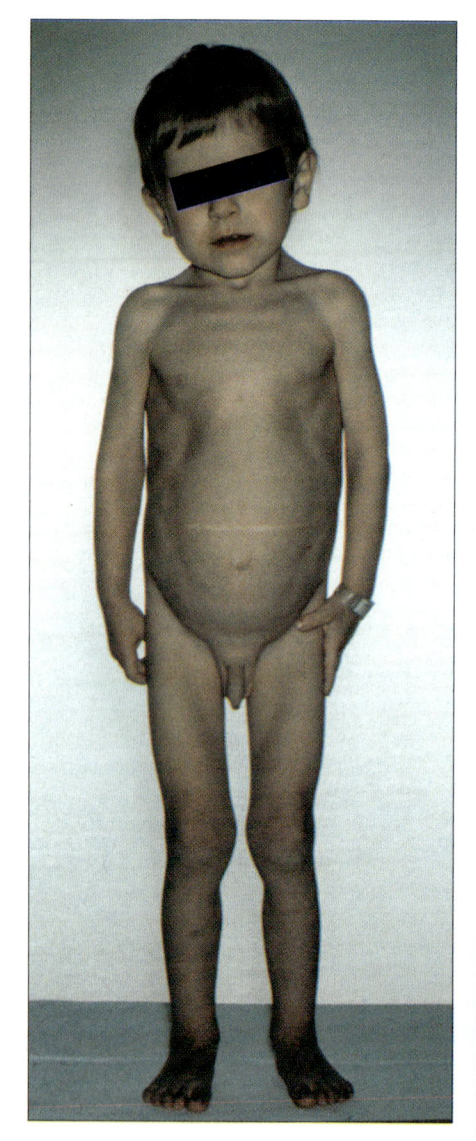

Fig. 10.13 Diagnosis. The diagnosis is made in the majority of children on the basis of recurrent chest infections, failure to thrive, and meconium ileus, and is confirmed by measurement of elevated sweat sodium. This boy presented with meconium ileus (see his abdominal scar); he is stunted and wasted with severe lung disease and a Harrison's sulcus.

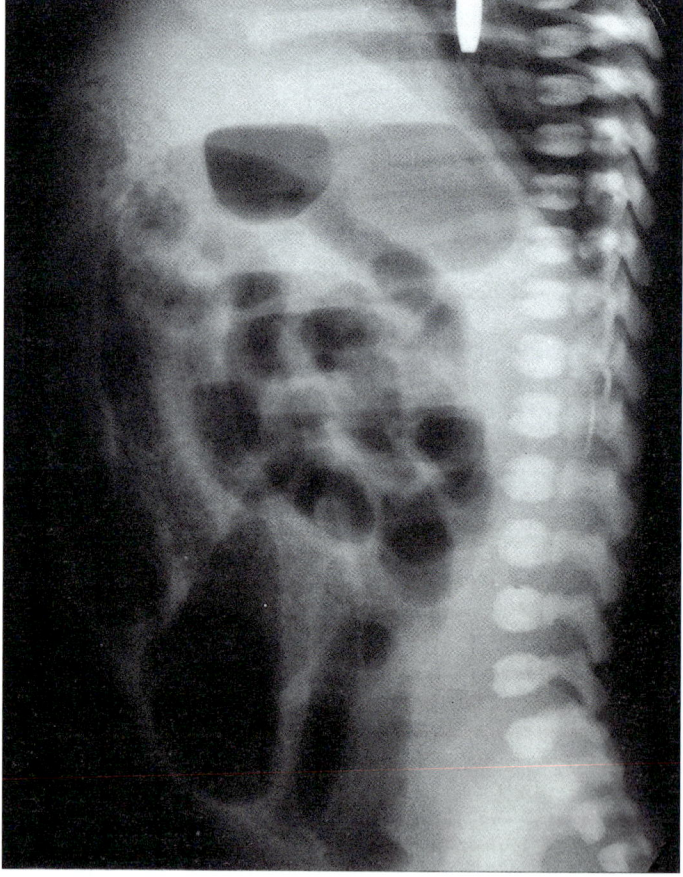

Fig. 10.14 Meconium ileus: pattern of intestinal obstruction. In 10–20% of patients with CF, presentation is in the neonatal period with intestinal obstruction due to meconium ileus. Thick sticky inspissated meconium blocks the intestinal lumen. Shown here is the pattern of intestinal obstruction, but in addition there is the 'foamy' appearance of inspissated meconium.

Pancreatic and Gallbladder Disease

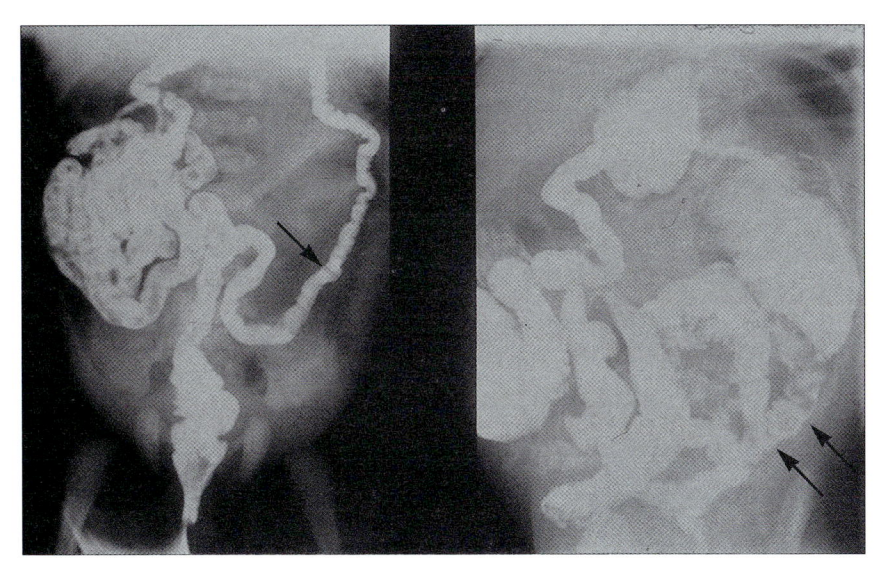

Fig. 10.15 Meconium ileus. These contrast studies using Gastrograffin demonstrate a microcolon (right, arrow) distal to inspissated meconium in the distal small bowel. There are filling defects (left, arrows) in the terminal ileum due to meconium pellets. The proximal small bowel is distended. In the management of meconium ileus a Gastrograffin enema is successful in relieving the intestinal obstruction.

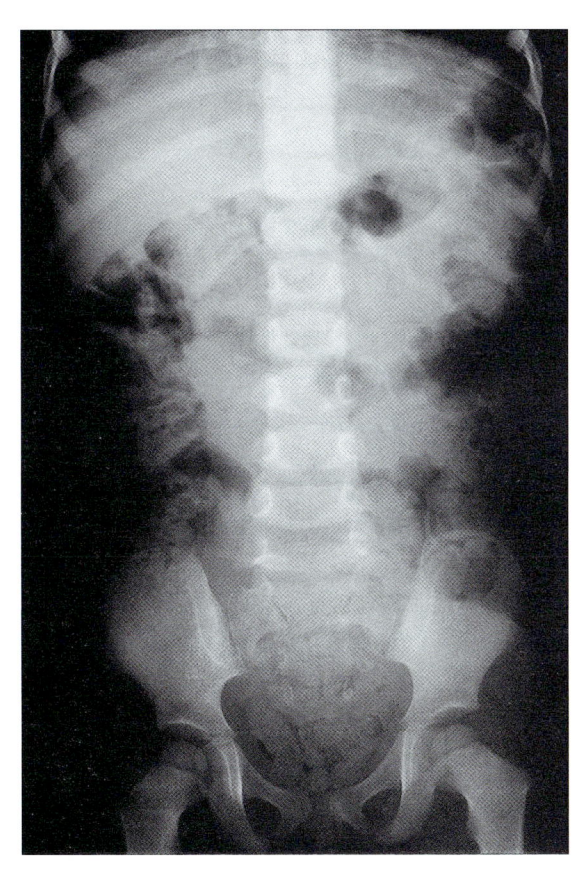

Fig. 10.16 Distal intestinal obstruction syndrome. Distal intestinal obstruction syndrome affects approximately 40% of older CF patients and is a form of partial intestinal obstruction which causes recurrent abdominal pain, constipation, vomiting, and abdominal distension with a right iliac fossa mass. This abdominal radiograph shows evidence of obstruction with gaseous distension of loops of bowel with fluid levels. Treatment is with *N*-acetylcysteine or oral Gastrograffin.

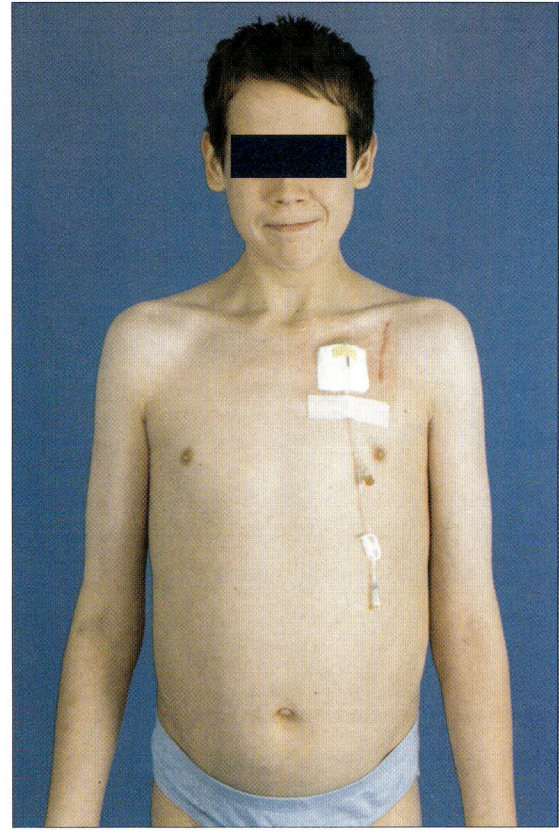

Fig. 10.17 Liver disease. The incidence of liver disease in children with CF is approximately 20%. It is more common in children with mild lung disease. They present with the gradual onset of abdominal distension, malnutrition, and bruising secondary to cirrhosis and portal hypertension. The clinical symptoms are related to portal hypertension. Hepatic dysfunction and liver failure are late features which may require liver transplantation.

Pediatric Gastroenterology and Hepatology

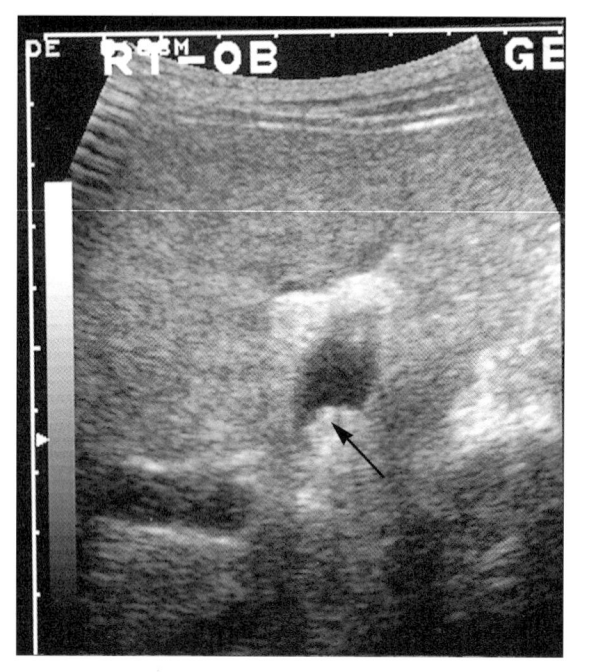

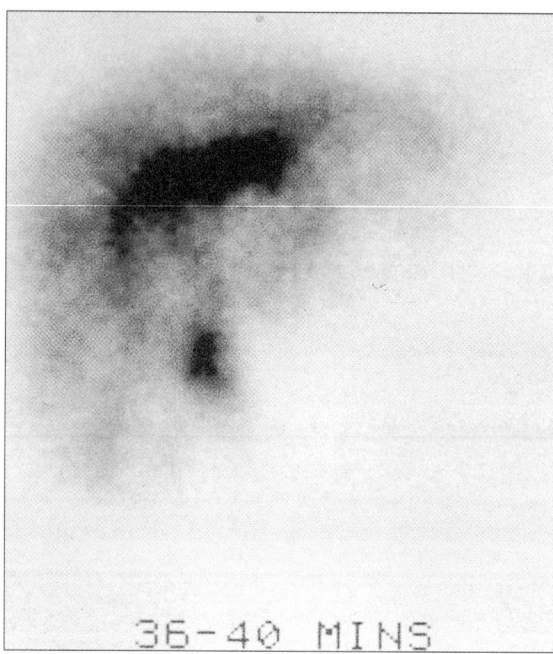

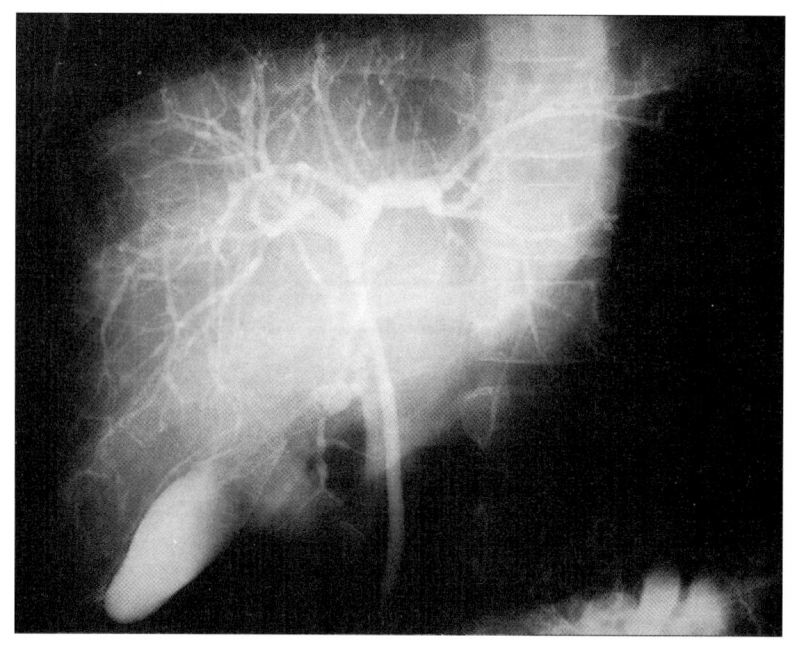

Figs 10.18–10.20 Early diagnosis of cystic fibrosis is difficult. Abdominal ultrasound may demonstrate heterogeneity of liver texture with a contracted gallbladder and gallstones (**10.18**, top left). Radioisotope scanning shows delayed excretion and pooling of dye in the bile ducts (**10.19**, top right). ERCP may show widespread abnormalities of the bile ducts, but biliary strictures are uncommon (**10.20**, bottom).

Pancreatic and Gallbladder Disease

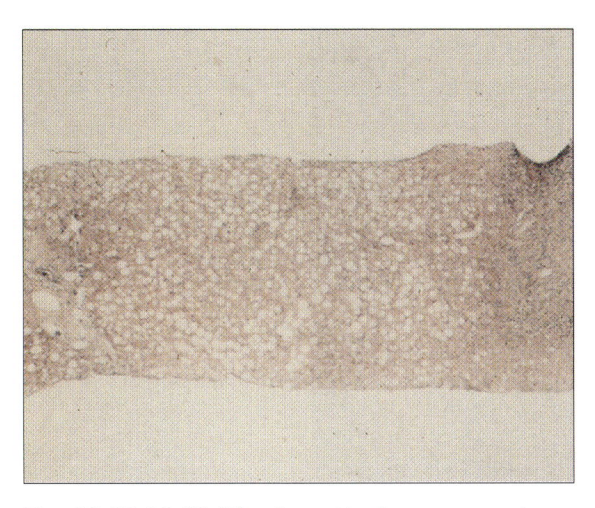

Figs 10.21–10.23 Histology. Histology may reveal a fatty liver (**10.21**, top left), focal biliary fibrosis (**10.22**, top right), or perivenular fibrosis (**10.23**, middle right).

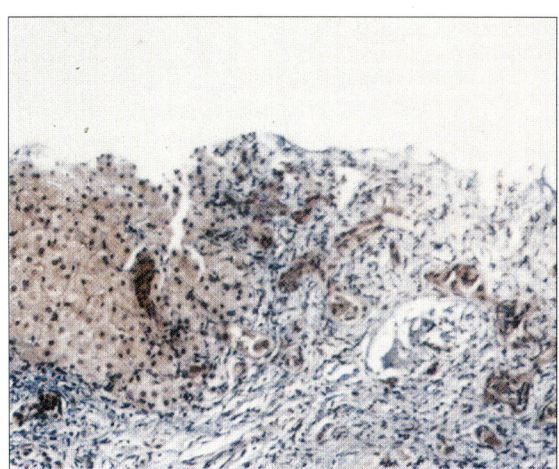

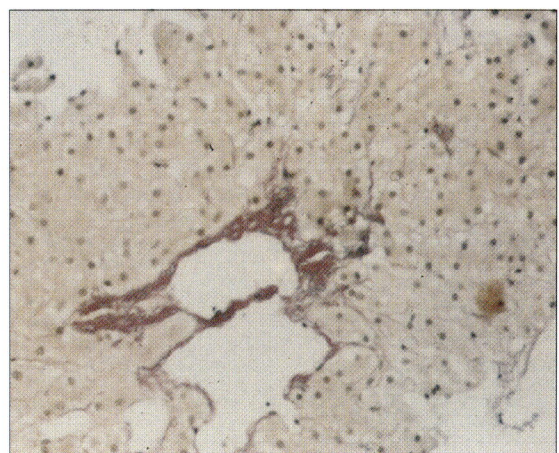

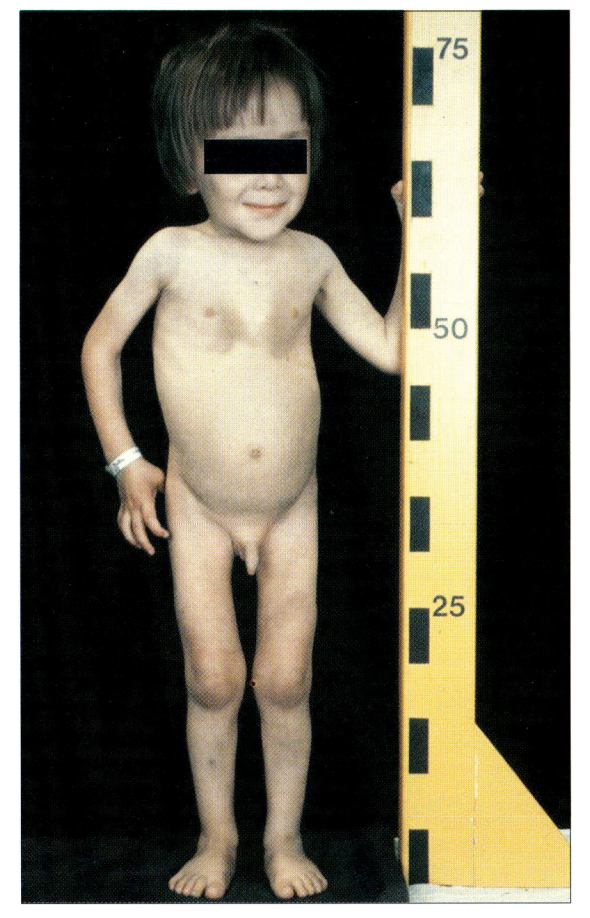

Fig. 10.24 Schwachman's syndrome. Schwachman's syndrome is an autosomal recessive disorder associated with failure to thrive, pancreatic acinar insufficiency, and neutropenia, secondary to bone marrow hypoplasia. The clinical features include abnormal thoracic configuration and hypotonia with recurrent chest infections secondary to abnormal neutrophil migration. Cutaneous involvement with dry skin and eczematous lesions are common.

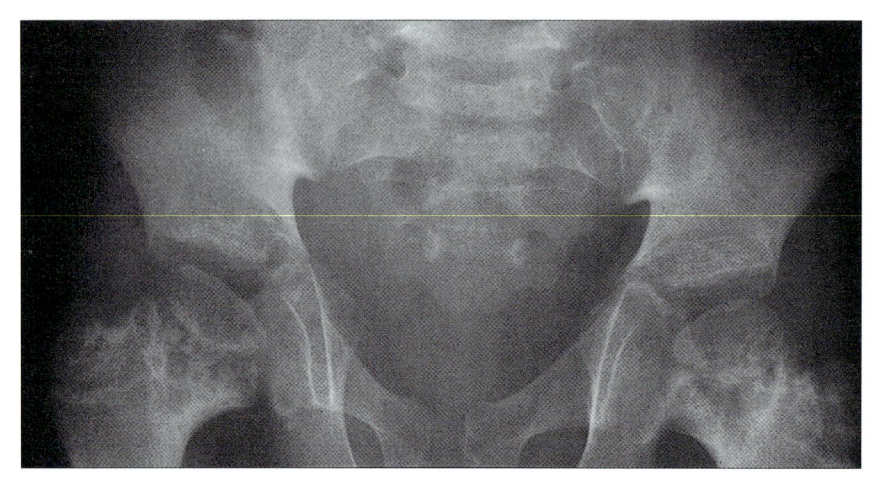

Fig. 10.25 Schwachman's syndrome: metaphyseal dysostosis. Metaphyseal dysostosis with multiple cystic areas may be severe at birth and persist, as in this child, although in some children the changes may improve with time.

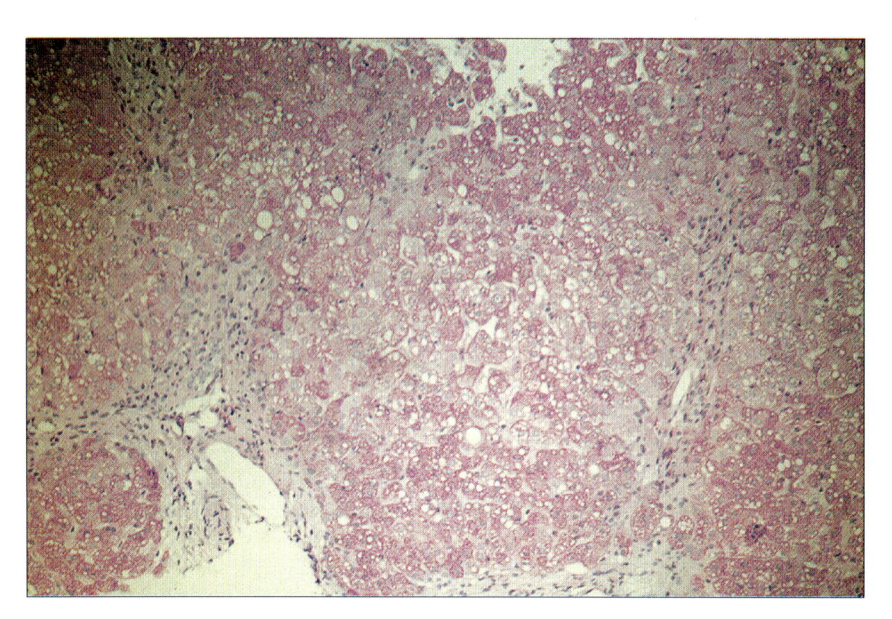

Fig. 10.26 Schwachman's syndrome: hepatic dysfunction. Hepatic dysfunction is associated with fatty infiltration and fibrosis. There may be progression to cirrhosis (Periodic Acid–Schiff, ×33).

Pancreatic and Gallbladder Disease

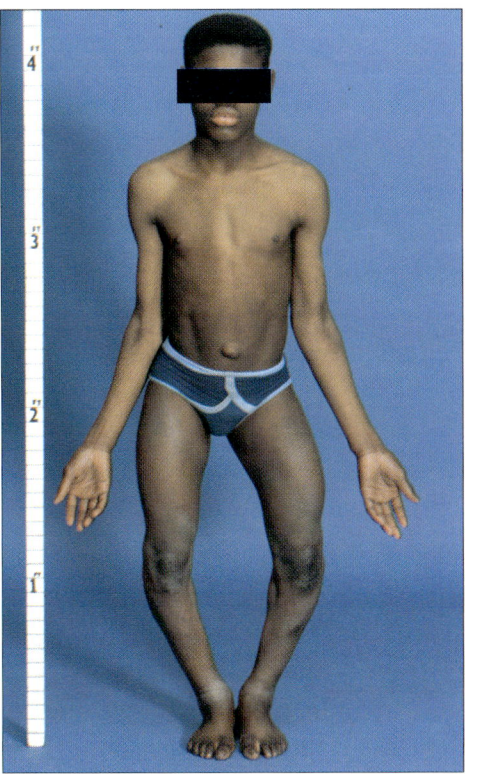

Fig. 10.27 Rickets Persistent steatorrhoea in Schwachman's syndrome may lead to severe rickets, as in this young man with genu valgum which he developed in infancy.

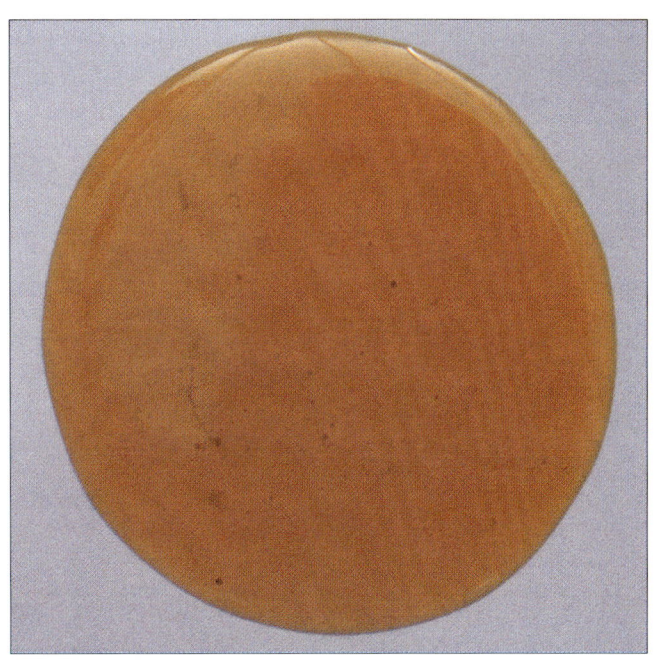

Fig. 10.28 Isolated lipase deficiency. The passage of oil per rectum, separate from stool, is the most striking feature of this rare disorder. Children complain of coloured, oily staining of their underclothes. Failure to thrive is not a feature. Pancreatic lipase activity is grossly reduced, but other pancreatic enzymes are normal. Treatment with pancreatin is effective in controlling the discharge of oil.

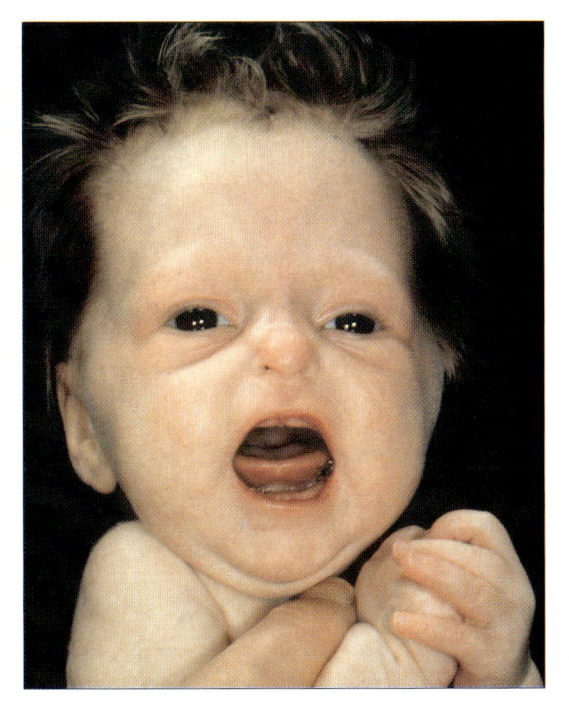

Fig. 10.29 Johanson Blizzard syndrome. Johanson Blizzard syndrome is characterised by pancreatic insufficiency, dwarfism, midline ectodermal scalp defects, hypoplasia or aplasia of the ala nasa, deafness, and dental anomalies. Some children have microcephaly and mental retardation.

11. Neonatal Liver Disease

INTRODUCTION

Neonatal jaundice which persists beyond 14 days should always be investigated, even in breast-fed babies. The differential diagnosis is between extrahepatic biliary disease (biliary atresia or choledocal cyst), the neonatal hepatitis syndrome, and intrahepatic biliary hypoplasia.

BILIARY ATRESIA

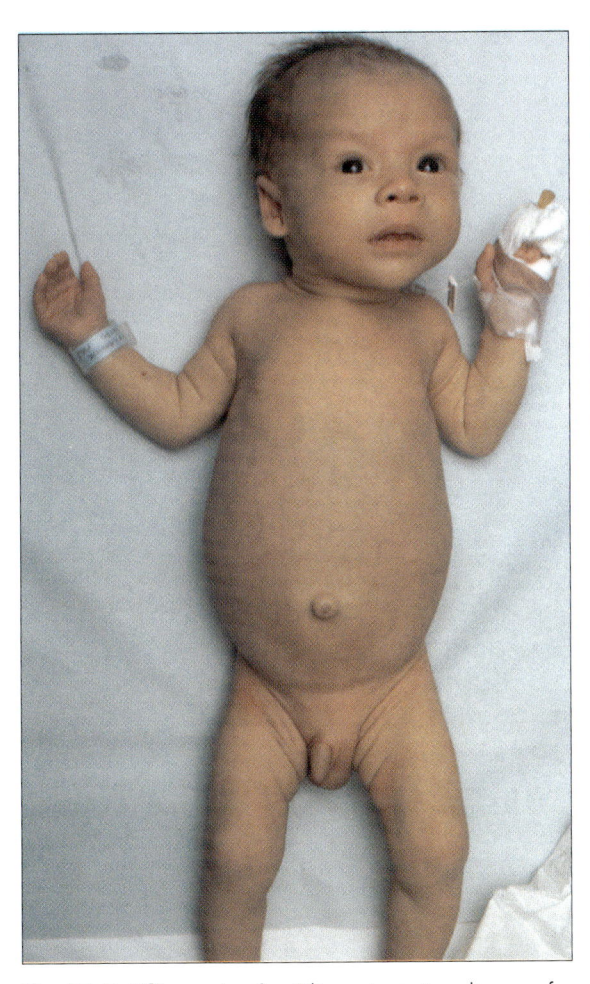

Fig. 11.1 Biliary atresia. Biliary atresia is a disease of unknown aetiology which occurs in about 1 in 14,000 live births. There is gradual fibrosis and destruction of the extra- and intra-hepatic biliary ducts and progressive cholestasis. Jaundice is apparent by the second day of life and hepatomegaly is obvious within 4 weeks.

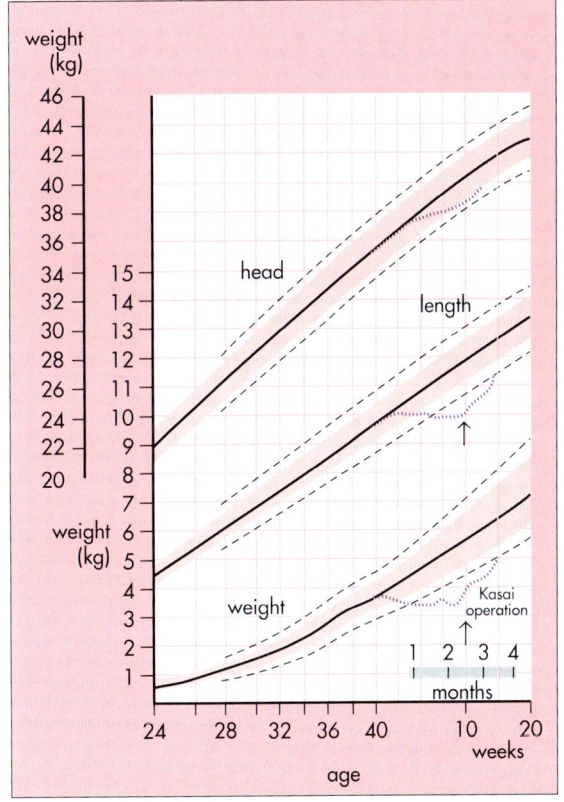

Fig. 11.2 Weight chart. Most babies with biliary atresia have a normal birth weight, but only gain weight slowly despite a good appetite. Some babies consume over 200 ml/kg of formula feed without appreciable weight gain. This weight chart demonstrates catch-up growth following a successful operation and supplemented feeds.

89

Pediatric Gastroenterology and Hepatology

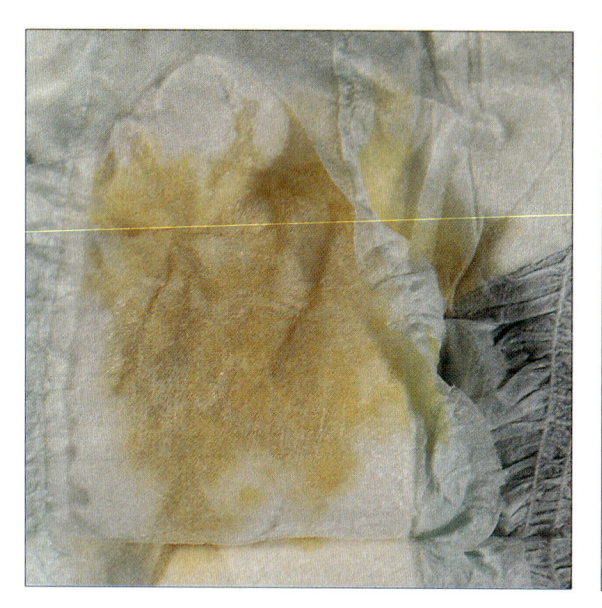

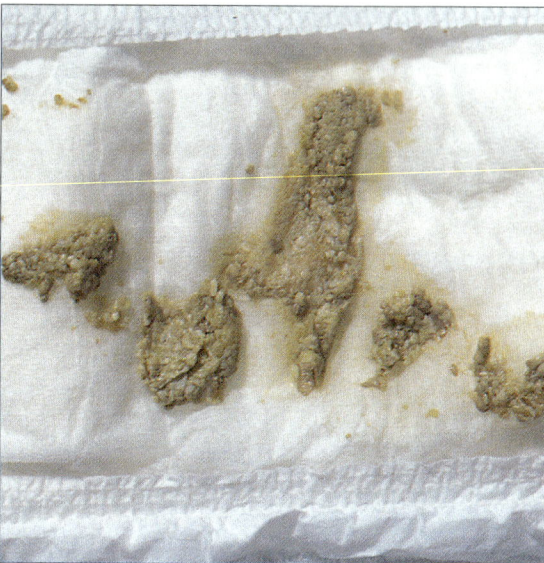

Figs 11.3, 11.4 White stool and dark urine. In babies with biliary atresia the urine is dark (**11.3**, left) and the stools become gradually paler (**11.4**, right), becoming completely white by 6 weeks of age.

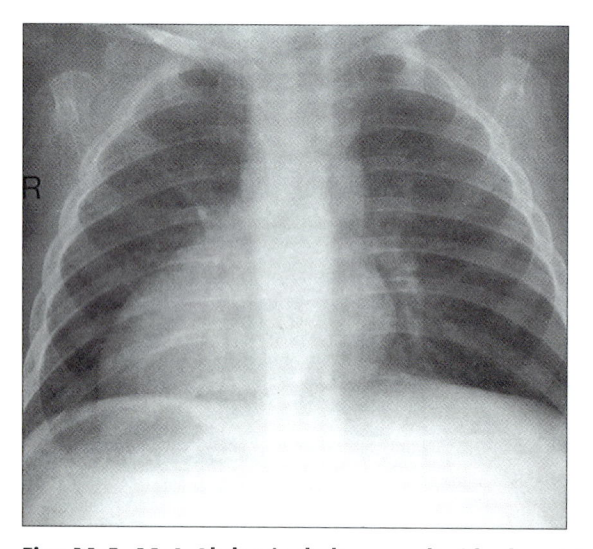

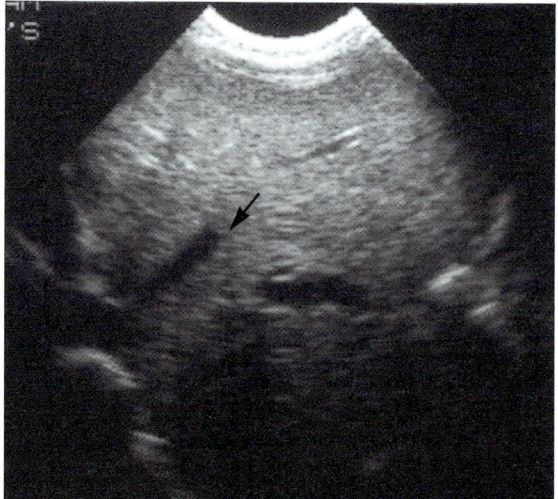

Figs 11.5, 11.6 Abdominal ultrasound with absent inferior vena cava (IVC). Of babies with biliary atresia, 25% have other congenital abnormalities, such as dextrocardia (**11.5**, left), ventricular septal defects, atrial septal defects, polysplenia, and the hypovascular syndrome in which there is abnormal hepatic vascular anatomy with a pre-duodenal portal vein, absent inferior vena cava, and azygous drainage from the liver. Ultrasound demonstrates the absent IVC in the liver, with the hepatic vein draining directly into the right atrium (arrow), which increases the surgical risk in liver transplantation (**11.6**, right).

Neonatal Disease

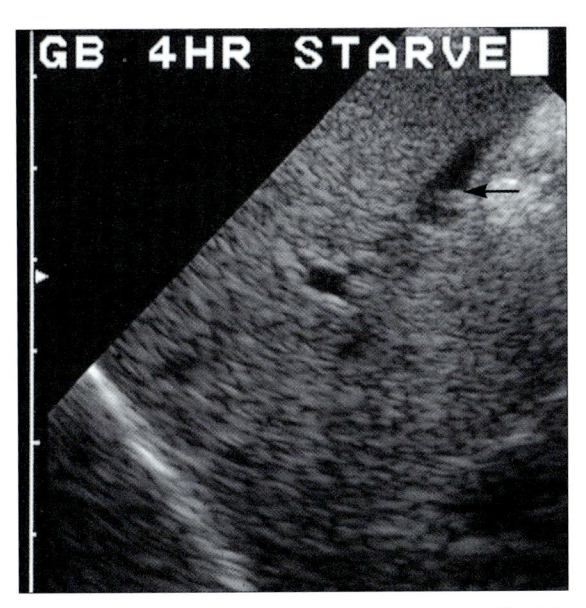

Fig. 11.7 Abdominal ultrasound. The normal gallbladder is large and easily demonstrated after a 4-hour fast. In babies with biliary atresia the gallbladder either cannot be visualised or is contracted as in this ultrasound scan.

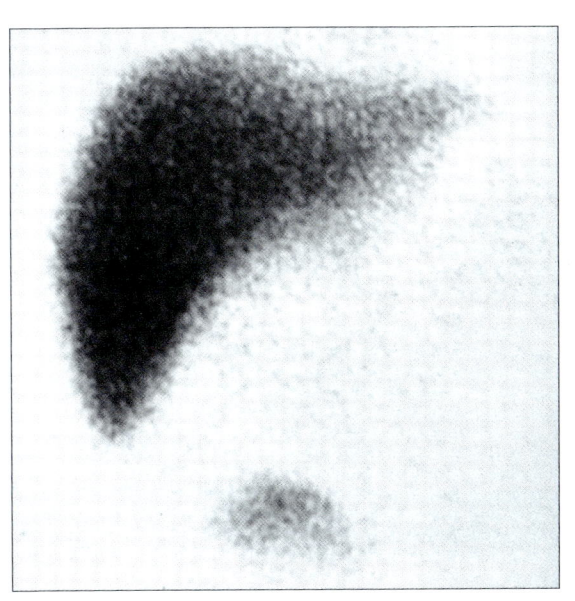

Fig. 11.8 TeBIDA scan. This radioisotope (99m technetium trimethyl 1-bromo-imino diacetic acid) is well taken up by liver cells, especially after pre-treatment with phenobarbitone (5 mg/kg for 5 days). In children with biliary atresia there is good hepatic uptake, but no excretion from the liver into the bowel within 24 hours.

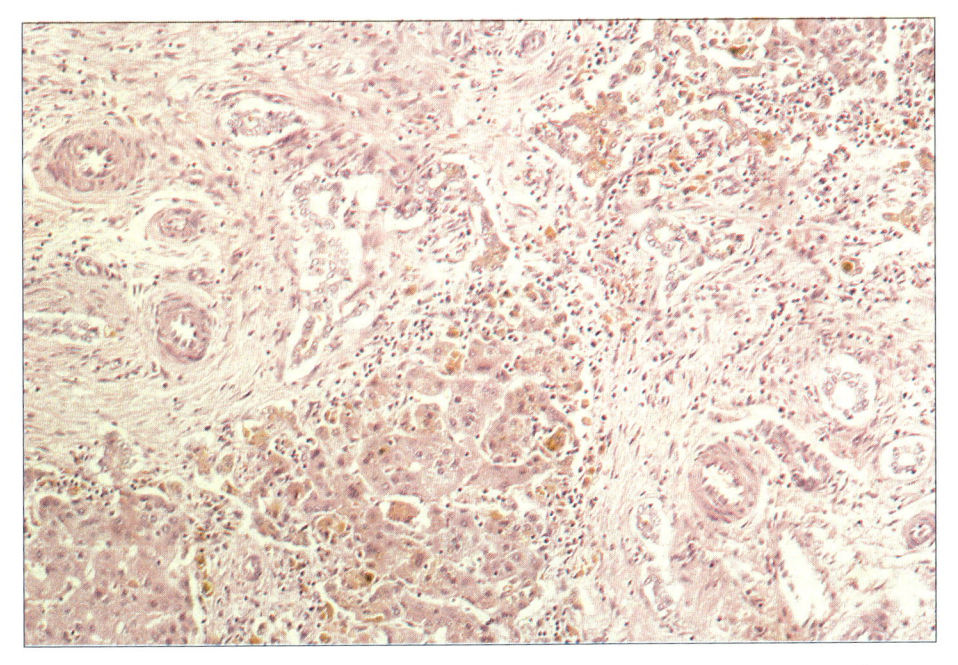

Fig. 11.9 Histology. The diagnosis of biliary atresia may be confirmed by demonstrating the characteristic findings of proliferation of bile ducts and ductules with bile plugs in the portal tracts, portal fibrosis, and oedema. There may be histological overlap with neonatal hepatitis if giant cells and extramedullary haemopoiesis are present. (Haematoxylin and Eosin, ×10.)

Pediatric Gastroenterology and Hepatology

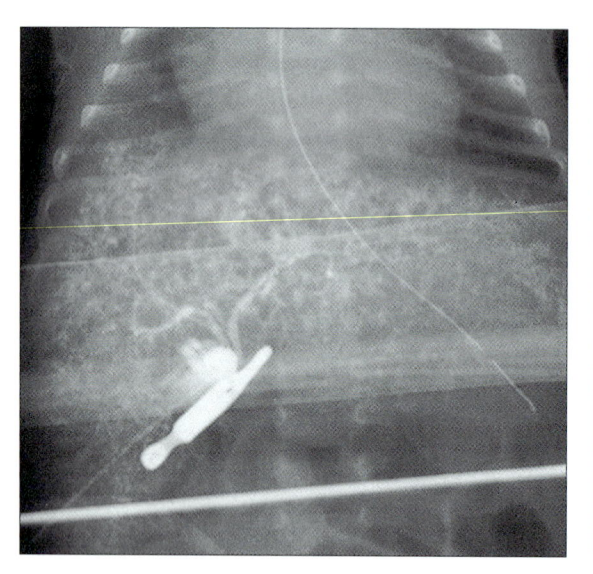

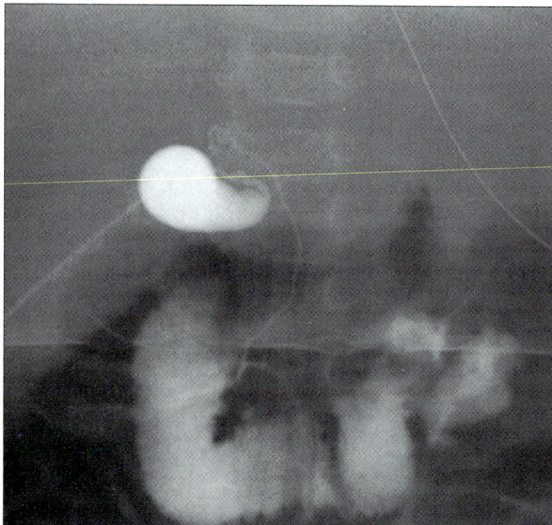

Figs 11.10, 11.11 Operative cholangiogram. As the diagnosis of biliary atresia may be difficult if histology is equivocal, it is usual to proceed to a laparotomy and operative cholangiogram. In contrast to the normal cholangiogram (**11.10**, left), **11.11** (right) demonstrates a small gallbladder with no filling of the biliary tree, suggestive of extensive destruction of the extrahepatic biliary tree that is characteristic of biliary atresia.

CHOLEDOCAL CYSTS

Choledocal cysts are localised cystic dilatation of all or part of the common bile duct. The cysts are more common in Japan (1 in 1000 live births) and in females (4:1). The cysts may present in infancy with prolonged jaundice or in older children with cholangitis and biliary fibrosis.

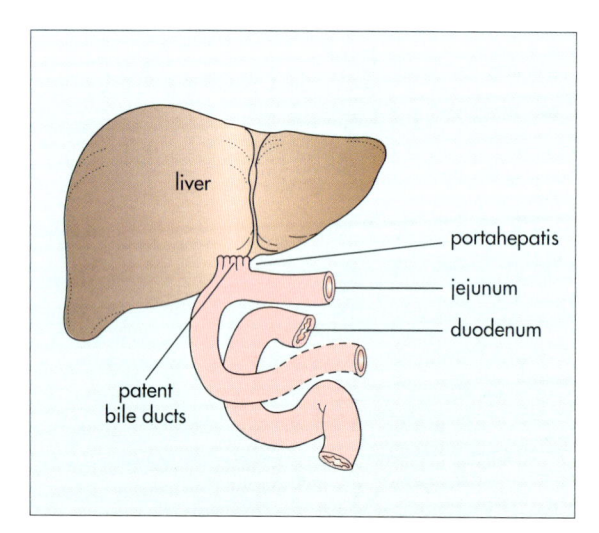

Fig. 11.12 Kasai portoenterostomy. Prior to the development of this operation children with biliary atresia died within 2 years. The fibrosed extrahepatic bile ducts and gallbladder are resected, and patent bile ducts are anastomosed to the jejunum to create a Roux-en-Y. If the operation is performed within 8 weeks of birth there is an 80% chance of achieving bile drainage. Complications include cholangitis, malabsorption, and progression of fibrosis to cirrhosis. An unsuccessful operation is an immediate indication for liver transplantation.

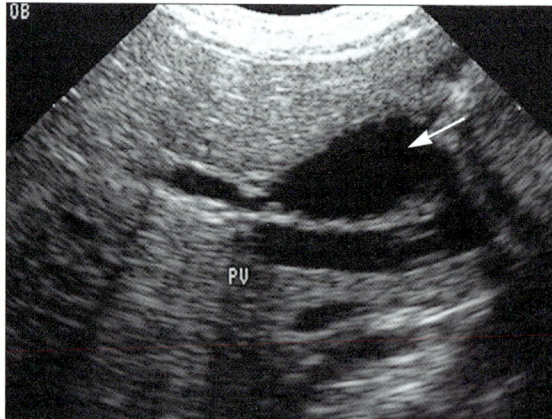

Fig. 11.13 Abdominal ultrasound. The diagnosis of a choledocal cyst is easily made by demonstrating a large cystic swelling below the liver. The cysts may be diagnosed antenatally by ultrasound.

Neonatal Disease

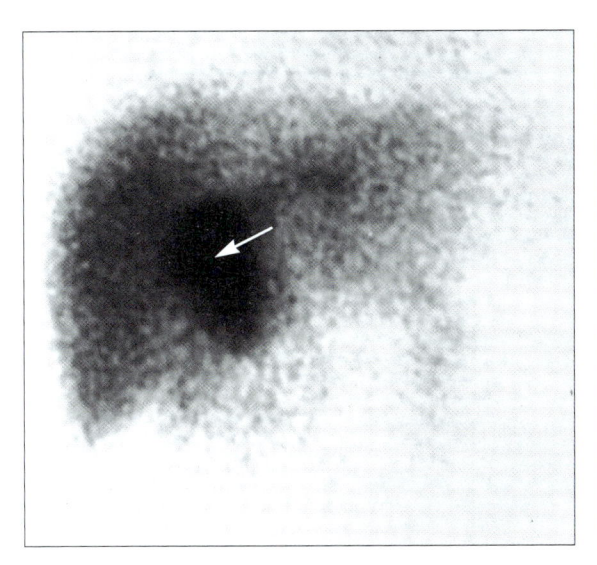

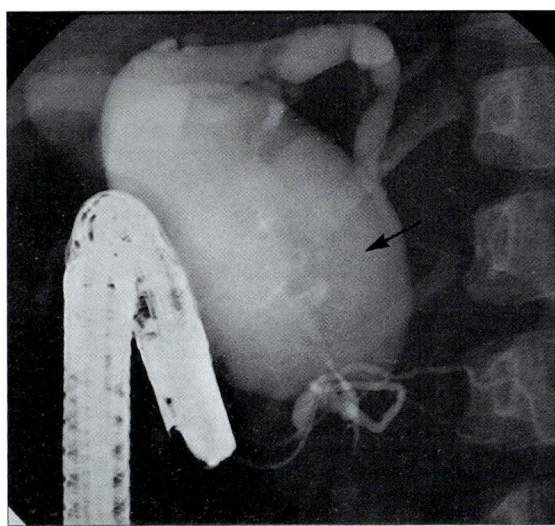

Figs 11.14, 11.15 Confirmation of diagnosis. The biliary nature of the cyst can be confirmed by a TeBIDA radioisotope scan (**11.14**, left) and the anatomy of the cyst can be defined by injecting dye through the liver into the dilated biliary tree (percutaneous transhepatic cholangiography) or endoscopically by endoscopic retrograde cholangiopancreatography (**11.15**, right).

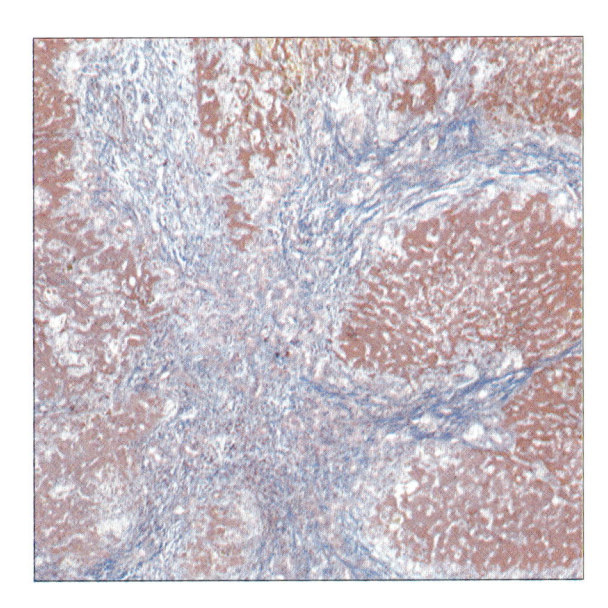

Fig. 11.16 Histology. The liver usually has evidence of biliary fibrosis, cholestasis, and bile plugs. The histological features are completely reversible after successful removal of the cyst and formation of a Roux-en-Y anastomosis with jejunum. Cholangitis is an occasional complication and there is a 2.5% risk of malignancy in the residual biliary tree in later years. (Masson Trichrome, ×4.)

NEONATAL HEPATITIS

In contrast to babies born with extrahepatic biliary atresia or choledocal cysts, babies with the neonatal hepatitis syndrome may be small for gestational dates and their stools contain some pigment, although the urine is dark. Dysmorphic features may be obvious. Standard liver function tests (**Fig. 11.17**) demonstrate hepatocyte damage, but are not diagnostic. The investigations required to differentiate between biliary atresia and neonatal hepatitis are given in **Fig. 11.18**.

Liver function tests

Investigation	Abnormality
Conjugated bilirubin <20 mmol/litre	Increased levels: Hepatocyte dysfunction or biliary obstruction
Aminotransferases • Aspartate (AST) <50 U/litre • Alanine (ALT) <40 U/litre	Increased levels: Hepatocyte inflammation/damage
Alkaline phosphatase • (ALP) <600 U/litre • Gammaglutamyltransferase • (GGT) <30 U/litre	Increased levels: Biliary damage/obstruction
Albumin 30–50 g/litre	Low levels: Chronic liver disease
Prothrombin time (PT) 12–15 seconds Partial thromboplastin time (PTT) 33–37 seconds	Prolonged: a, Vitamin K deficiency b, Poor hepatic synthesis
Ammonia <50 mmol/litre protein	Increased if: Abnormal catabolism/urea cycle defect
Glucose >4 mmol/litre	Low in: Acute or chronic liver failure

Fig. 11.17 Liver function tests.

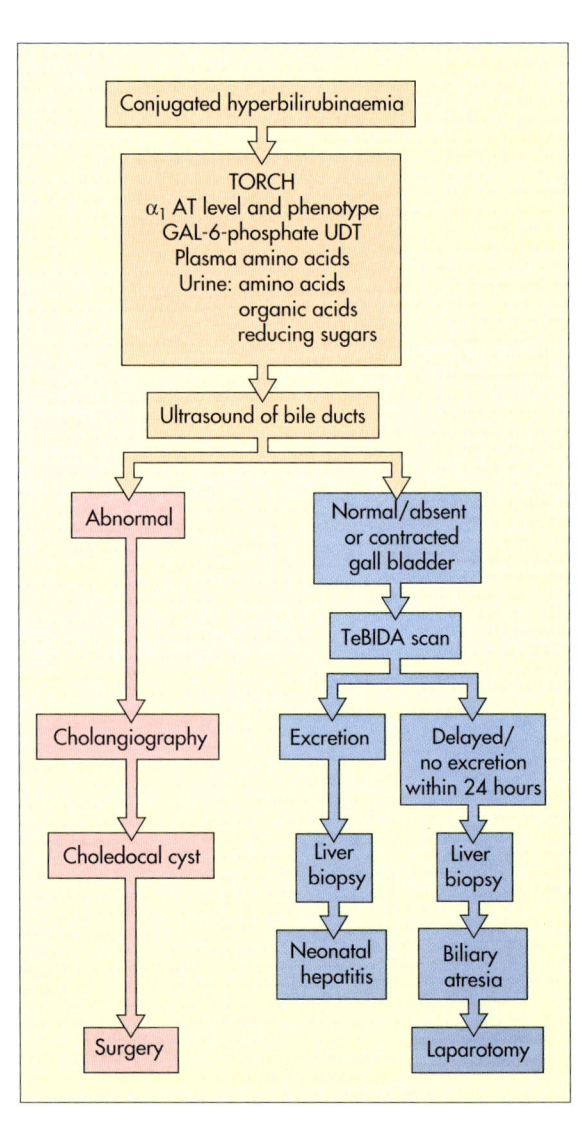

Fig. 11.18 Investigations to differentiate biliary atresia and neonatal hepatitis.

Neonatal Disease

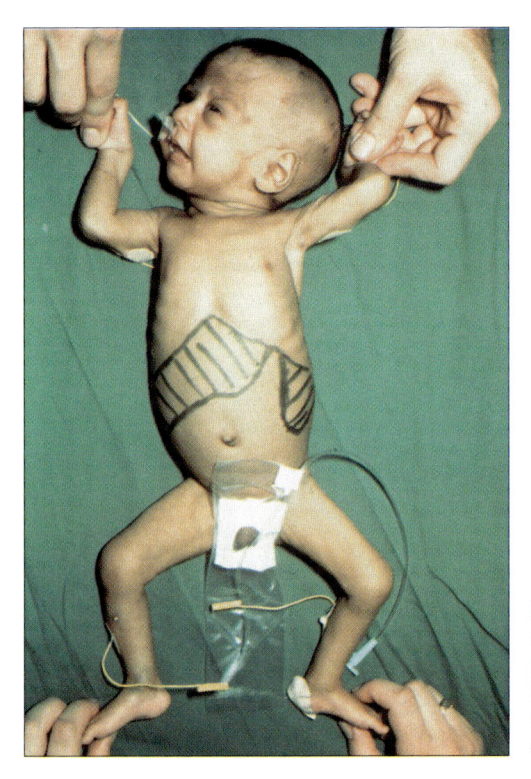

Fig. 11.19 Neonatal hepatitus. This baby was born at 37 weeks' gestation with obvious intrauterine retardation. He was jaundiced with hepatosplenomegaly, and malnourished with loss of fat and muscle stores. The most likely differential diagnosis is neonatal hepatitis secondary to an intrauterine infection or an inborn error of metabolism.

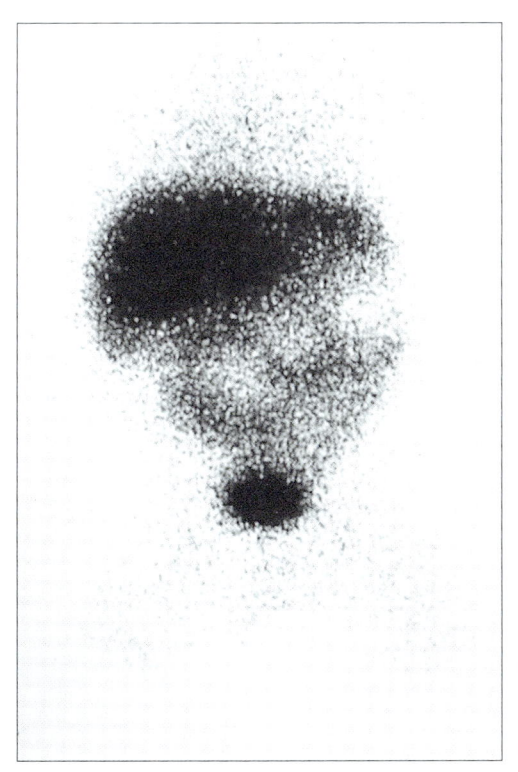

Fig. 11.20 Diagnosis. The abdominal ultrasound demonstrated a homogeneous liver with a normal sized gallbladder after a 4-hour fast, suggesting normal biliary excretion; this was confirmed by a TeBIDA radioisotope scan which demonstrated good hepatic uptake of the isotope and prompt excretion into the bowel within 4 hours, suggestive of neonatal hepatitis.

Pediatric Gastroenterology and Hepatology

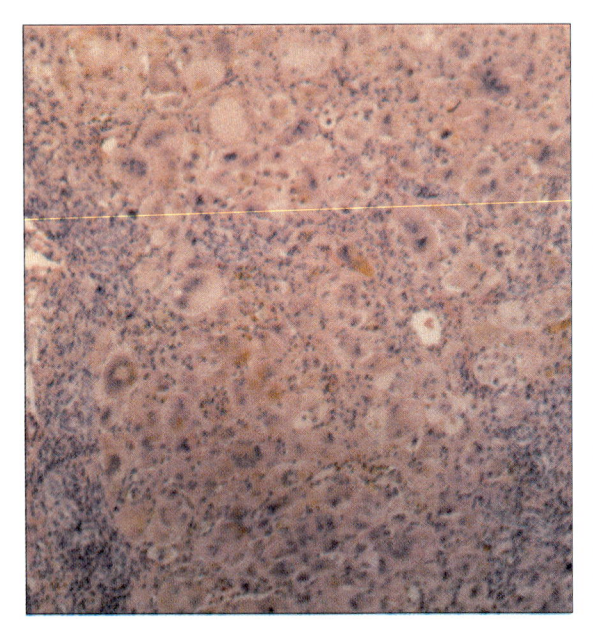

Fig. 11.21 Biopsy. The liver biopsy demonstrated typical, but non-specific, features of neonatal hepatitis. There is extramedullary haemopoiesis, cholestasis, giant cell, and rosette formation of the hepatocytes (Haematoxylin and Eosin ×25).

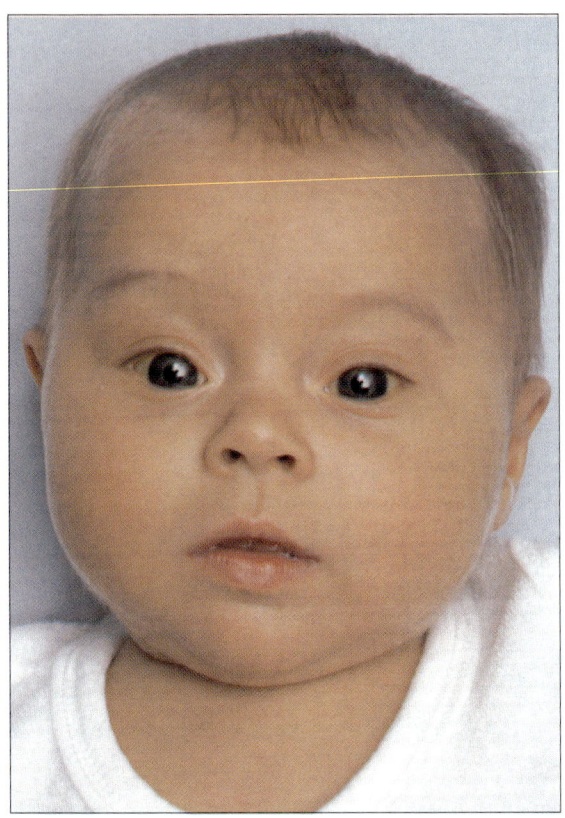

Fig. 11.22 Neonatal hepatitis. This condition occurs in 30% of babies with trisomy 13, 18 or 21. The hepatitis may be overlooked in Down's syndrome if babies have coexistent cardiac disease. The liver disease normally resolves spontaneously but may contribute to failure to thrive in the early months..

CYTOMEGALOVIRUS HEPATITIS

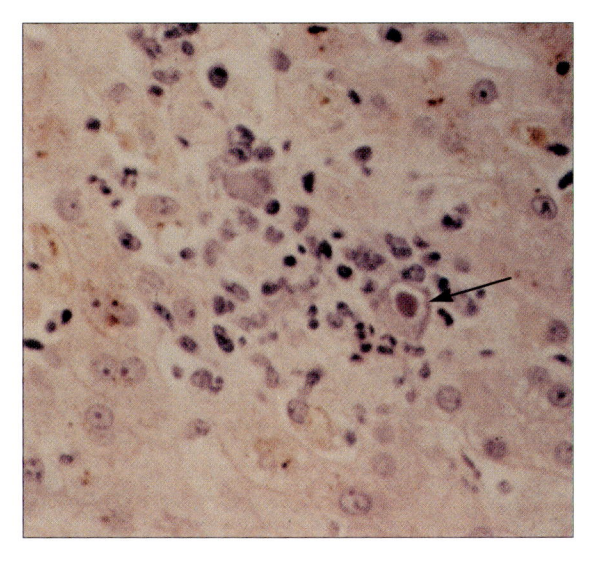

Fig. 11.23 Cytomegalovirus (CMV) hepatitis. CMV infection is the most common intrauterine infection to cause neonatal hepatitis. The diagnosis is usually made by demonstration of IgM antibodies to CMV or from evidence of active infection (CMV in the urine). Babies with this infection usually present with microcephaly, hepatosplenomegaly, chorioretinitis, or retinitis pigmentosa. The pathognomonic inclusion bodies of CMV are only occasionally demonstrated on liver histology (Immunoperoxidase ×40).

RUBELLA HEPATITIS

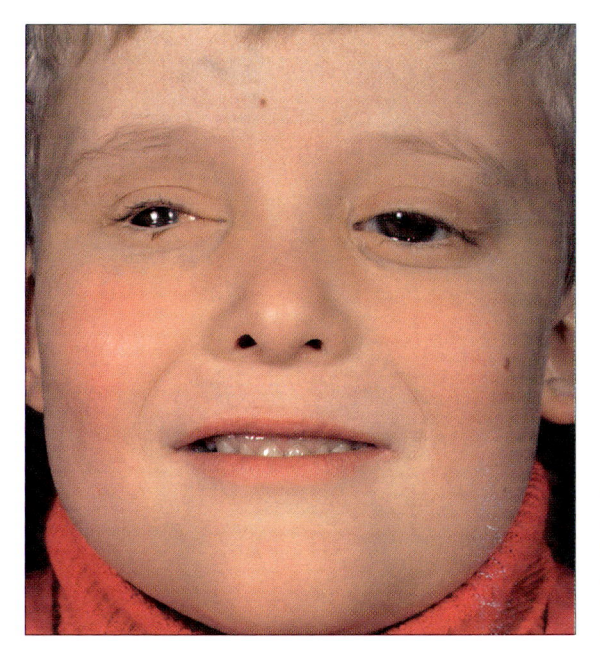

Fig. 11.24 Rubella hepatitis. Rubella hepatitis is now rare as a result of widespread immunisation. This 14-year-old boy was born with a severe neonatal hepatitis and developed cataracts, deafness, progressive liver disease, and vitamin E neuropathy following an intrauterine infection with rubella.

TOXOPLASMOSIS

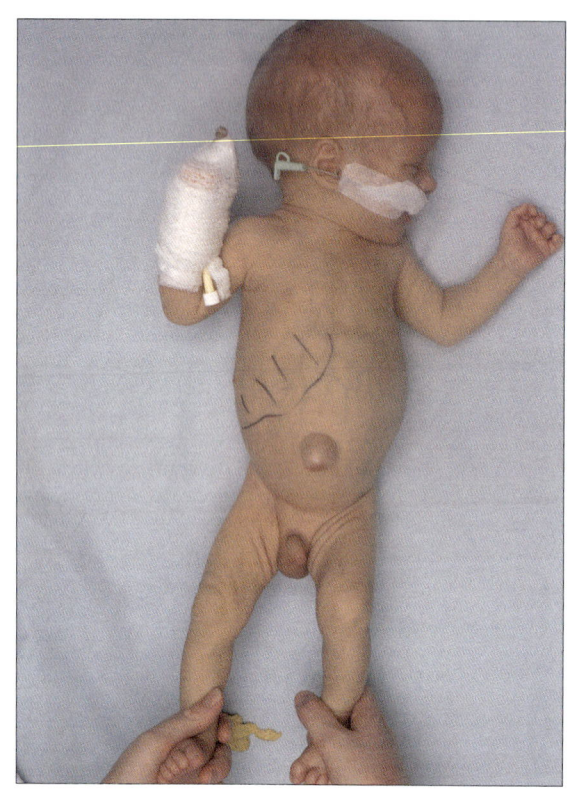

Fig. 11.25 Toxoplasmosis. Toxoplasmosis is a rare cause of neonatal hepatitis. The mother of this 6-week-old baby was IgM positive for toxoplasmosis at her antenatal booking. The baby had persistent neonatal jaundice, failure to thrive, hepatosplenomegaly, and hydrocephalus.

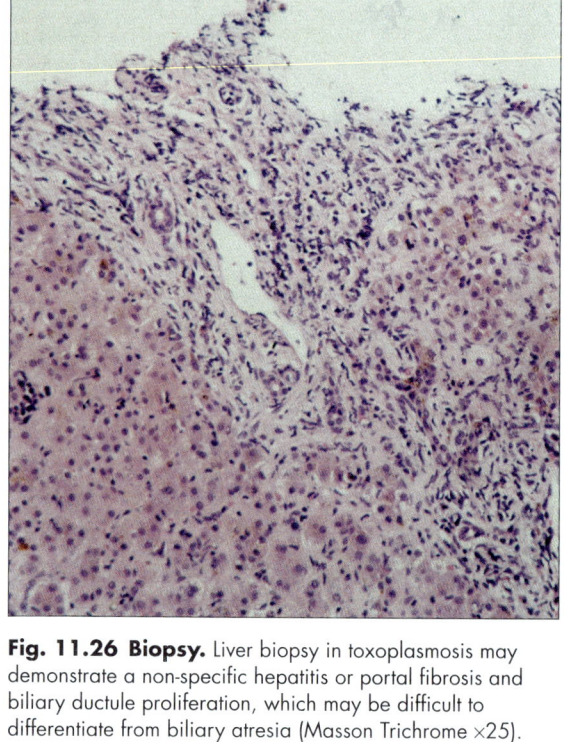

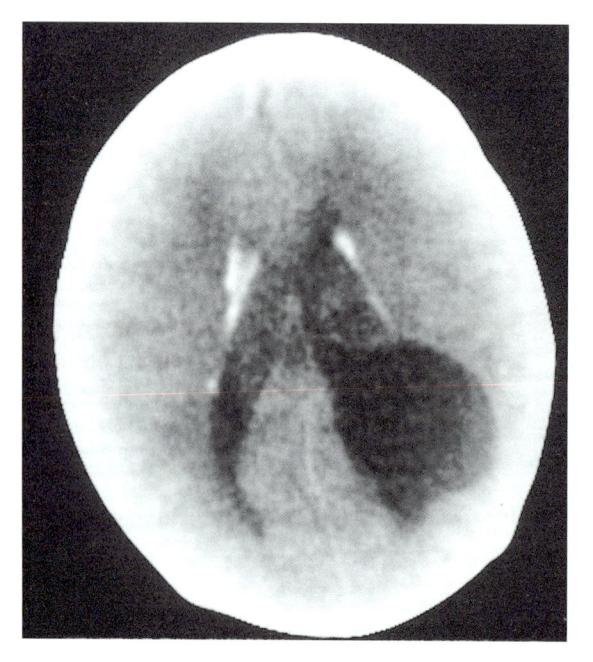

Fig. 11.26 Biopsy. Liver biopsy in toxoplasmosis may demonstrate a non-specific hepatitis or portal fibrosis and biliary ductule proliferation, which may be difficult to differentiate from biliary atresia (Masson Trichrome ×25).

Fig. 11.27 CT scan. The CT scan in toxoplasmosis demonstrates calcification and a large cyst. The baby later developed optic atrophy, despite treatment with spiramycin.

12. Inherited Metabolic Disease

ALPHA-1-ANTITRYPSIN DEFICIENCY

This autosomal recessive disorder is the most common inherited liver disease, with an incidence of 1:7000. The deficiency of the hepatic enzyme alpha-1-antitrypsin may lead to neonatal liver disease, chronic liver disease, or emphysema in adults.

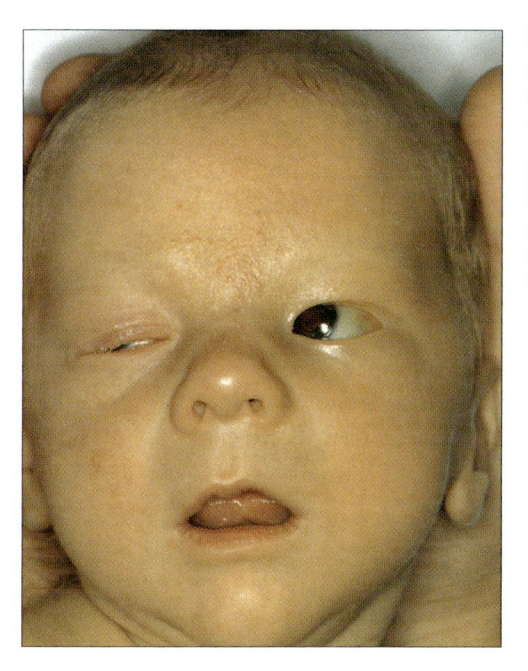

Fig. 12.1 Presentation. Alpha-1-antitrypsin deficiency may present with persistent neonatal jaundice and a vitamin K responsive coagulopathy (late haemorrhagic disease of the newborn). It is more common in breast-fed babies and in babies who did not receive prophylactic vitamin K at birth. This 6-week-old baby with persistent jaundice had abnormal bleeding around his umbilicus and following his Guthrie heel prick test. He presented with a left hemiparesis, 6th and 7th nerve palsies, and a right 3rd nerve palsy. His prothrombin time was unrecordable, but returned to normal following a single intravenous injection of vitamin K.

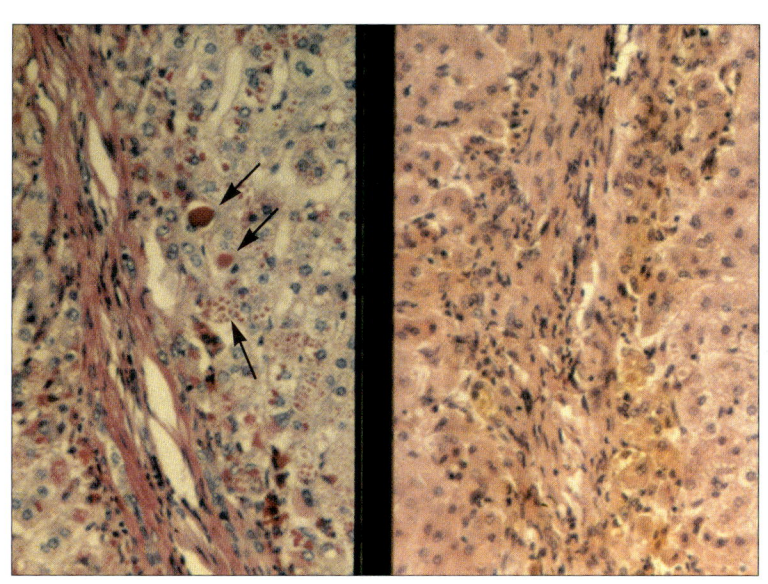

Fig. 12.2 Diagnosis. The diagnosis was made by identifying a reduced level of alpha-1-antitrypsin in the serum (normal, >1.0 g/litre) and estimating the phenotype (protein inhibitor ZZ, PIZZ) which is associated with liver disease. Liver biopsy demonstrated the characteristic PAS-positive granules in the hepatocytes (left, Periodic Acid–Schiff, diastase resistant, ×10). Note the cholestasis around portal tracts (right, Haematoxylin and Eosin, ×10).

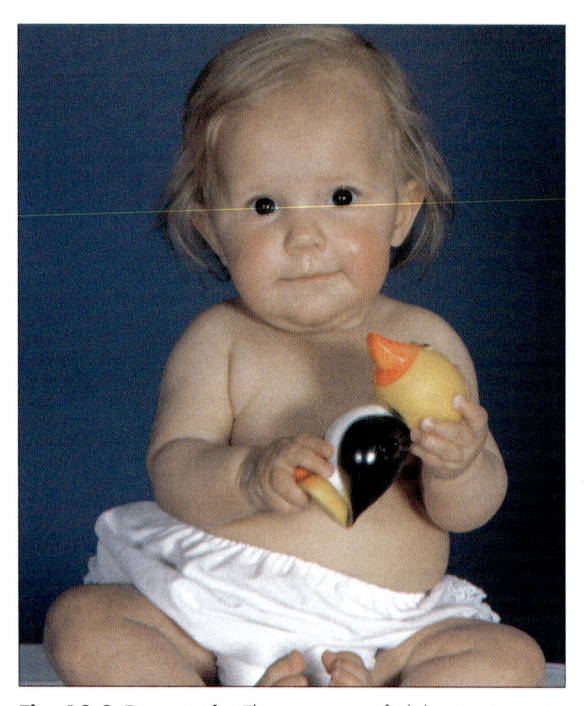

Fig. 12.3 Prognosis. The prognosis of alpha-1-antitrypsin deficiency is very variable. Approximately 30% of babies make an almost complete recovery with nutritional support and fat-soluble vitamin supplementation.

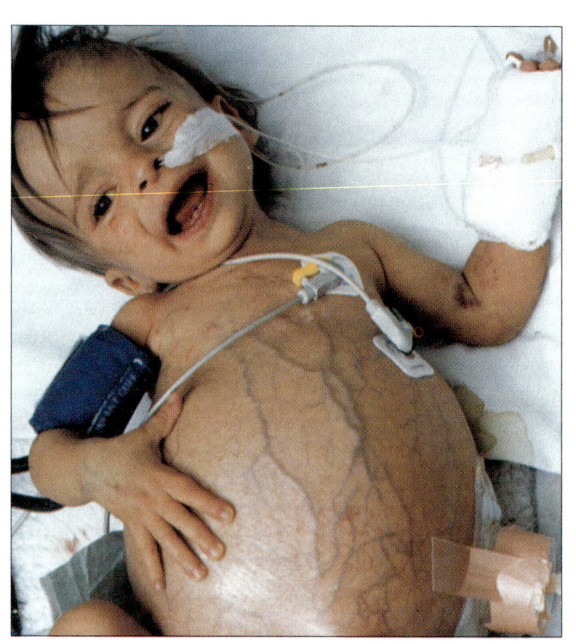

Fig. 12.4 Prognosis. In contrast, approximately 60% of children who present in infancy with alpha-1-antitrypsin deficiency will develop cirrhosis and portal hypertension, and 30% will develop liver failure in the first year of life. This baby developed cirrhosis, portal hypertension, ascites, and gross malnutrition by 6 months of age without being obviously jaundiced.

TYROSINAEMIA TYPE I

Tyrosinaemia Type I is an autosomal recessive disorder with an incidence of 1:15,000. The clinical presentation varies from acute liver failure with coagulopathy and encephalopathy to chronic liver disease with rickets. Ascites may be present at birth. The disorder is secondary to deficiency of the hepatic enzyme fumarylacetoacetase, which leads to an accumulation of tyrosine, methionine, and toxic metabolites which cause cardiac, liver, renal, and neurological abnormalities. The diagnosis is confirmed by identifying the toxic metabolite succinylacetone in the urine. Management consists of strict dietary control of protein; this controls the biochemical features, but not the progression of liver disease. A new drug—2-(2-nitro-4-trifluoromethylbenzoyl)-1,3-cyclonexanedione (NTBC)—which prevents the formation of toxic metabolites may change the natural history.

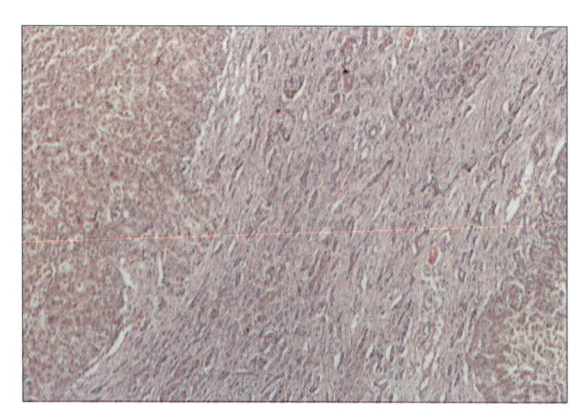

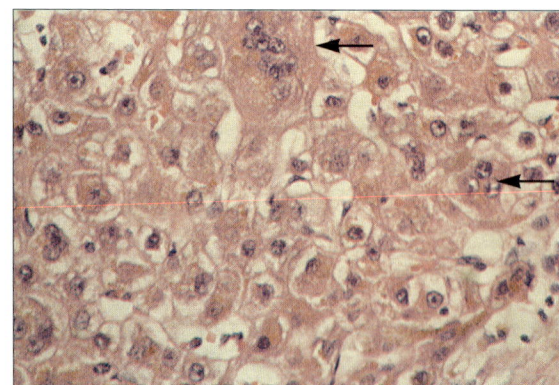

Figs 12.5, 12.6 Histology. The liver histology is non-specific with fatty infiltration and hepatitis (**12.5**, left, Haematoxylin and Eosin, ×4). Cirrhosis may be present *in utero*. Hepatic dysplasia (**12.6**, right, Haematoxylin and Eosin, ×25) leads inevitably to hepatocellular carcinoma.

Inherited Metabolic Disease

COMPLICATIONS OF TYROSINAEMIA

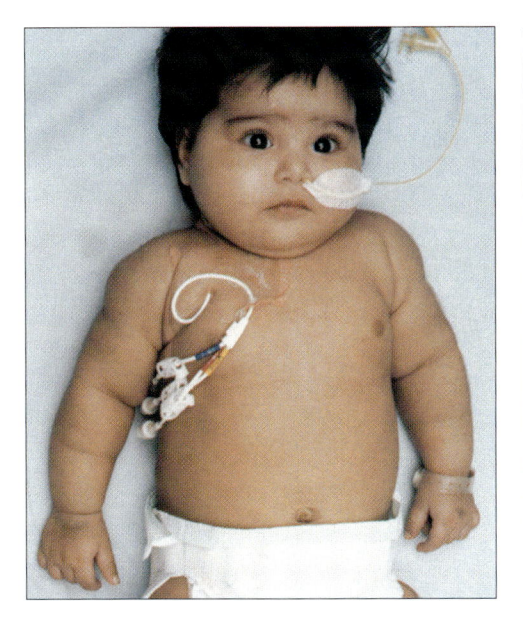

Fig. 12.7 Hypoglycaemia. Tyrosinaemia Type I is associated with severe hypoglycaemia secondary to either acute liver failure or islet cell hyperplasia with hyperinsulinism. These conditions may be differentiated by measuring insulin and C-peptide levels during hypoglycaemia. Hyperinsulinism leads to abnormal growth with an excess of fat deposits, as in this baby. It is controlled by oral diazoxide, although fluid retention may be a problem.

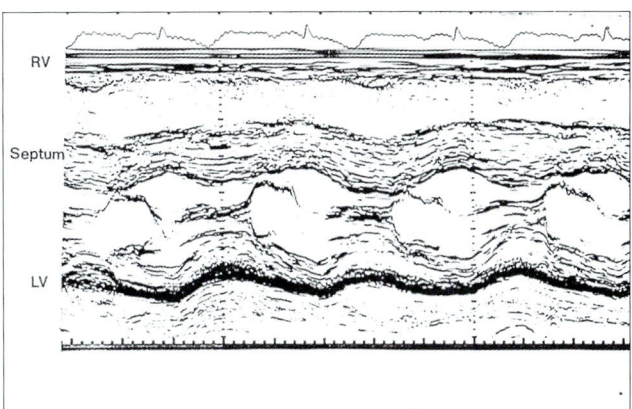

Fig. 12.8 Cardiac complications. Cardiac complications include a hypertrophic cardiomyopathy (HOCM) which affects the septum. It is reversible following liver transplantation or treatment with NTBC.

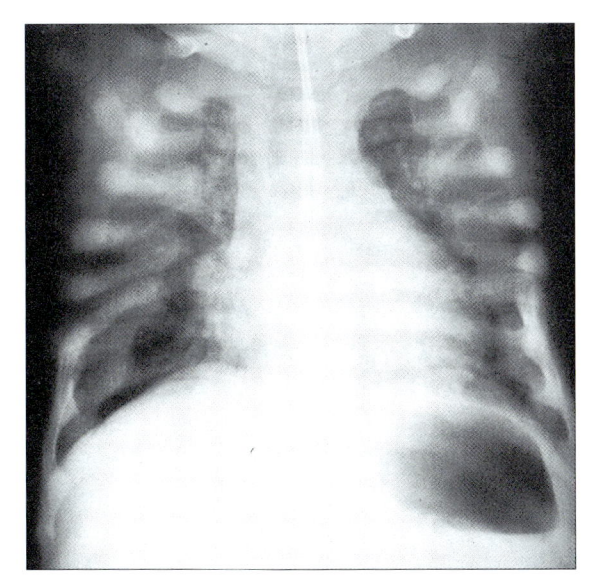

Fig. 12.9 Renal tubular acidosis. Renal tubular acidosis may exacerbate rickets, as in this child with severe vitamin D resistant rickets.

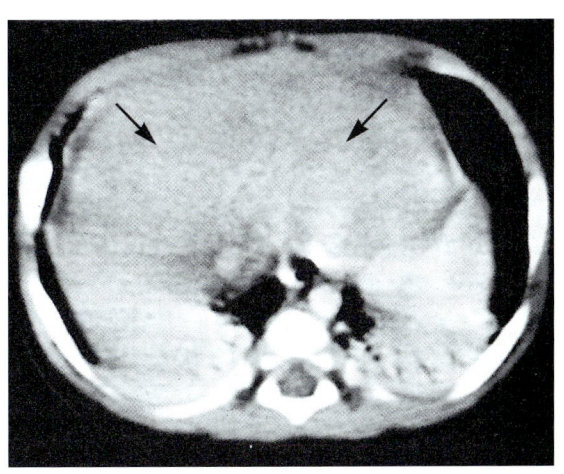

Fig. 12.10 Hepatocellular carcinoma. Screening for the early detection of hepatocellular carcinoma is essential. Ultrasound and CT scans may demonstrate irregular nodules, while a rise in alphafetoprotein level suggests malignancy.

Pediatric Gastroenterology and Hepatology

CYSTIC FIBROSIS

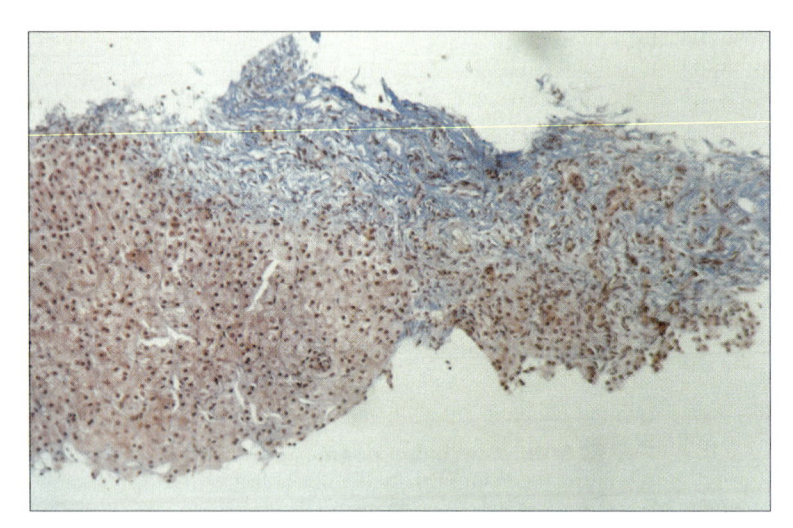

Fig. 12.11 Cystic fibrosis. Very occasionally cystic fibrosis presents as neonatal hepatitis. Babies develop progressive jaundice and failure to thrive with recurrent chest infections. The characteristic histological features are cholestasis, bile plugs, biliary fibrosis, and fatty infiltration. The neonatal hepatitis resolves in the majority of babies. (Masson Trichrome, ×10.)

WILSON'S DISEASE

Wilson's disease is an inborn error of metabolism in which there is abnormal biliary copper excretion and accumulation of copper in the liver, brain, kidney, and cornea. The disorder is autosomal recessive with an incidence of 1:30,000. It may present with any form of liver disease in children older than 3 years. Neurological symptoms usually do not develop until adolescence.

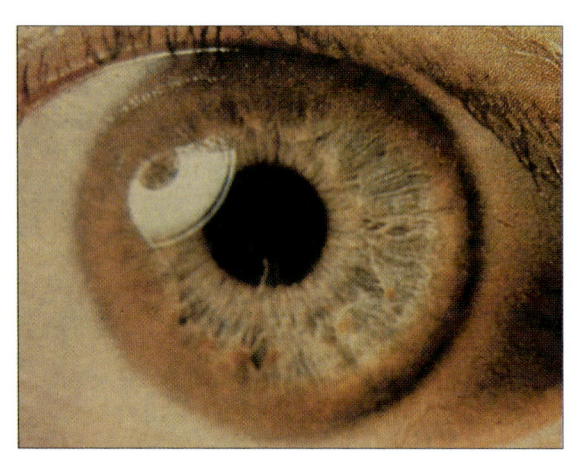

Fig. 12.12 Wilson's disease. The characteristic Kayser–Fleischer rings are not usually visible before the age of 7 years.

Fig. 12.13 Diagnosis. The diagnosis is usually made on the basis of low serum copper (< 10 μmol/litre) and ceruloplasmin (< 200 mg/litre), and an elevated urinary copper (> 1.0 μmol/24 h), particularly after penicillamine challenge. Children with Wilson's disease may have normal serum levels, as in this boy with a non-specific hepatitis for 6 months. The diagnosis was made on the basis of abnormal urinary copper and an elevated hepatic copper (> 250 mg/g dry weight). Treatment with penicillamine (20 mg/kg) is effective if started early enough.

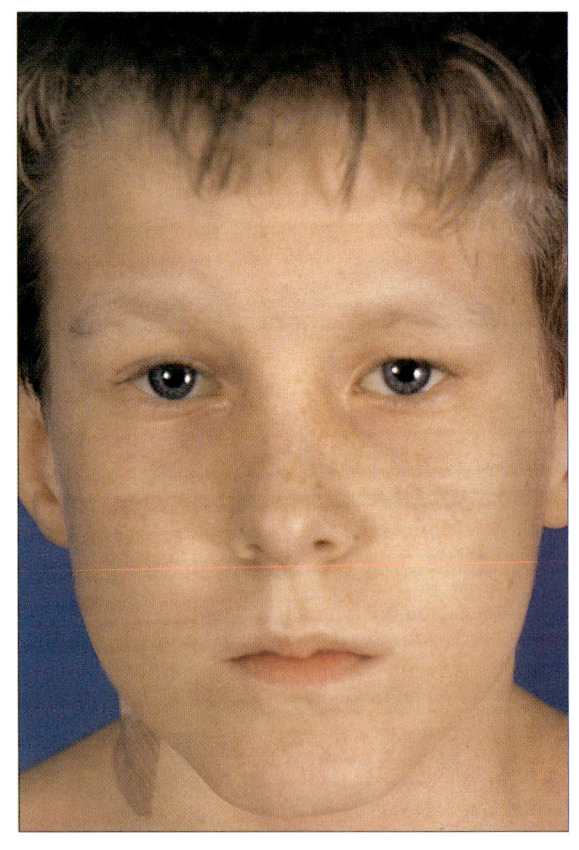

Inherited Metabolic Disease

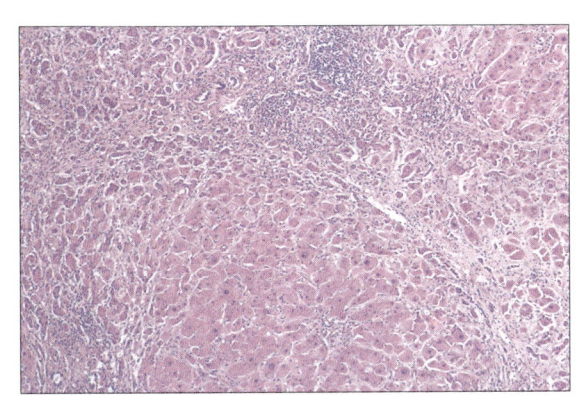

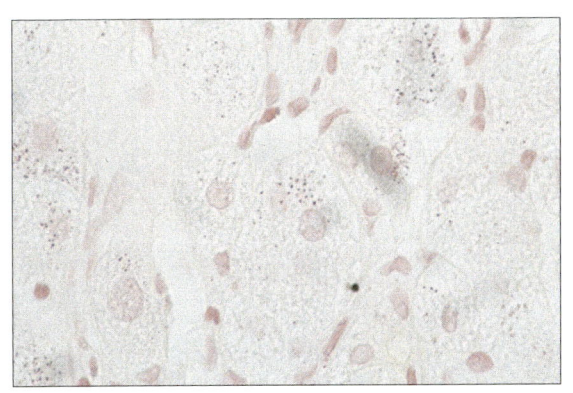

Figs 12.14, 12.15. Fulminant Wilson's disease This liver biopsy from a child with fulminant Wilson's disease demonstrates severe hepatitis and fibrosis (**12.14**, left, Haematoxylin and Eosin, ×4). Liver histology is non-specific, but copper storage may be demonstrated using an orcein stain (**12.15**, right, orcein, ×40) or by measuring total liver copper.

INTRAHEPATIC BILIARY HYPOPLASIA

Intrahepatic biliary hypoplasia or paucity of interlobular bile ducts (PIBD) is considered to be present when the ratio of interlobular bile ducts and arterioles in the portal tracts is less than 0.6. Clinical features include cholestasis, hepatomegaly, pruritus, and failure to thrive. There is gradual progression to cirrhosis and portal hypertension and an eventual requirement for liver transplantation. PIBD may be syndromic (Alagille's syndrome) or non-syndromic.

ALAGILLE'S SYNDROME

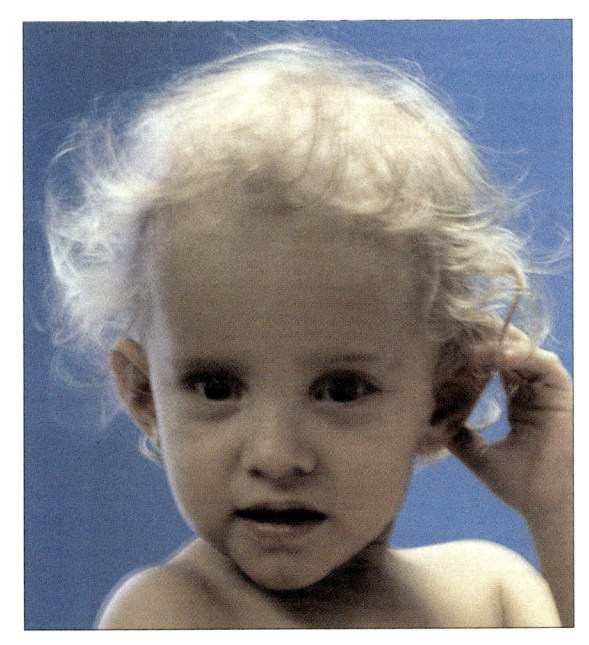

Fig. 12.16 Alagille's syndrome. This autosomal dominant condition has an incidence of 1:100,000 births. It is associated with cardiac, facial, renal, ocular, and skeletal abnormalities. The facial features include a triangular face with a high forehead and frontal bossing, deep-set widely spaced eyes, and a saddle-shaped nasal bridge.

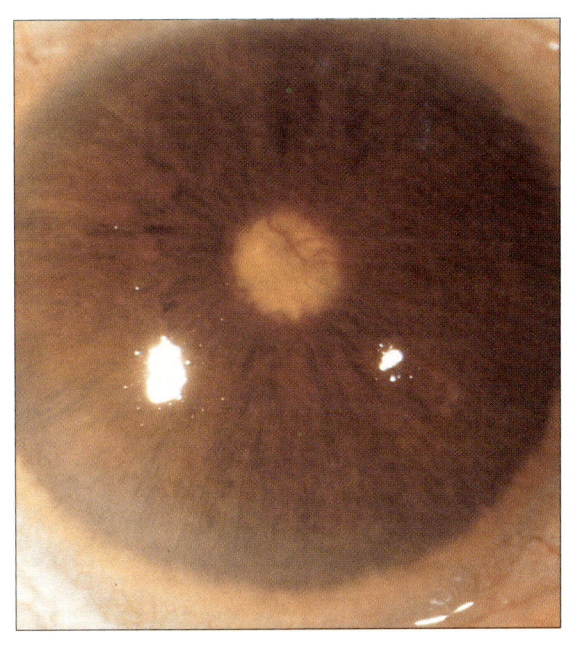

Fig. 12.17 Posterior embryotoxin. Posterior embryotoxin is present in 90% of patients with Alagille's syndrome, compared with 10% of the general population. There may also be retinal pigmentation on fundoscopy.

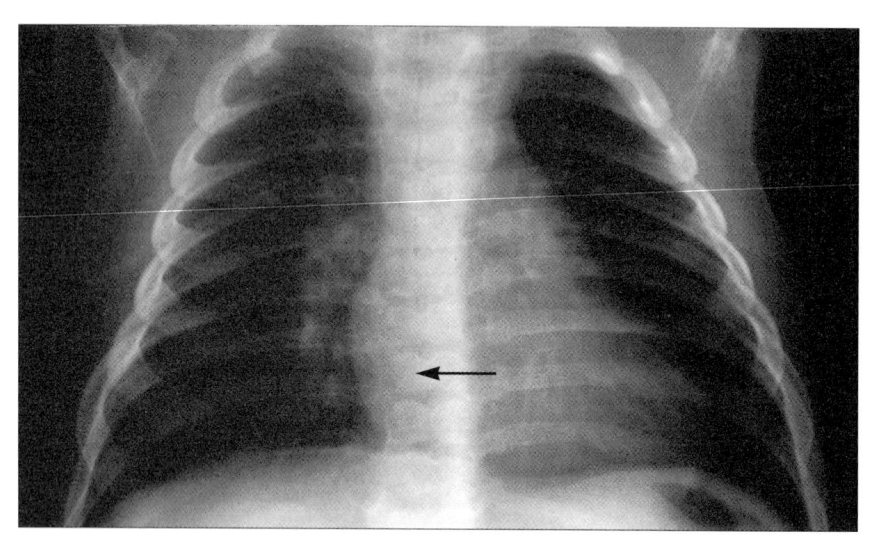

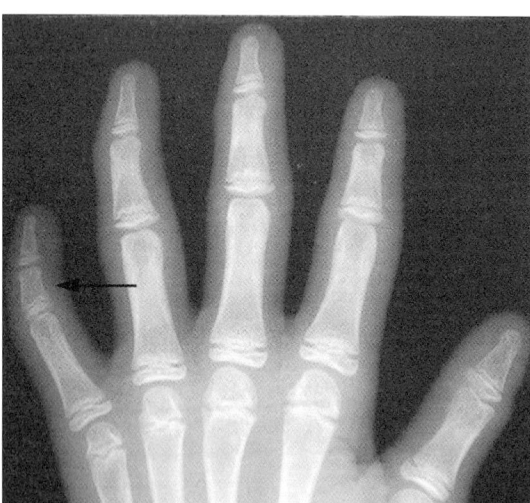

Figs 12.18, 12.19 Alagille's syndrome. Skeletal abnormalities include abnormal thoracic vertebra (**12.18**, top, butterfly vertebra) and curving of the proximal digits (**12.19**, left).

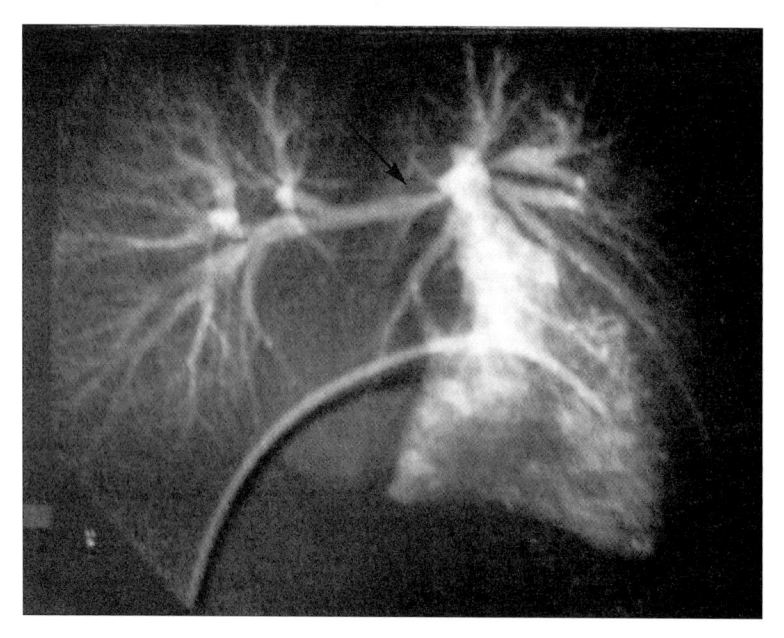

Fig. 12.20 Alagille's syndrome. The most common cardiac abnormality is peripheral pulmonary stenosis. Electrocardiography may demonstrate right bundle branch block or right ventricular hypertrophy. Echocardiography may be completely normal. The diagnosis is suspected clinically and confirmed by angiography. The prognosis of peripheral pulmonary stenosis is variable and the condition may regress after liver transplantation.

Inherited Metabolic Disease

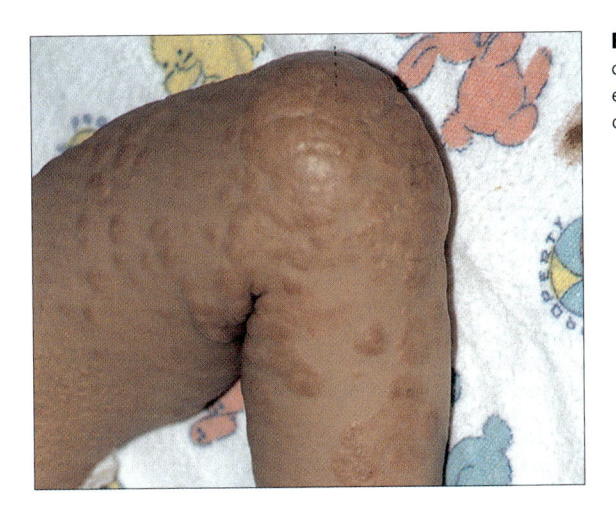

Fig. 12.21 Cholesterol catabolism. The associated defect in cholesterol catabolism in this syndrome leads to elevated plasma cholesterol and xanthomata, which regress after liver transplantation.

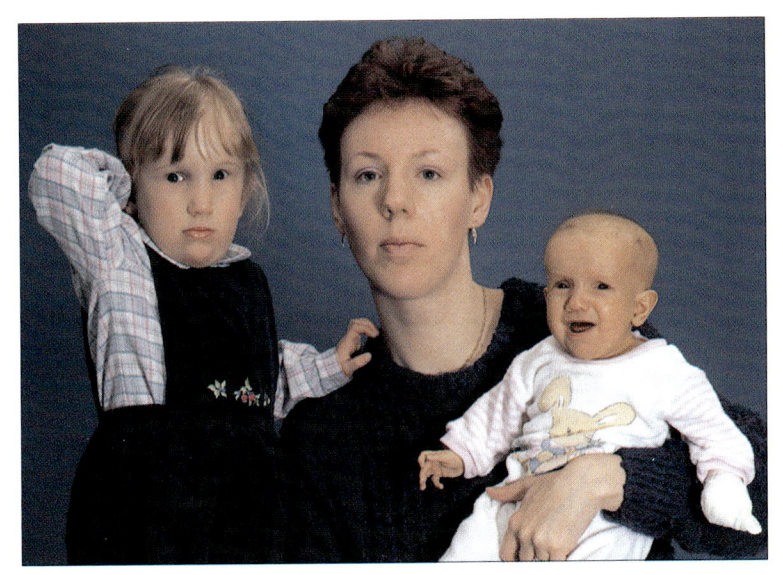

Fig. 12.22 Heterogeneity. The heterogeneity of this autosomal dominant condition is demonstrated by this family. The mother displays the characteristic facial features, but is otherwise physically normal. The eldest daughter has the characteristic facial features and severe peripheral pulmonary stenosis, but no liver or renal disease. The baby has the characteristic facial features, peripheral pulmonary stenosis, biliary hypoplasia, and renal tubular acidosis. She had severe failure to thrive and distressing pruritus, cirrhosis, and portal hypertension. She underwent a successful transplant operation following cardiac surgery for her pulmonary stenosis.

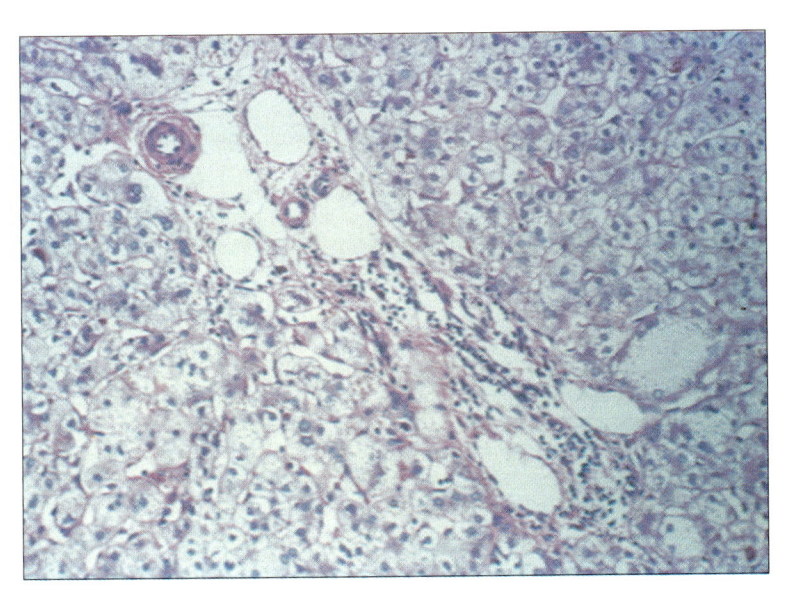

Fig. 12.23 Histology. Liver histology may be non-specific and careful examination is required to identify the paucity of interlobular bile ducts. In the first 3 months of life; the predominant features may be cholestasis and giant cell transformation with visible interlobular ducts. The biopsy may be differentiated from extrahepatic biliary atresia by the absence of portal fibrosis and extrahepatic biliary ductule proliferation. (Haematoxylin and Eosin, ×10.)

NON-SYNDROMIC BILIARY HYPOPLASIA

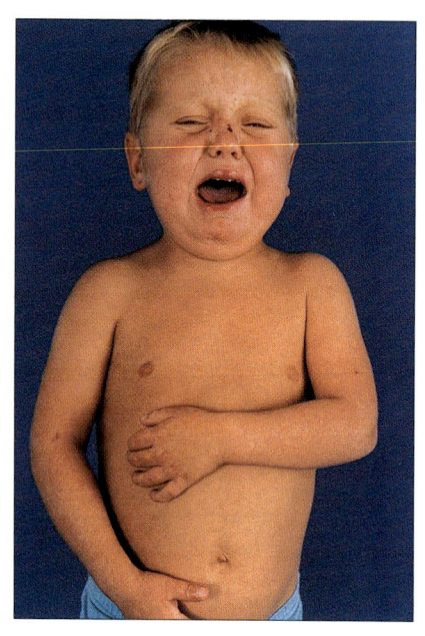

Fig. 12.24 Non-syndromic biliary hypoplasia. Paucity of intrahepatic bile ducts may occur in a variety of familial cholestatic syndromes without the characteristic features described above in Alagille's syndrome. These diseases include progressive fibrosing intrahepatic cholestasis and Bylers' disease. These diseases generally have a worse prognosis and are characterised by intense pruritus which may be an indication for biliary diversion or liver transplantation.

INBORN ERRORS OF BILE ACID METABOLISM

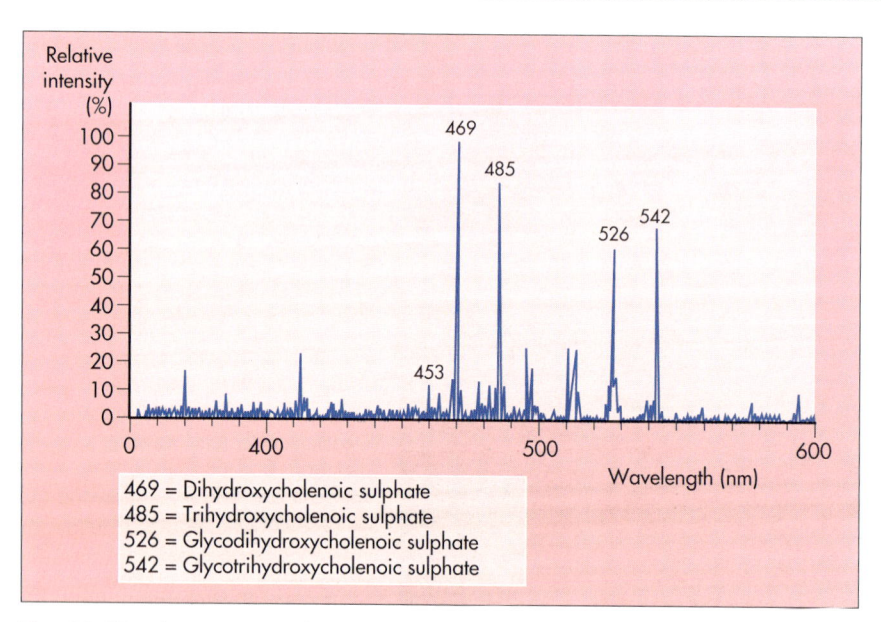

469 = Dihydroxycholenoic sulphate
485 = Trihydroxycholenoic sulphate
526 = Glycodihydroxycholenoic sulphate
542 = Glycotrihydroxycholenoic sulphate

Fig. 12.25 Inborn errors of bile acid metabolism. The diagnosis of these rare autosomal recessive disorders of bile acid metabolism has been revolutionised by the development of fast atom bombardment ionisation mass spectrometry (FAB-MS) which detects bile acid metabolites in urine. The FAB-MS spectrum indicates a defect in the synthesis of 3-β-hydroxysteroid dehydrogenase isomerase enzymes. Babies present with persistent jaundice and cholestasis; they rapidly develop liver failure, so require liver transplantation. The condition may be reversible with treatment with oral bile acids (cholic acid or chenodeoxycholic acid) and hence early diagnosis is essential.

Inherited Metabolic Disease

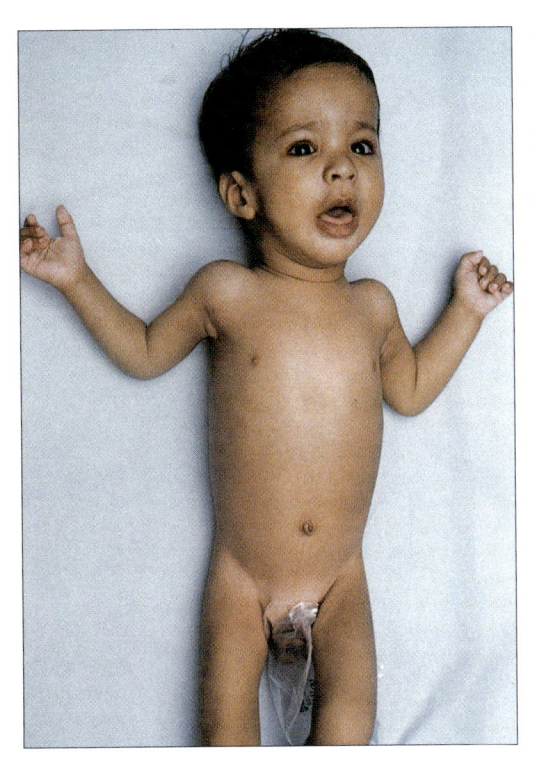

Fig. 12.26 Zellweger's syndrome. Zellweger's syndrome is a rare disorder which is associated with absent or dysfunctional peroxisomes leading to multi-organ failure. The incidence is 1:100,000 live births and it affects the sexes equally. Babies may be small for gestational dates and have severe hypotonia with feeding difficulties. Dysmorphic features include epicanthic folds, Brushfield's spots, and a high forehead. There is severe failure to thrive and psychomotor retardation. The diagnosis may be suspected by demonstration of abnormal urinary bile salt metabolites using FAB-MS or the detection of very long chain fatty acids in serum. Treatment with oral bile acids may produce some clinical improvement, but death is inevitable within 2 years. Note this baby's hypotonic posture, characteristic facial features, and associated malnutrition.

NIEMANN–PICK DISEASE TYPE C

Niemann–Pick disease Type C (NPC) is a rare neurovisceral storage disorder which may present with fetal ascites or neonatal hepatitis. There is a defect in cholesterol esterification which leads to hepatosplenomegaly and neurological disease. The diagnosis is confirmed by the detection of foamy storage cells in liver and bone marrow and by measuring cholesterol esterification in fibroblast culture.

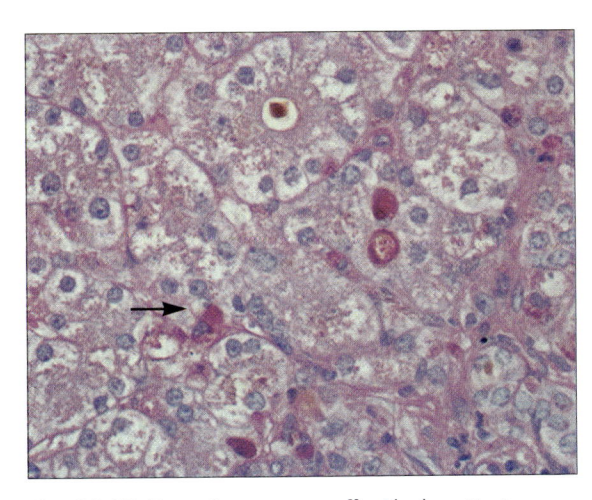

Fig. 12.27 Hepatic storage cells. The hepatic storage cells may be difficult to differentiate from Kupffer cells in babies with neonatal hepatitis. The hepatitis usually resolves to leave an inactive fibrosis or cirrhosis with persistent splenomegaly. (Periodic Acid–Schiff, diastase, ×100.)

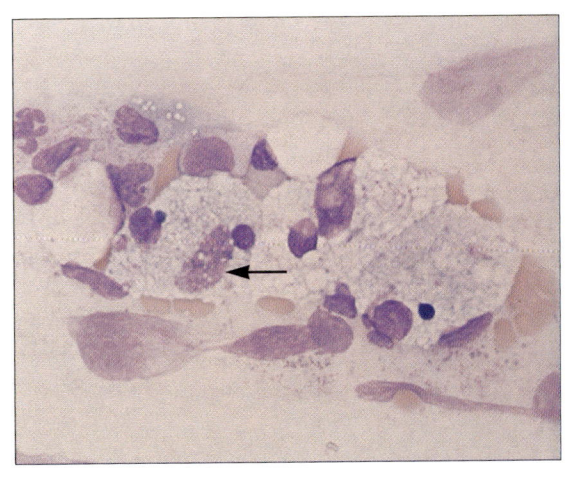

Fig. 12.28 Foamy storage cells. The foamy storage cells are best demonstrated in bone marrow aspirate. (May-Grünwald-Giemsa stain, ×160.)

Pediatric Gastroenterology and Hepatology

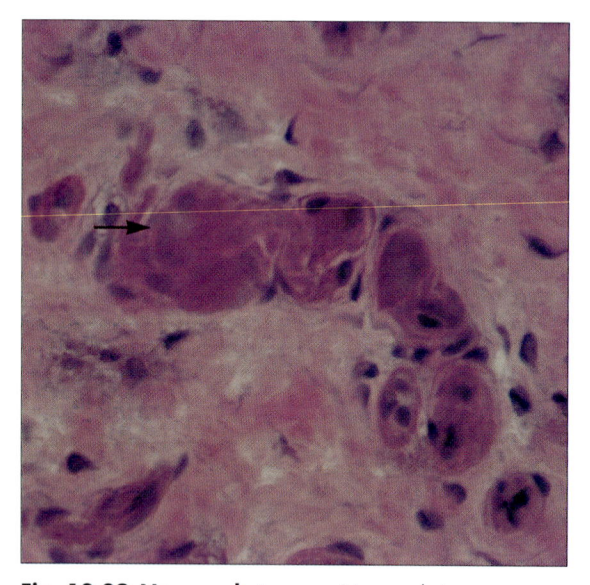

Fig. 12.29 Neuronal storage. Neuronal storage secondary to NPC is demonstrable in stillborn babies and is best seen in the ganglion cells of a suction rectal biopsy. Although most babies who present with neonatal hepatitis do not develop neurological symptoms until the age of 5 years, neurological disease is inevitable and leads to ataxia and dementia. (Periodic Acid Schiff, ×160.)

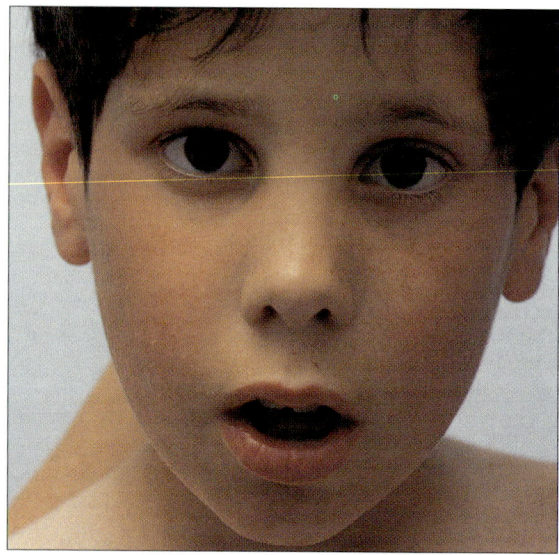

Fig. 12.30 Supranuclear ophthalmoplegia. The pathognomonic neurological sign of NPC is a supranuclear ophthalmoplegia. This child is able to move his eyes laterally, but not vertically. Note how hypotonic his face is. Most children become increasingly disabled and die of respiratory infection in mid-adolescence. The disease is not cured by liver or bone marrow transplantation.

GAUCHER'S DISEASE

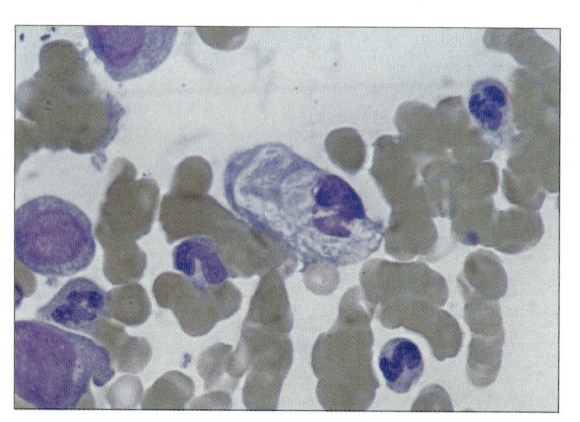

Figs 12.31–12.33 Gaucher's Disease. This autosomal recessive disorder is secondary to a deficiency of glucose ceramide, which leads to hepatosplenomegaly and neurological and bone disease. The diagnosis is confirmed by the identification of large multinucleated cells in bone marrow aspirate (**12.31**, top left, Masson Trichrome, ×4). It may now be cured by bone marrow transplantation. Enzyme replacement and gene therapy are future therapeutic possibilities. The liver biopsy demonstrates fibrosis (**12.32**, bottom left, Haematoxylin and Eosin, ×10) and the pink Gaucher's cells (**12.33**, bottom right, Haematoxylin and Eosin, ×25).

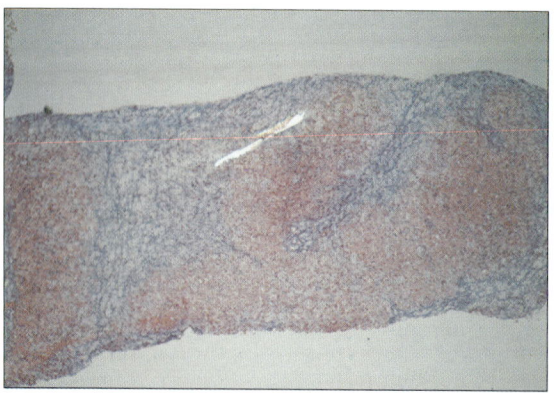

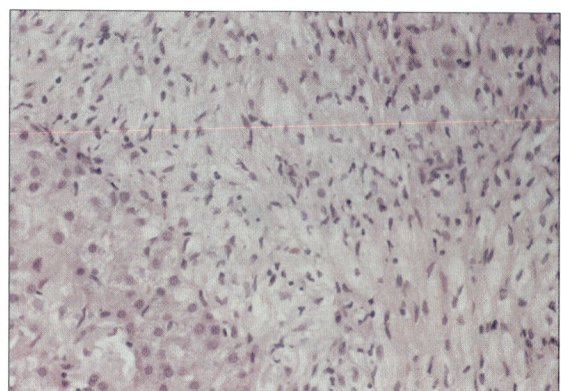

GALACTOSAEMIA

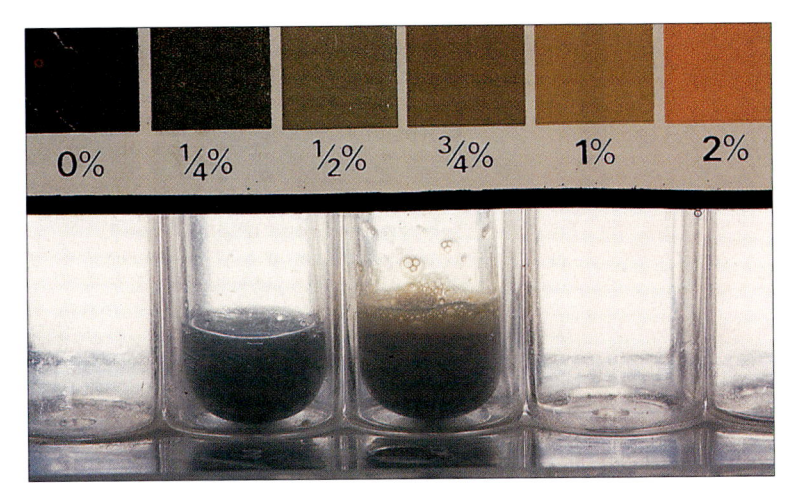

Fig. 12.34 Galactosaemia. This rare autosomal recessive disorder has an incidence of 1:40,000 live births. The presentation may be acute with hypoglycaemia, jaundice, hepatomegaly, coagulopathy, and cataracts. The diagnosis is suspected by identifying reducing substances in the urine, which are only present if the child is fed with a lactose-containing feed. It may be confirmed by measurement of the red cell enzyme galactose-6-phosphate uridyl transferase. The disease is reversible with a galactose-free diet, although the long-term prognosis should be guarded.

FRUCTOSE INTOLERANCE

Hereditary fructose intolerance is an autosomal recessive disease due to a deficiency of fructose-1-phosphate aldolase. Clinical features do not become obvious until sucrose is introduced to the diet. In the young infant vomiting, hypoglycaemia, hepatomegaly, failure to gain weight, jaundice, abnormal liver function tests, and coagulopathy are the presenting symptoms. Renal tubular acidosis is associated in all cases. Older children have a strong aversion to sugar. The diagnosis is confirmed by identifying the genetic mutation or establishing that the enzyme is deficient on liver biopsy. Avoidance of fructose-containing feeds produces a remarkable improvement in symptoms and clinical signs.

Fructose 1,6-diphosphatase deficiency may have a similar presentation with hypoglycaemia, ketosis, and hepatomegaly, which is associated with fructose intolerance. The diagnosis is confirmed by enzyme assay in the liver.

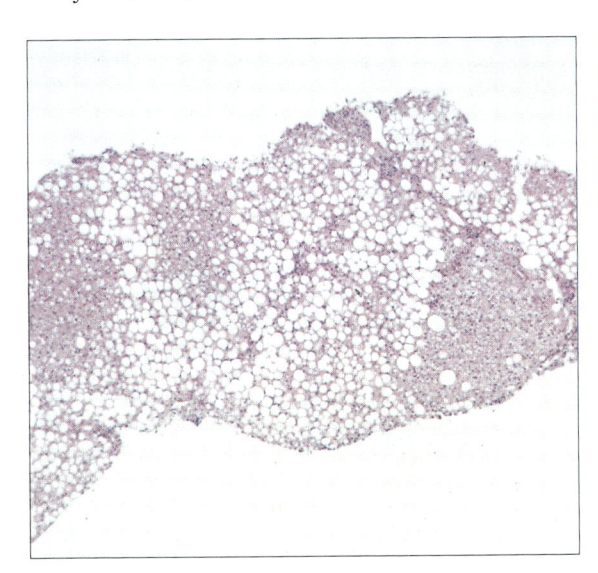

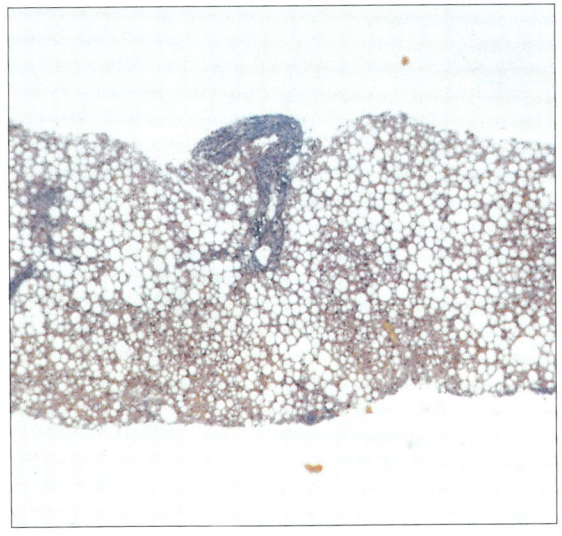

Figs 12.35, 12.36 Fructose intolerence. The liver histology usually demonstrates considerable fatty infiltration (**12.35**, left, Haematoxylin and Eosin, ×10) with fibrosis (**12.36**, right, Masson Trichrome, ×10), which may progress to cirrhosis if untreated.

GLYCOGEN STORAGE DISEASE

There are many different variants of glycogen storage disease in which the concentration, molecular structure, or function of glycogen is abnormal in the liver, heart, kidney, and skeletal muscle. It is an autosomal recessive disorder with an incidence of 1:50,000.

GLYCOGEN STORAGE DISEASE TYPE I

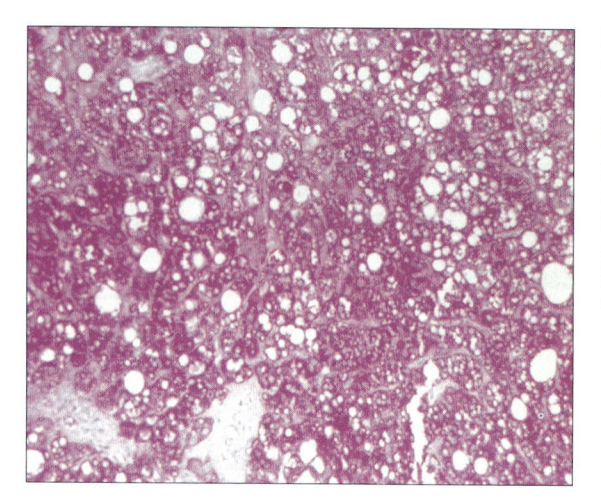

Fig. 12.37 Glycogen storage disease Type I.
Glycogen storage disease Type I (GSD Type I) is due to a deficiency of glucose-6-phosphatase in the liver, kidney, pancreas, and gut. There are a number of variants (Types 1A–1D). Increased glycogen storage leads to hepatomegaly. Hypoglycaemia secondary to the inability to utilise glycogen may be life-threatening. The diagnosis is confirmed histologically by demonstrating the absence of glucose-6-phosphatase on liver biopsy or by measuring the enzyme in the liver. Demonstrated here are glycogen-laden hepatocytes with some fatty infiltration. (Periodic Acid–Schiff, ×25.)

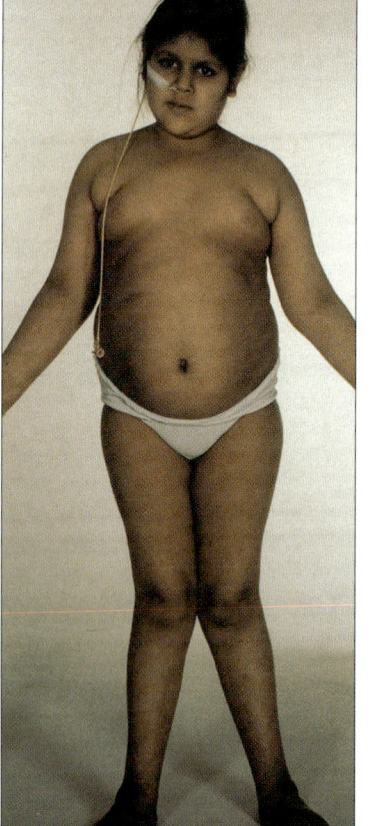

Figs 12.38, 12.39 Management of GSD Type I. Management of GSD Type I includes continuous enteral feeding of glucose and/or slow-release glucose preparations (corn starch). This Asian girl with gross hepatomegaly, hyperlipidaemia, stunting, and muscle weakness was initially referred for liver transplantation (**12.38**, left). Instigation of continuous enteral feeds produced a dramatic improvement in height and weight (**12.39**, bottom) and 5 years later she was able to discontinue nasogastric feeding and assume a near-normal lifestyle.

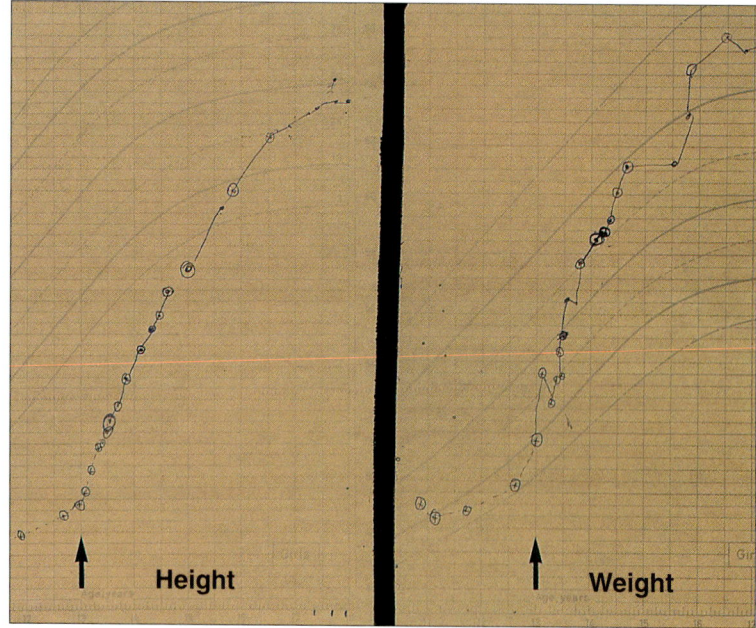

Inherited Metabolic Disease

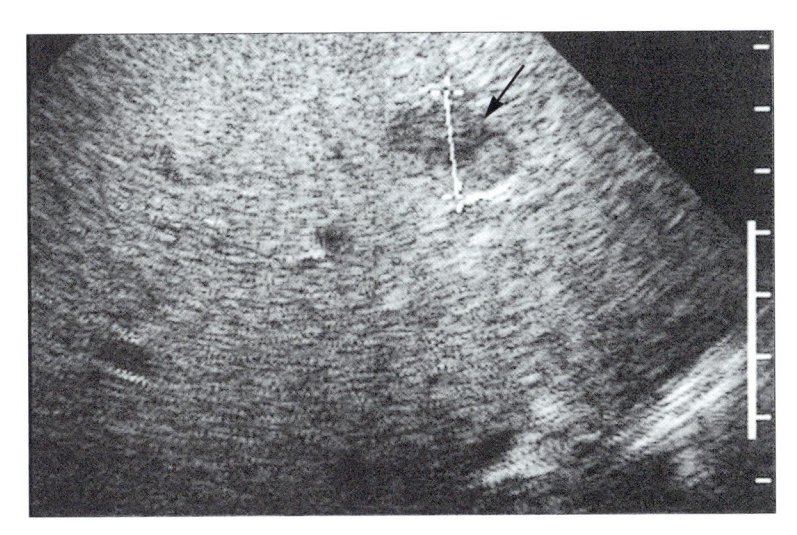

Figs 12.40, 12.41 Management of GSD Type I. It is important to monitor cardiac and renal function and screen for hepatic adenomas using ultrasound (**12.40**, top) and CT scan (**12.41**, middle).

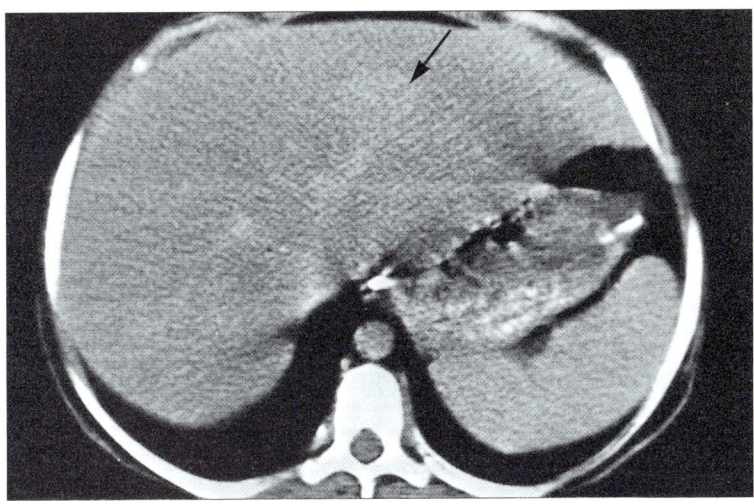

GLYCOGEN STORAGE DISEASE TYPE III (AMYLO-1,6-GLUCOSIDASE DEFICIENCY)

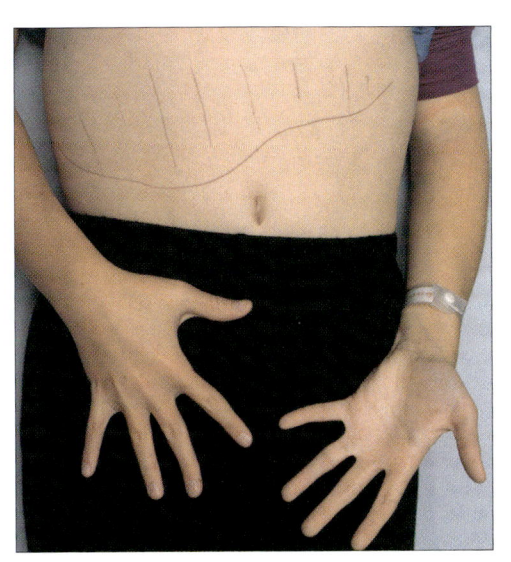

Fig. 12.42 Clinical features. The clinical features of glycogen storage Type III are similar to those of GSD Type I, but hypoglycaemia tends to be less severe. Peripheral muscle weakness develops later and is managed by increasing the protein content of the diet. Hepatic fibrosis leading to cirrhosis is a potential complication, as in this 14-year-old girl with hepatomegaly (note marks on the abdomen), early cirrhosis, and myopathy of the small muscles of the hand.

NEONATAL HAEMOCHROMATOSIS

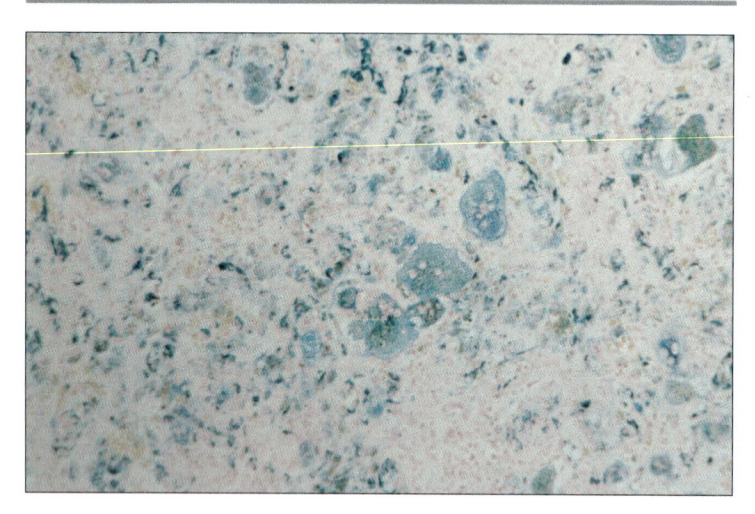

Figs 12.43, 12.44 Neonatal haemochromatosis. This rare inherited disease presents with acute liver failure in infancy. The diagnosis is confirmed by demonstrating an elevated serum iron (> 50 mmol/litre) and an elevated serum ferritin (> 1000 µg/litre). Liver histology may demonstrate submassive fatty necrosis with excess iron storage (**12.43**, top left, Perls, ×10). The disease is fatal unless transplantation is performed This child received a transplant at 15 days of age and made a complete recovery (**12.44**, top right).

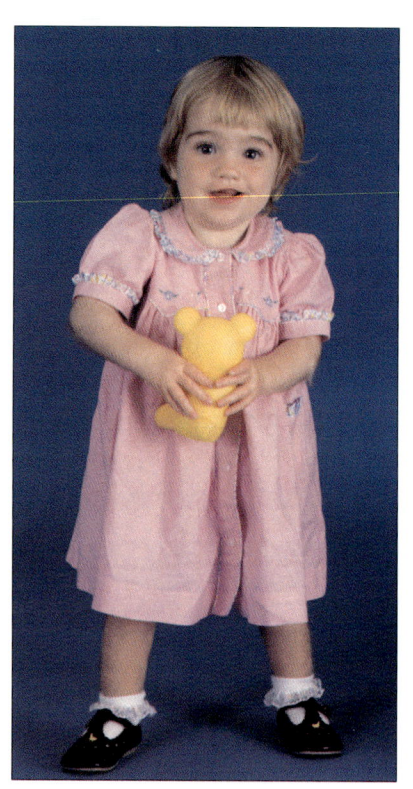

FATTY ACID OXIDATION DEFECTS

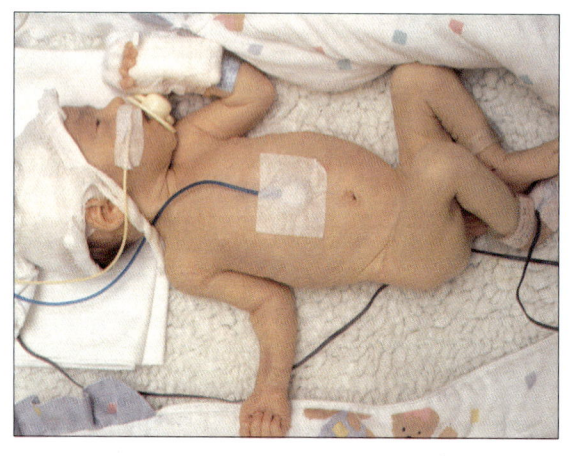

Fig. 12.45 Fatty acid oxidation defects. These rare inherited disorders may present with neonatal hepatitis or acute liver failure. They are characterised by the development of multi-organ failure, including neurological and hepatic disease, as in this baby who died from acute liver failure. The diagnosis is suggested by identifying microvesicular fatty infiltration in hepatocytes. Fatty acid oxidation products in the urine are rarely demonstrated. The prognosis is poor, and for patients with acute liver failure the disease proves fatal. These disorders may be associated with electron chain transport defects secondary to mitochondrial deletions or depletions.

ALPERS' DISEASE (PROGRESSIVE NEURONAL DEGENERATION WITH LIVER DISEASE)

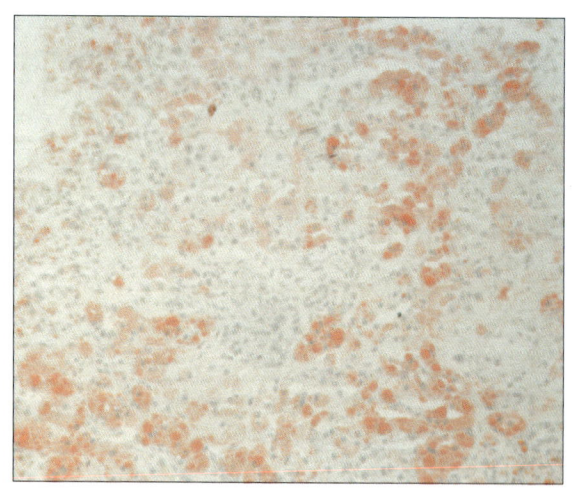

Fig. 12.46 Alpers' disease. Alpers' disease is a familial disorder which presents with developmental delay, intractable convulsions, and acute liver failure. It may be associated with sodium valproate ingestion. The disease is fatal and is not cured by liver transplantation. There may be an underlying defect in fatty acid oxidation and/or electron chain transport. The liver histology demonstrates microvesicular fatty infiltration of the hepatocytes. (Oil red-O, ×10.)

13. Chronic Liver Disease in Childhood

The main causes of chronic liver disease in childhood are indicated in **Fig. 13.1** with the relevant biochemical investigations.

CHRONIC VIRAL HEPATITIS

HEPATITIS B

Hepatitis B is transmitted vertically (70% of non-vaccinated babies born to carrier mothers are infected), horizontally from close family members, or parenterally from blood products. The incidence of chronic liver disease in childhood is unknown, but at least 10% of children will develop cirrhosis and/or hepatocellular carcinoma. Most hepatitis B carriers are asymptomatic, but have evidence of mild chronic hepatitis biochemically and histologically.

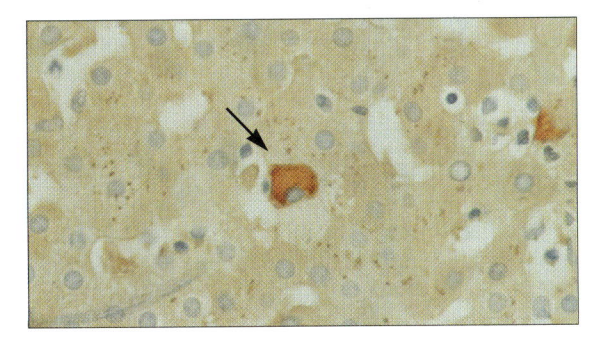

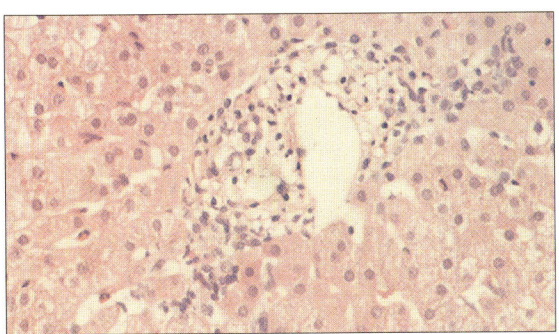

Chronic liver disease in childhood	
Disease	**Diagnostic investigations**
Chronic hepatitis	Inflammatory infiltrate in portal tracts on histology
Hepatitis B, C, EBV, CMV	Viral serology
Autoimmune hepatitis	IgG >20 g/litre, ↓C3, C4 levels Positive: • Liver–kidney microsomal antibodies • Antinuclear factor antibodies • Smooth muscle antibodies
Primary sclerosing cholangitis	ERCP, Liver biopsy
Wilson's disease	Low serum copper/ceruloplasmin Increased urinary copper
Alpha-1-antitrypsin deficiency	Alpha-1-antitrypsin level phenotype PIZZ
Cystic fibrosis	Sweat test, liver biopsy
Tyrosinaemia type 1	Urinary succinylacetone
Congenital hepatic fibrosis	Liver histology

Fig. 13.1 Chronic Liver disease in childhood.

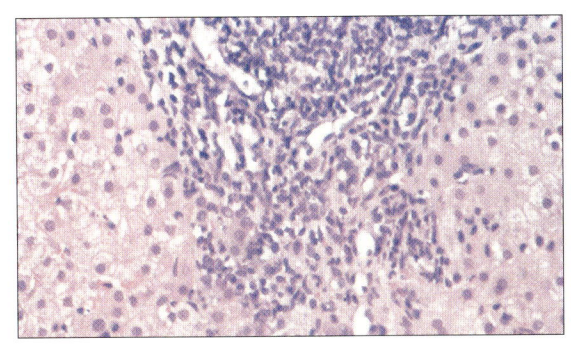

Figs 13.2–13.4 Hepatitis B surface antigen. Hepatitis B surface antigen may be demonstrated in hepatocytes (**13.2**, top left, orcein stain, ×40). This does not necessarily correlate with inflammation, which may be mild (**13.3**, bottom left, Haematoxylin and Eosin, ×25) when the inflammatory cells are limited to the portal tract or more aggressive when they spill over into the liver parenchyma (**13.4**, bottom right, Haematoxylin and Eosin, ×25). Treatment with interferon-α is effective in 30–50% of children.

113

HEPATITIS C

Hepatitis C is transmitted parenterally from blood products, although horizontal infection is common in Europe. Vertical transmission is rare unless the mother is co-infected with human immunodeficiency virus (HIV). The incidence of chronic liver disease secondary to hepatitis C is thought to be higher than that with hepatitis B, with at least 30% of children progressing to cirrhosis with a risk of hepatocellular carcinoma.

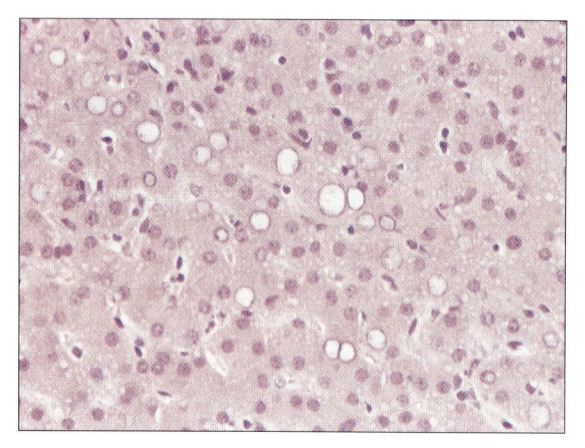

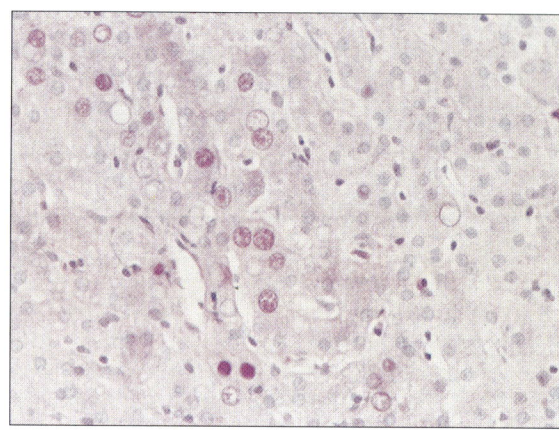

Fig. 13.5, 13.6 Hepatitis C. The biopsy findings indicate fatty change (**13.5,** left), glycogenated nuclei, and cytoplasmic eosinophilia (**13.6,** right). (Haematoxylin and Eosin, ×25.)

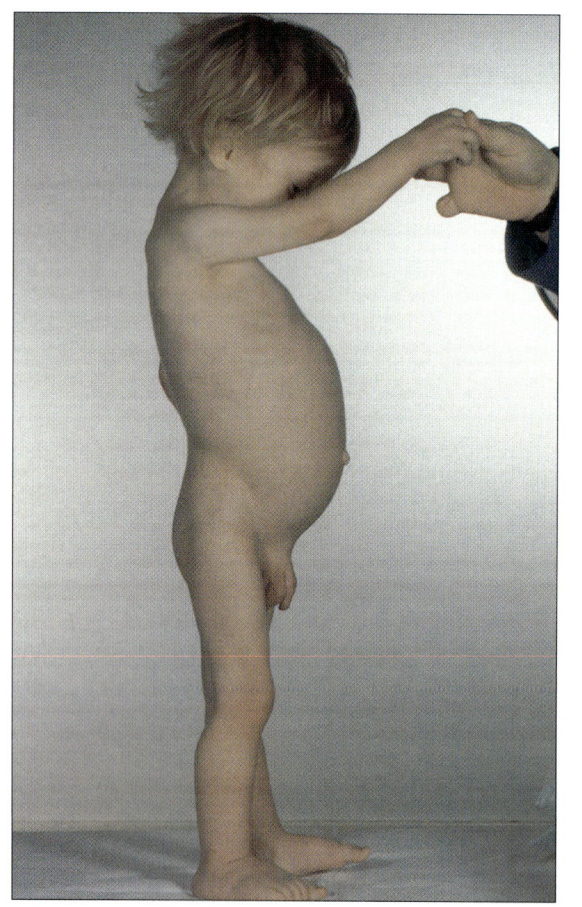

AUTOIMMUNE HEPATITIS

Autoimmune hepatitis is more common in girls than in boys. Type I has positive antinuclear factor and smooth muscle antibodies and may be associated with primary sclerosing cholangitis. Type II is associated with positive liver and kidney microsomal antibodies.

Fig. 13.7 Autoimmune hepatitis. Autoimmune hepatitis may present in an insidious way, with the gradual onset of cirrhosis and portal hypertension. This 2-year-old boy presented with malnutrition, haemolytic anaemia, cirrhosis, and portal hypertension due to Type I autoimmune hepatitis.

Chronic Liver Disease in Childhood

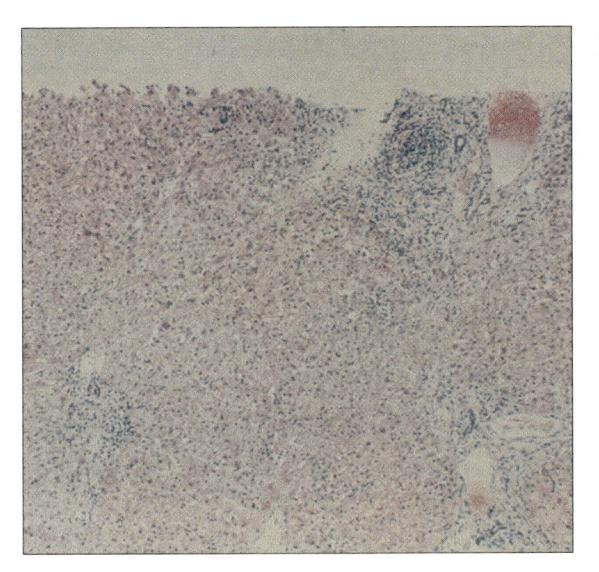

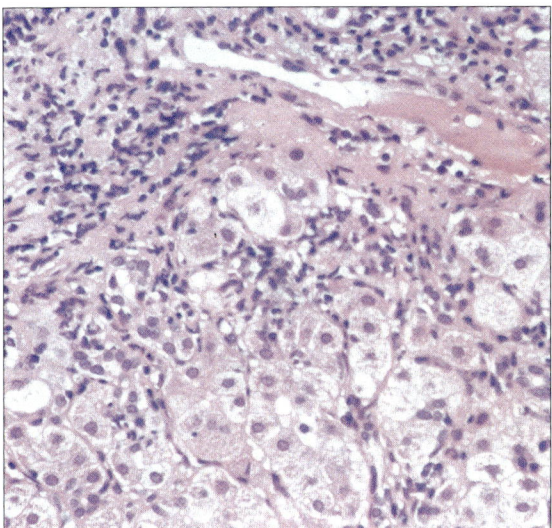

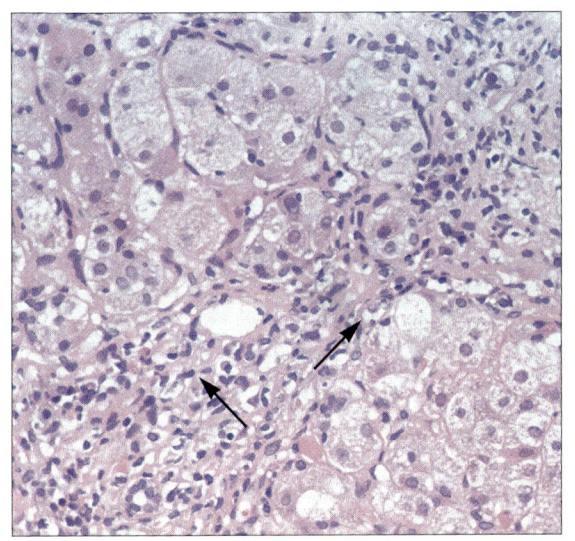

Figs 13.8–13.10 Histology. Histology demonstrates an increase in inflammatory cells in the portal tracts (**13.8**, top left, Haematoxylin and Eosin, ×10), which extend beyond the limiting plate (piecemeal necrosis), causing damage to periportal hepatocytes (**13.9**, top right, Haematoxylin and Eosin, ×25), leading to bridging fibrosis (**13.10**, middle right, Haematoxylin and Eosin, ×25).

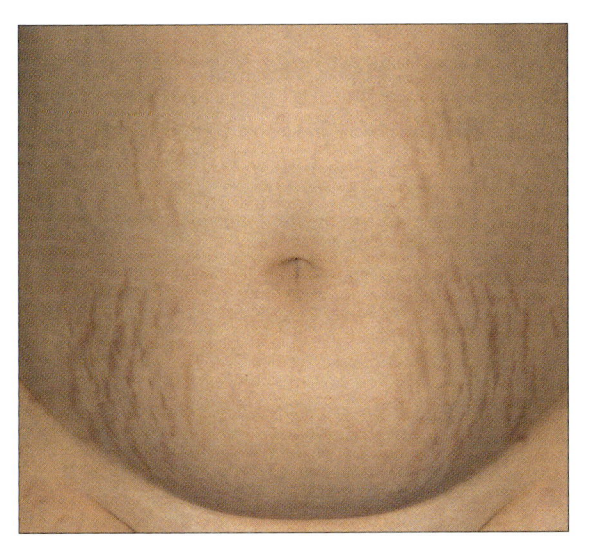

Fig. 13.11 Immunosuppression. Most children respond to immunosuppression with prednisolone (2 mg/kg) and azathioprine (0.5–2 mg/kg). Therapy may be required indefinitely and is associated with stunting and cutaneous striae.

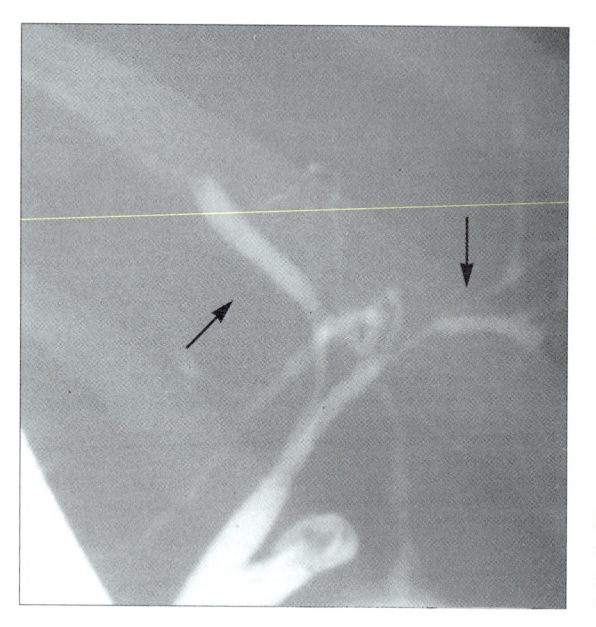

PRIMARY SCLEROSING CHOLANGITIS

Primary sclerosing cholangitis is a condition of unknown aetiology which may be associated with ulcerative colitis or Type I autoimmune hepatitis. The presentation varies from the insidious onset of chronic liver disease to the development of obstructive jaundice and hepatic dysfunction.

Fig. 13.12 Diagnosis. The diagnosis is made by the characteristic endoscopic retrograde cholangiopancreatography (ERCP) findings, which indicate irregular narrowing and dilatation of the intra- and extra-hepatic biliary tree.

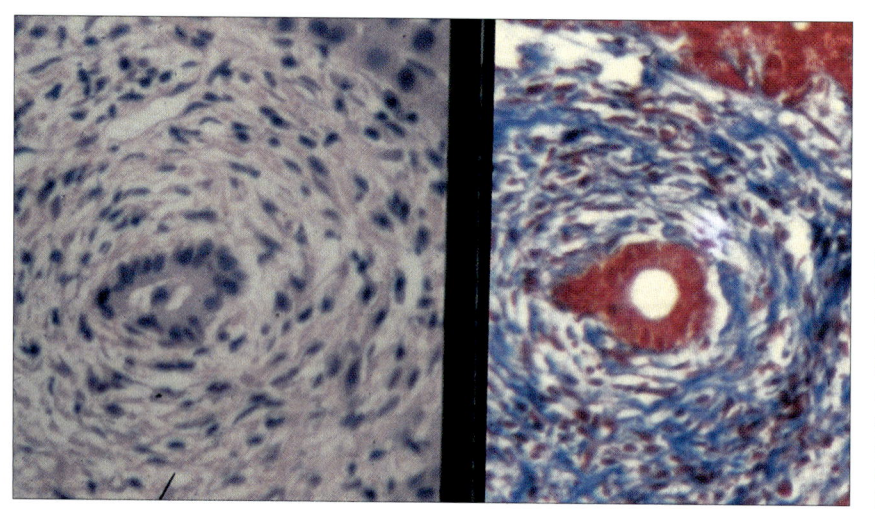

Fig. 13.13 Biopsy. The liver biopsy demonstrates severe fibrosis around bile ducts (onion skinning of the bile ducts) and there may be overlap with the features of chronic active hepatitis (13.9). (Left, Haematoxylin and Eosin, ×40; right, Masson Trichrome, ×40.)

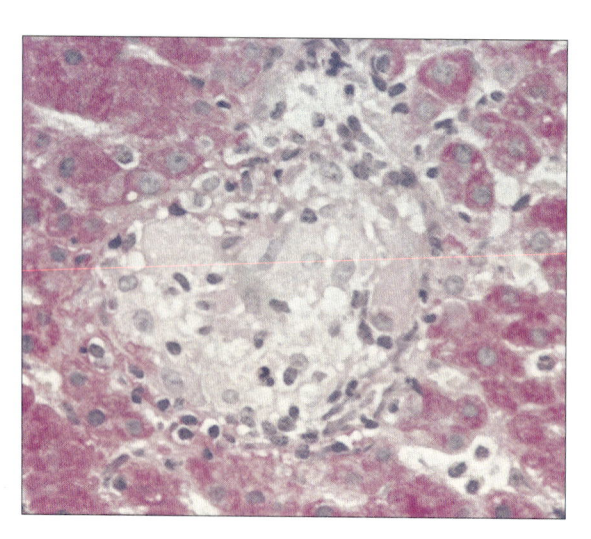

GRANULOMATOUS HEPATITIS

In childhood, granulomata in the liver may be secondary to infectious disease (tuberculosis, brucellosis, fungal infections, parasitic infections, cytomegalovirus, and Epstein–Barr virus), malignant disease (Hodgkin's disease), or sarcoid or chronic granulomatous disease. The treatment and outcome depend on the underlying cause.

Fig. 13.14 Granulomatous hepatitis. Here is demonstrated a well-defined epithelioid non-caseating granuloma. (Periodic Acid–Schiff, ×40.)

Chronic Liver Disease in Childhood

FIBROPOLYCYSTIC DISEASE

Fibropolycystic disease has a wide spectrum, ranging from congenital hepatic fibrosis to congenital intrahepatic biliary dilatation (Caroli's disease) with or without polycystic kidneys.

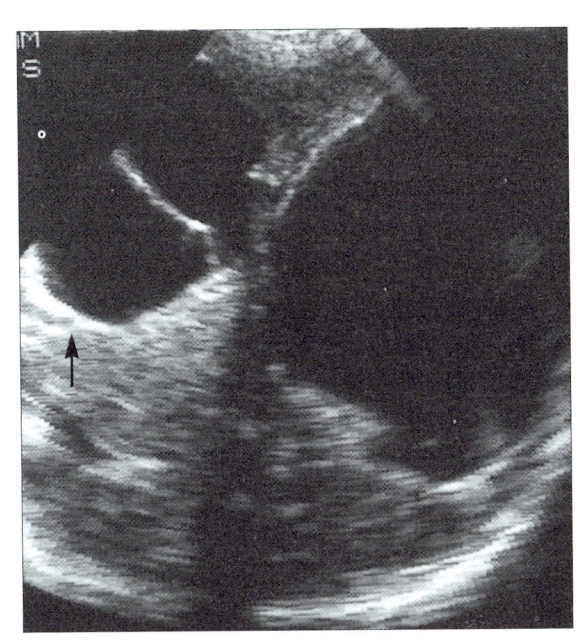

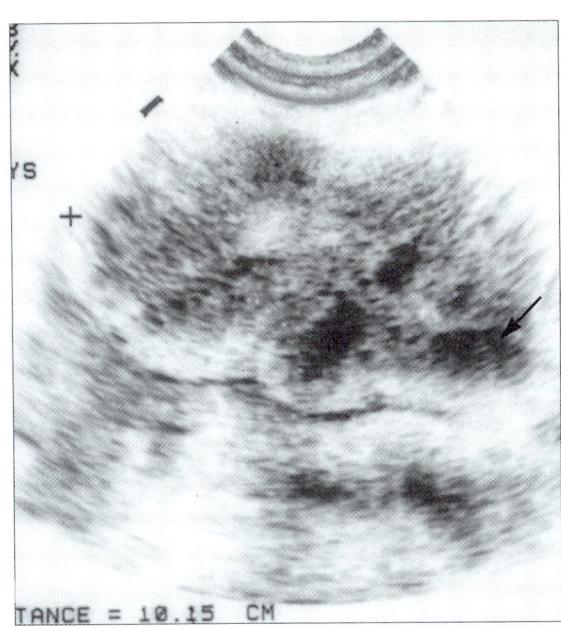

Figs 13.15, 13.16 Diagnosis. The diagnosis is suggested by firm hepatosplenomegaly with normal liver function tests. It is confirmed by abdominal ultrasound, which demonstrates hepatic (**13.15**, left) or renal (**13.16**, right) cysts.

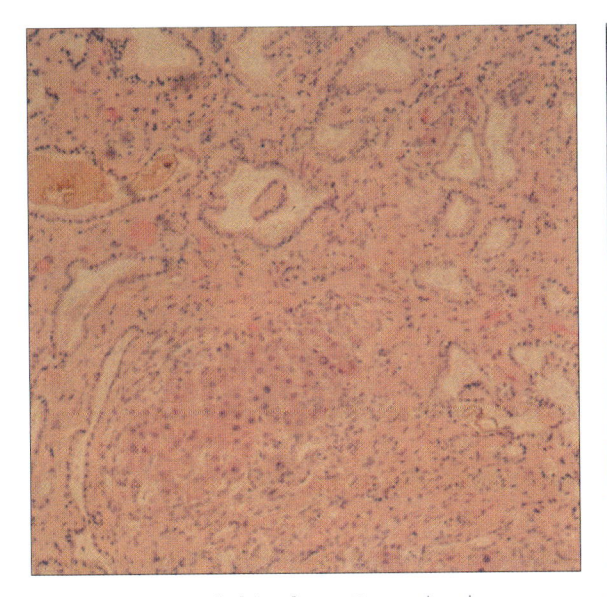

Fig. 13.17 Hepatic histology. Hepatic histology demonstrates broad bands of fibrous tissue which are clearly differentiated from hepatic parenchyma. Portal tracts are widened and linked by bands of fibrous tissue. Bile ducts are prominent, dilated, and abnormal. Management depends on the severity of the renal disease and portal hypertension. (Haematoxylin and Eosin, ×40.)

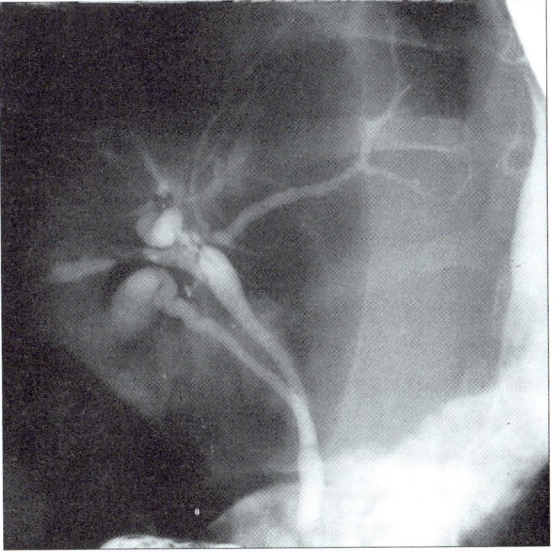

Fig. 13.18 Caroli's disease. Caroli's disease, or intrahepatic biliary dilatation, is associated with recurrent cholangitis and the development of cholangiocarcinoma in adult life. The diagnosis is confirmed by ERCP, which demonstrates the abnormal biliary tree. Gallstones may develop in the dilated intrahepatic bile ducts.

117

CARDIAC CIRRHOSIS

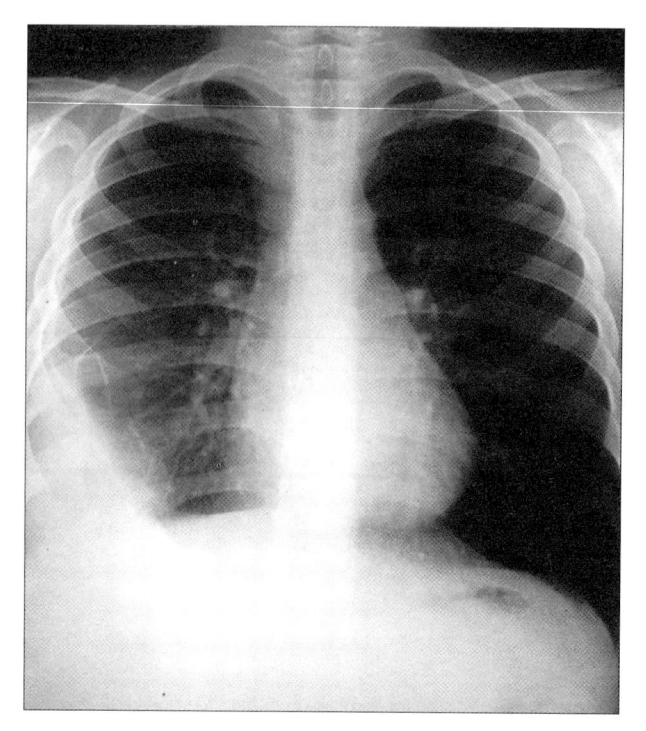

Figs 13.19, 13.20 Cardiac cirrhosis. This young man presented with a pleural effusion, cirrhosis, and ascites (**13.19**, left). Abdominal ultrasound demonstrated abnormal hepatic veins (**13.20**, bottom), secondary to chronic tuberculous constrictive pericarditis. There was complete resolution following pericardiectomy.

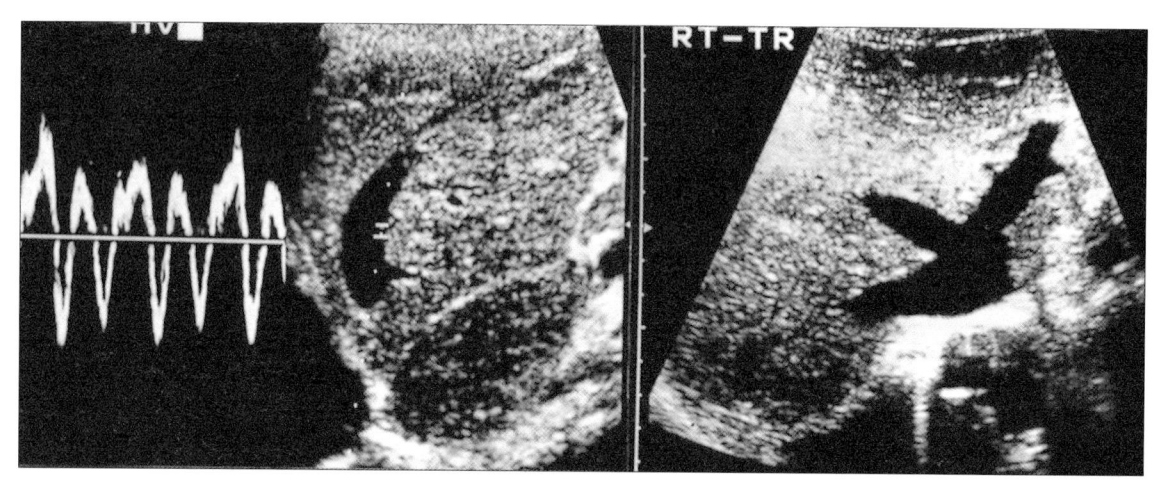

Chronic Liver Disease in Childhood

CIRRHOSIS AND PORTAL HYPERTENSION

Cirrhosis with portal hypertension is the inevitable outcome for untreated or unresponsive chronic liver disease. The clinical signs are described in **Figs 13.21–13.36**.

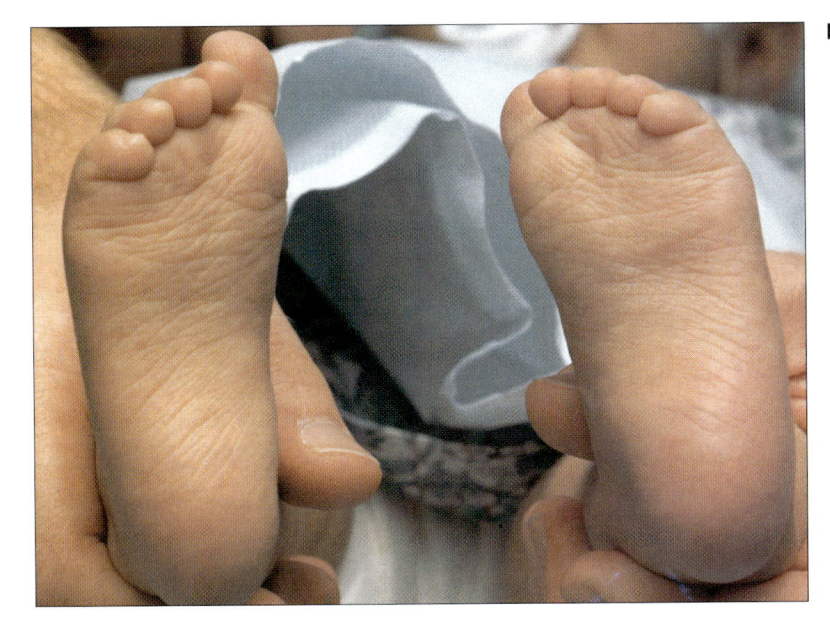

Fig. 13.21 Plantar erythema.

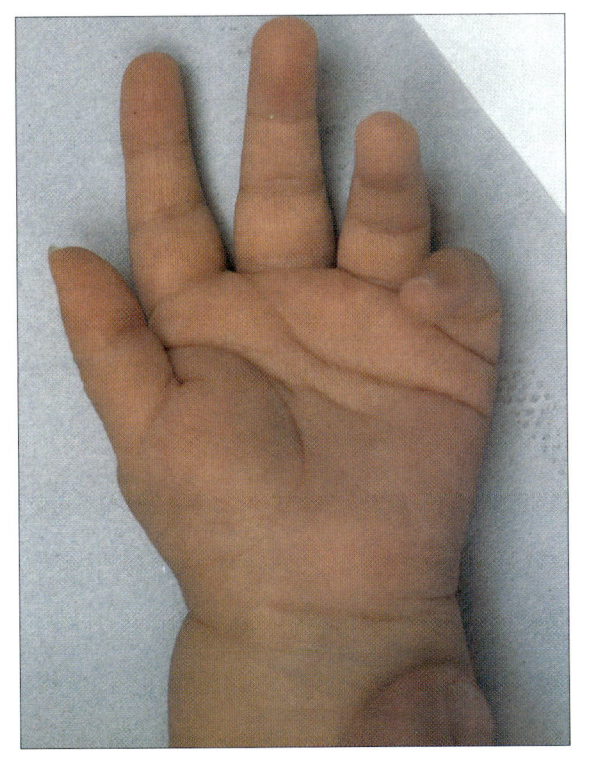

Fig. 13.22 Palmar erythema.

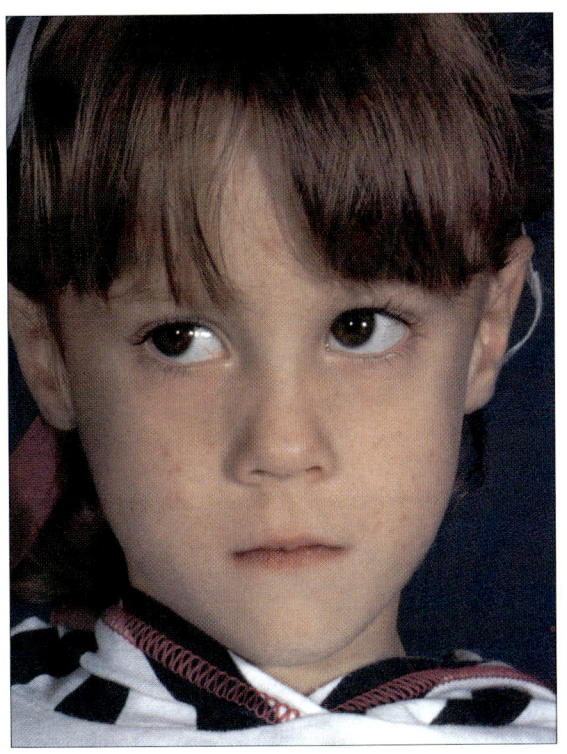

Fig. 13.23 Facial telangiectasia.

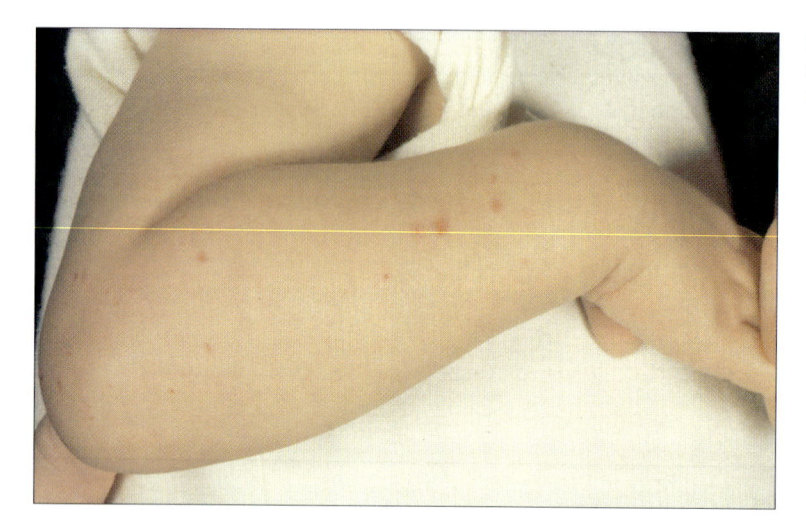

Fig. 13.24 Spider naevi. Although common in normal children, there are usually more than five in liver disease.

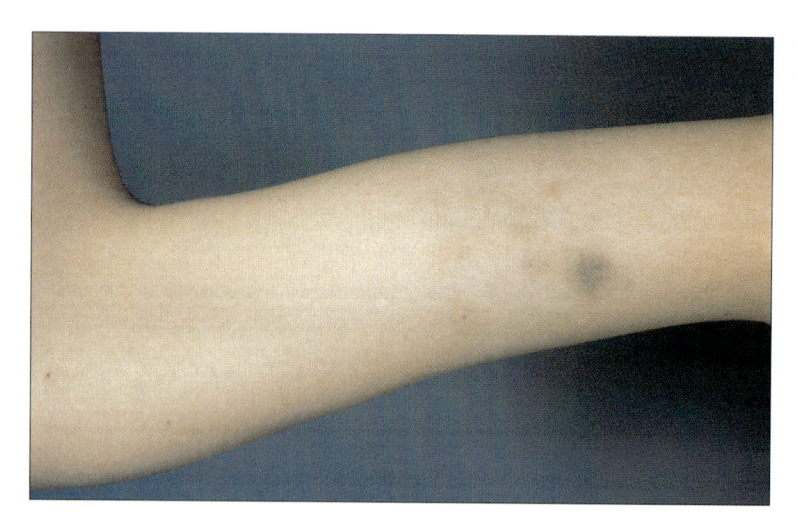

Fig. 13.25 Bruising. Increased bruising develops secondary to reduced synthesis of coagulation factors and hypersplenism.

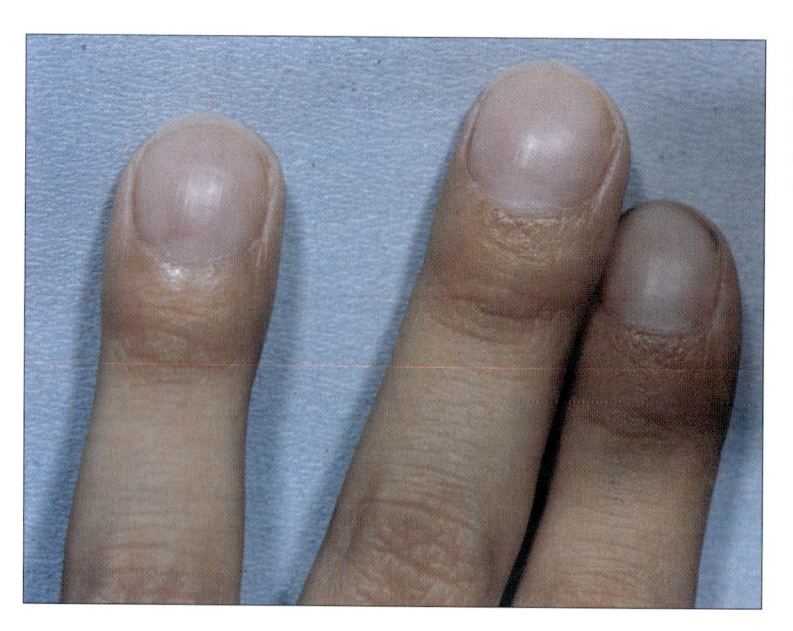

Fig. 13.26 Clubbing. Severe clubbing is common in children with cirrhosis. Some children also develop peripheral and central cyanosis secondary to pulmonary arteriovenous shunting.

Chronic Liver Disease in Childhood

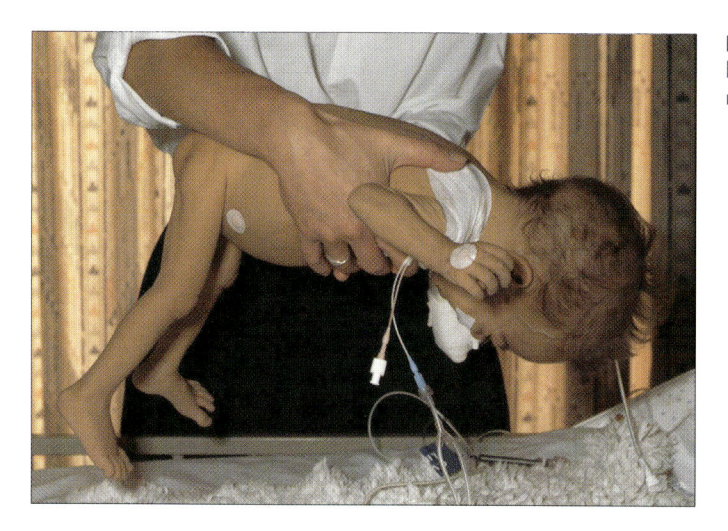

Fig. 13.27 Hypotonia. Chronic liver disease leads to hypotonia and delayed motor development, which are reversed post-transplantation.

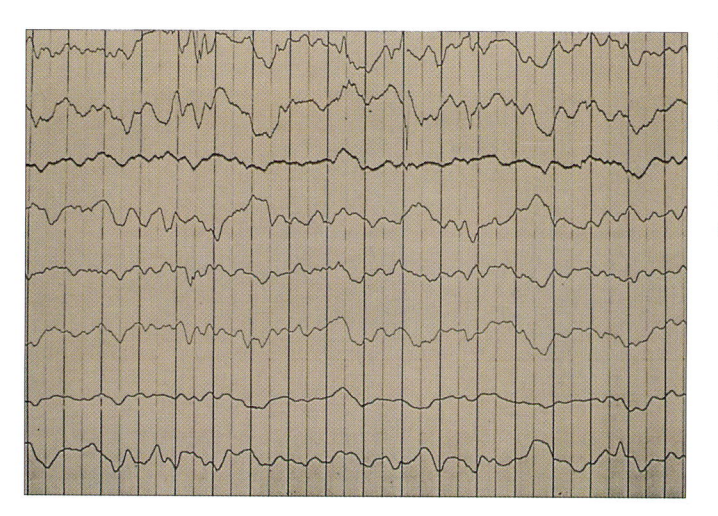

Fig. 13.28 Hepatic encephalopathy. Chronic hepatic encephalopathy leads to drowsiness, impaired concentration, and reversal of sleep patterns. The electroencephalogram demonstrates reduced amplitude waves (delta waves) with slow rhythm (3 cycles/second). Treatment is by reducing protein intake to less than 2 g/kg/day and oral lactulose.

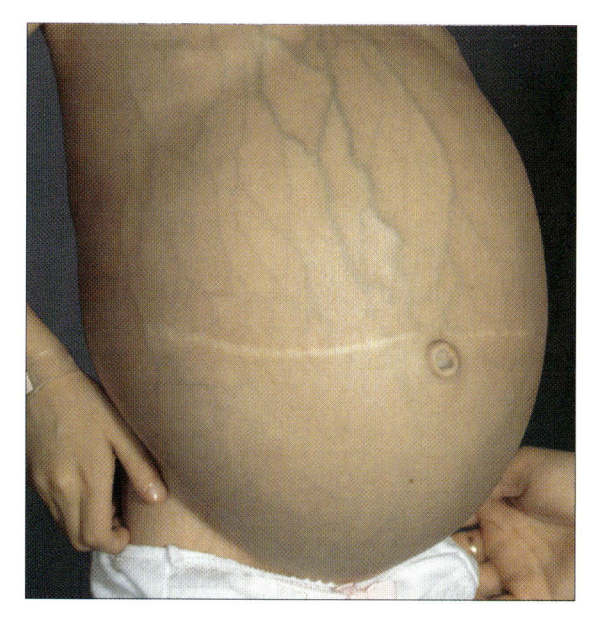

Fig. 13.29 Ascites. Ascites is a common complication and presents with abdominal distension and dilated abdominal veins. Treatment is with fluid- and salt-restriction and diuretics.

Pediatric Gastroenterology and Hepatology

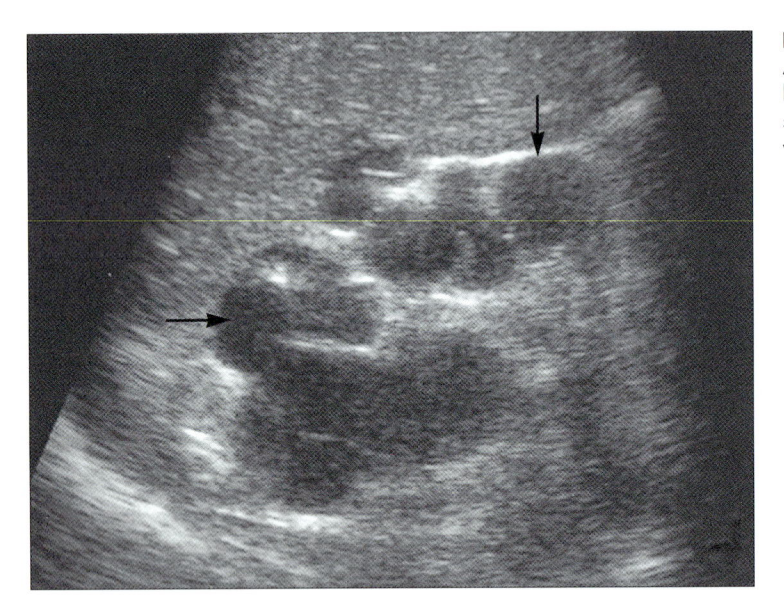

Fig. 13.30 Abdominal ultrasound. Abdominal ultrasound may detect portal hypertension by identifying splenomegaly or splenic or mesenteric varices.

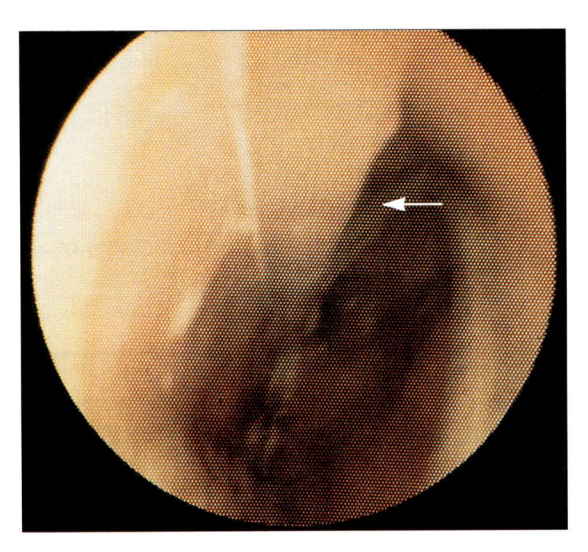

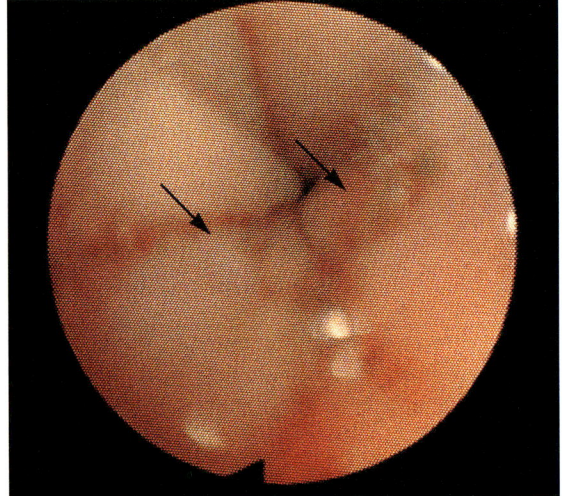

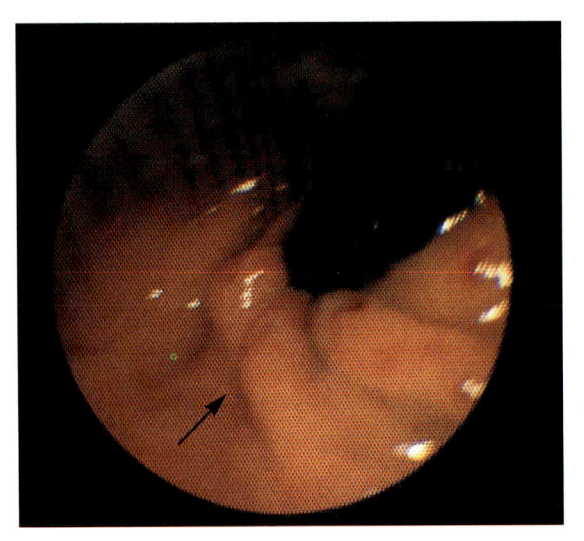

Figs 13.31–13.33 Varices. Oesophageal (**13.31**, middle left, **13.32**, right) and gastric (**13.33**, bottom left) varices are best detected at endoscopy. This inevitable complication of portal hypertension may lead to life-threatening haematemesis, which is initially managed with endoscopic sclerotherapy.

Chronic Liver Disease in Childhood

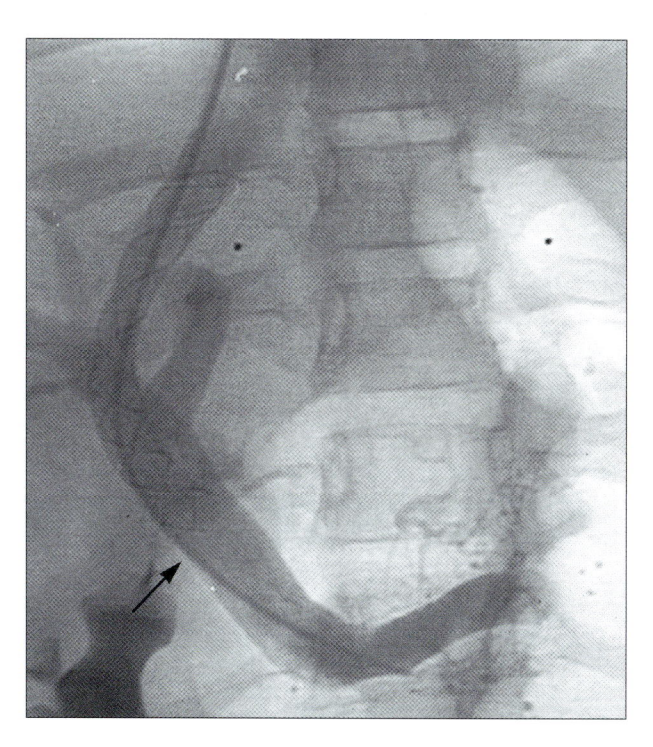

Fig. 13.34 Variceal bleeding. Persistent variceal bleeding, particularly from gastric varices, requires more definitive measures and may be an indication for liver transplantation. Transjugular intrahepatic portal systemic shunting (TIPS) is a new technique in which the hepatic veins are cannulated via the internal jugular vein and a shunt (arrow) is placed between the hepatic veins and the portal vein. This technique may act as a 'bridge to transplantation', as in this 9-year-old boy with intractable variceal bleeding.

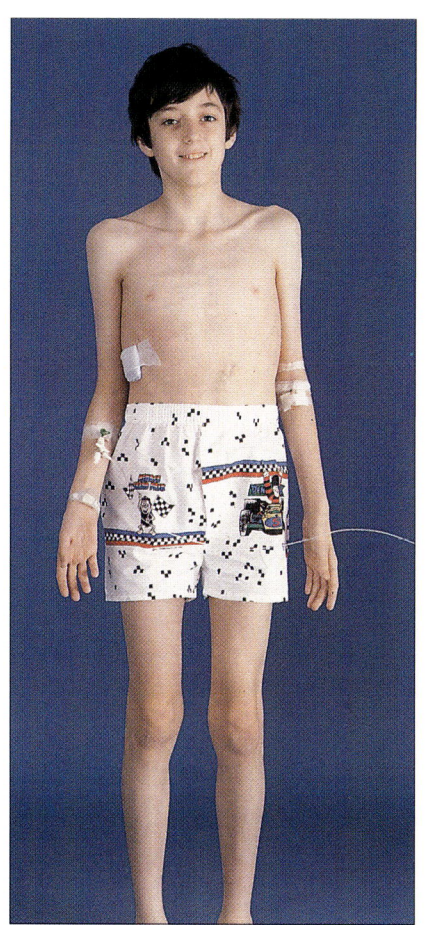

Fig. 13.35 Severe hepatic dysfunction. Chronic liver disease with severe hepatic dysfunction leads to growth failure with malnutrition, stunting, and delayed puberty, as in this 16-year-old boy. He developed cirrhosis, portal hypertension, and bleeding oesophageal varices secondary to biliary atresia, despite a successful Kasai portoenterostomy.

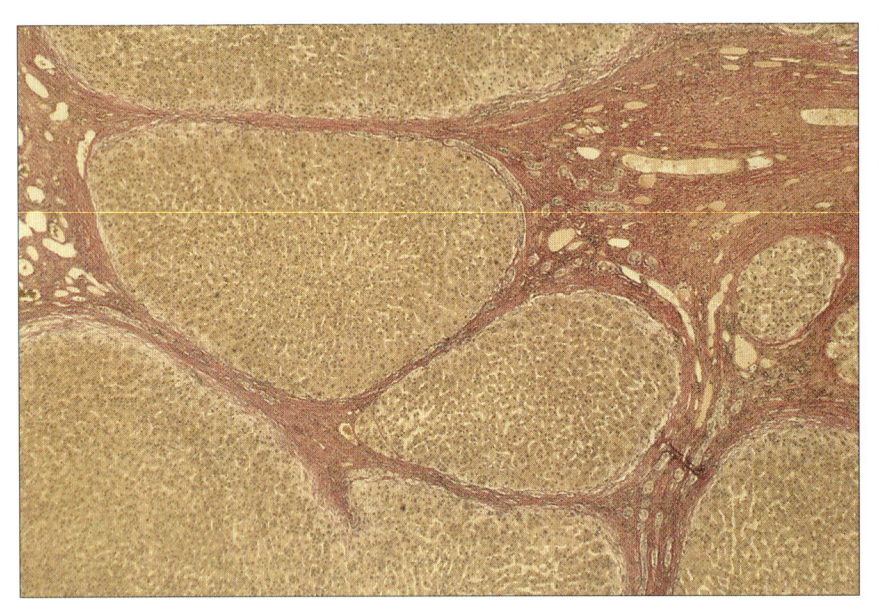

Fig. 13.36 Histology. The diagnosis of cirrhosis may be confirmed histologically by demonstrating increased fibrosis, nodular formation, and hepatic regeneration (Haematoxylin and Eosin, ×10).

EXTRAHEPATIC PORTAL VEIN OBSTRUCTION

Extrahepatic portal vein obstruction may be due to a congenital abnormality or secondary to thrombosis from inherited coagulation disorders (protein C, protein S deficiency) or from severe neonatal sepsis and dehydration. Children usually present with haematemesis and splenomegaly.

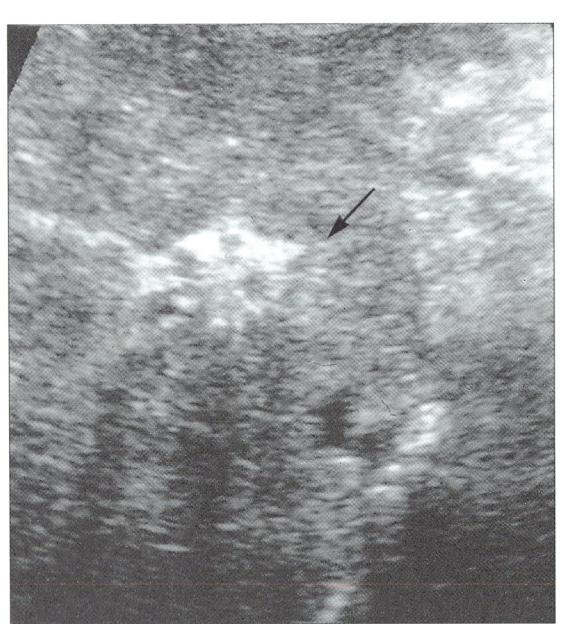

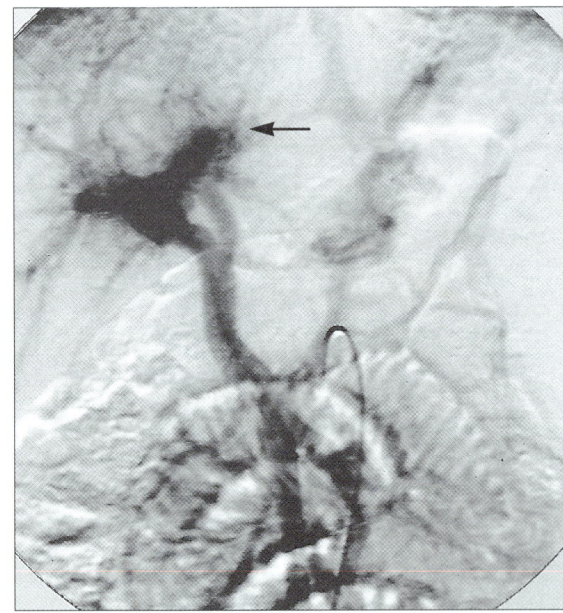

Figs 13.37, 13.38 Diagnosis. Abdominal ultrasound demonstrates a portal cavernoma (**13.37**, left) and confirmation is by angiography, which demonstrates a thrombosed portal vein with portal cavernoma and collateral blood flow (**13.38**, right). Initially, medical management is with endoscopic sclerotherapy for variceal bleeding, but occasionally splenorenal shunt is indicated if there are gastric varices.

14. Hepatic Tumours

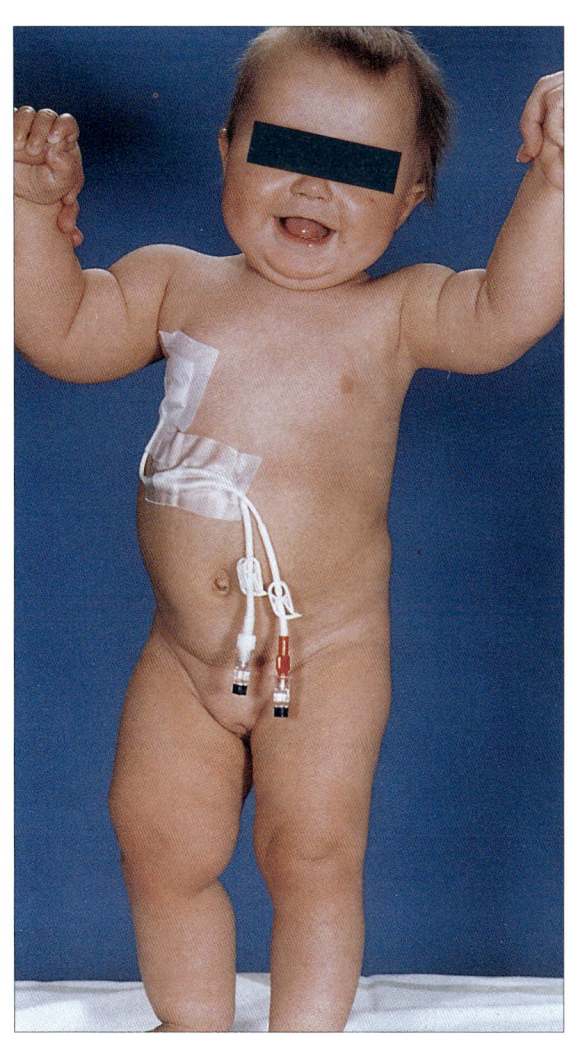

Fig. 14.1 Hepatic tumours in childhood. The most common hepatic tumours in childhood are metastases from neuroblastoma, Wilms' tumour, lymphoma, or leukaemia. Primary liver tumours account for less than 2% of paediatric malignancies. Hepatoblastoma develops in children less than 5 years old and may be associated with hemihypertrophy (as in this child). Hepatocellular carcinoma develops in older children and may be associated with hepatitis B infection, tyrosinaemia type I, or cirrhosis from any cause.

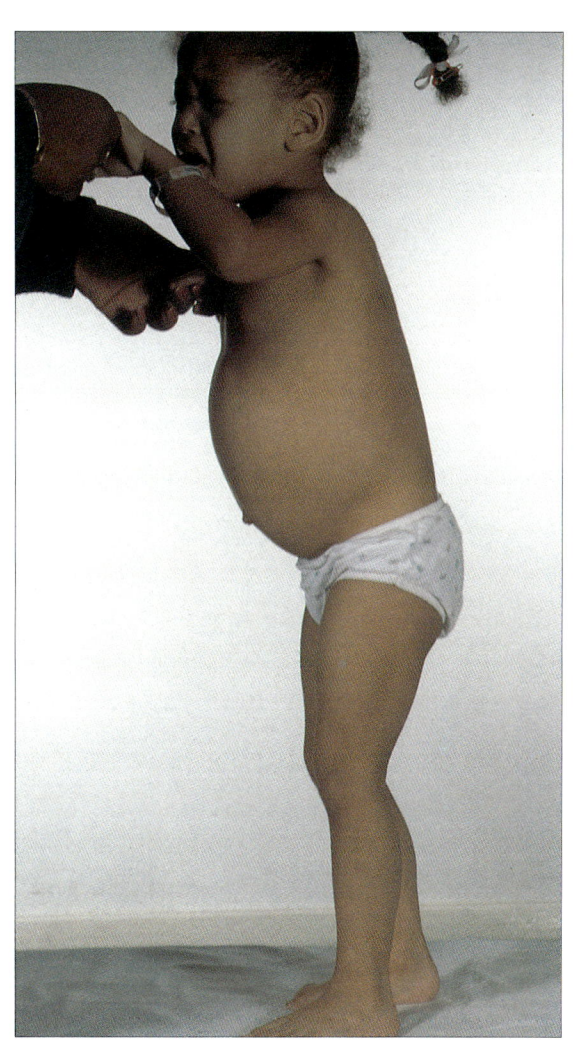

Fig. 14.2 Clinical presentation. The clinical presentation is usually with asymptomatic liver enlargement.

Pediatric Gastroenterology and Hepatology

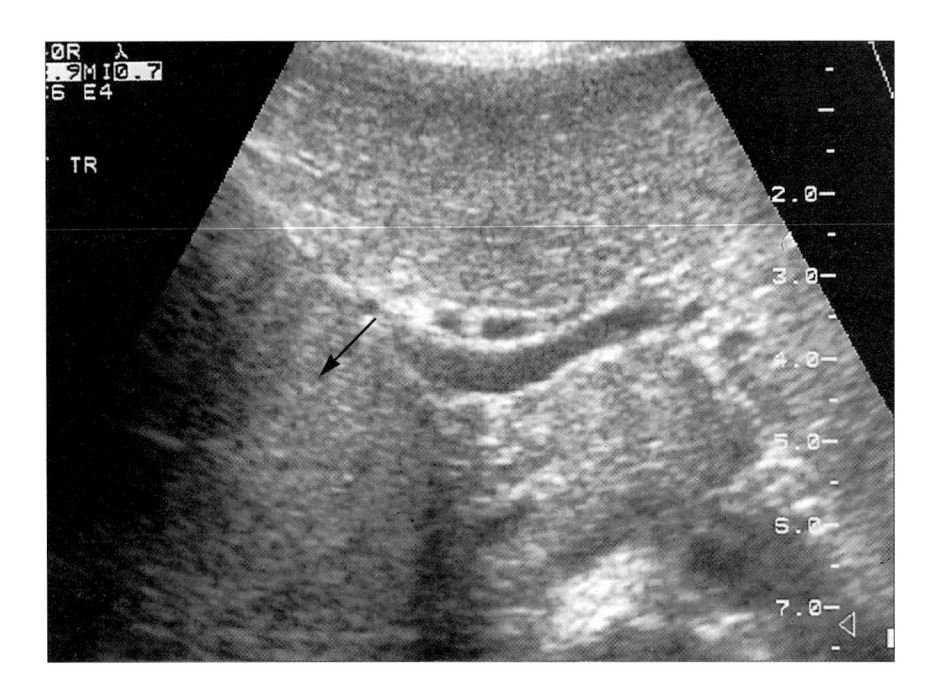

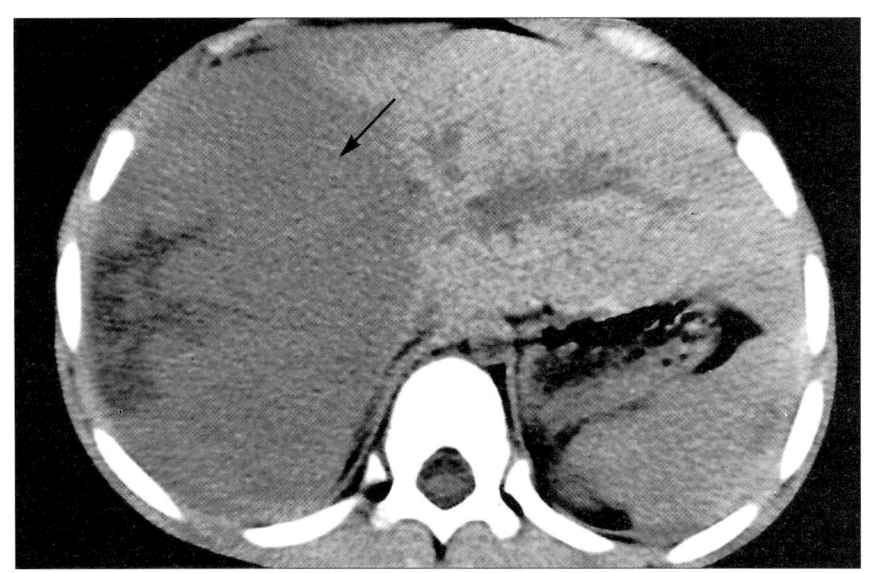

Figs 14.3–14.5 Imaging the tumour: ultrasound and CT scan. A hepatic mass may be demonstrated by abdominal ultrasound (**14.3**, top), CT scan (**14.4**, bottom), and angiography (**14.5**, top, opposite page).

Hepatic Tumours

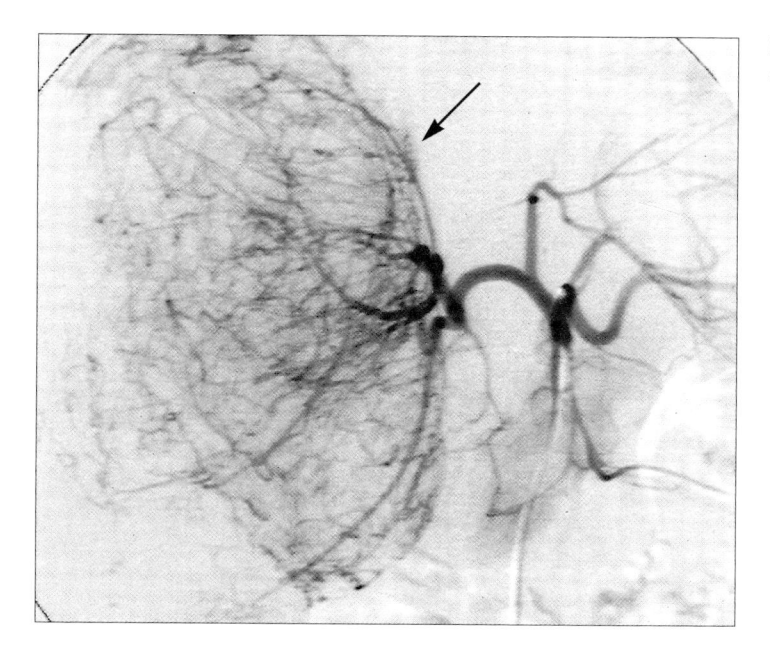

Fig. 14.5 Imaging the tumour: angiography. (See opposite page.)

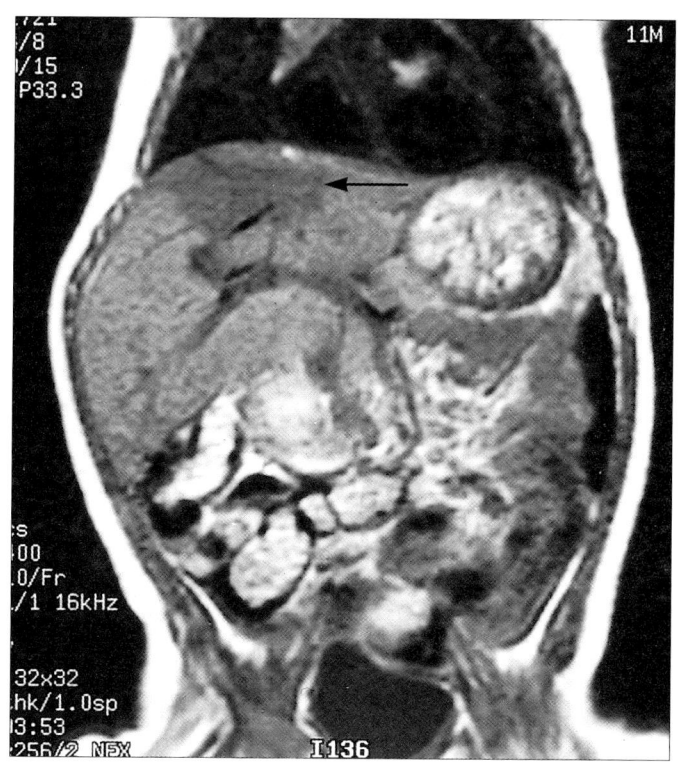

Fig. 14.6 Imaging the tumour and vascular supply. MRI may demonstrate both the tumour and the vascular supply, which is essential if surgery is planned.

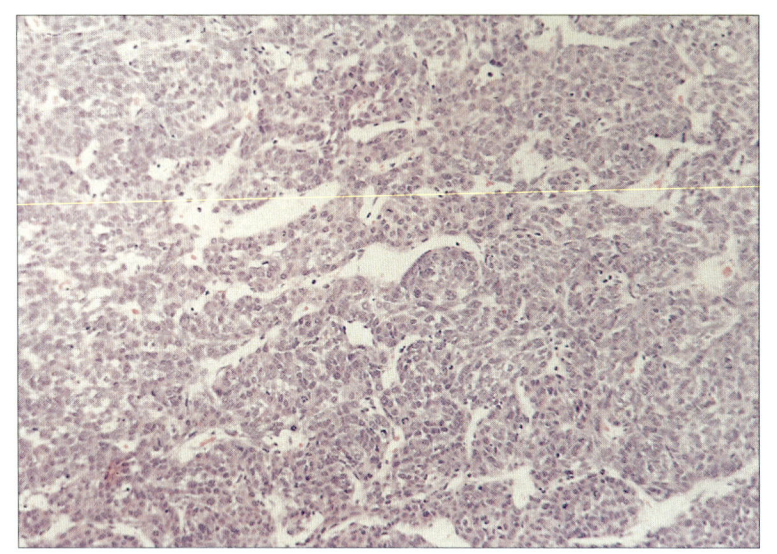

Fig. 14.7 Hepatoblastoma. The histology of hepatoblastoma is characterised by malignant cells, which may be fetal, embryonal, or anaplastic. Most tumours respond to chemotherapy and may then be resected surgically. Unresectable hepatoblastomas without metastases are an indication for liver transplantation. (Haematoxylin and Eosin, ×33.)

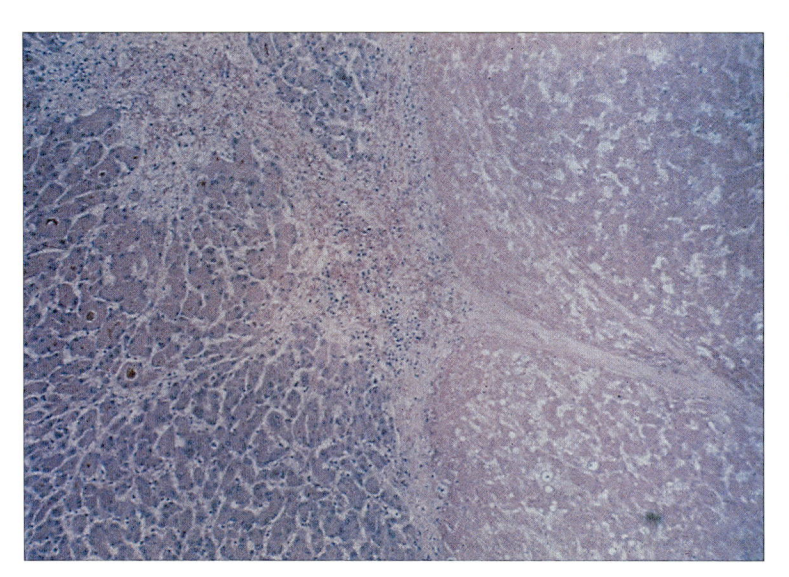

Fig. 14.8 Hepatocellular carcinoma. The tumour cells in hepatocellular carcinoma are of varying size, with hyperchromatic nuclei and frequent mitoses. The tumour is relatively unresponsive to chemotherapy. (Haematoxylin and Eosin, ×40)

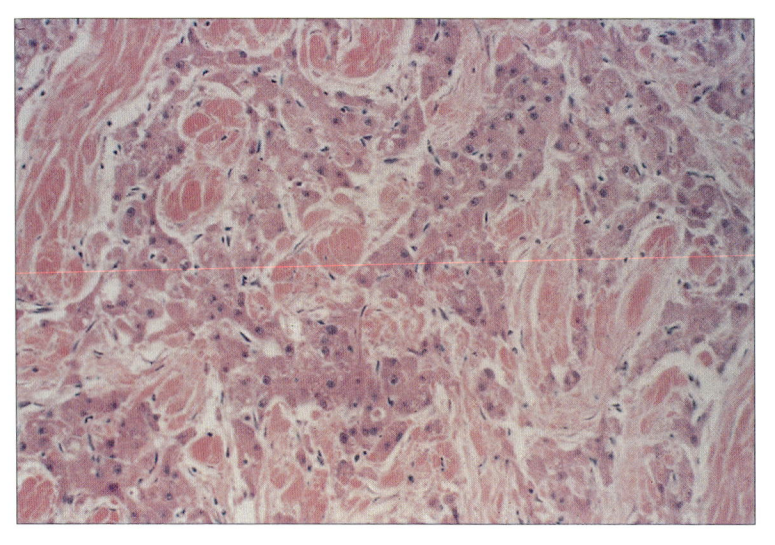

Fig. 14.9 Fibrolamellar hepatocellular carcinoma. The fibrolamellar variant of hepatocellular carcinoma has acidophilic cytoplasm and prominent nucleoli separated by bands of collagen. It is a slow-growing tumour with a longer course. (Haemotoxylin and Eosin, ×20.)

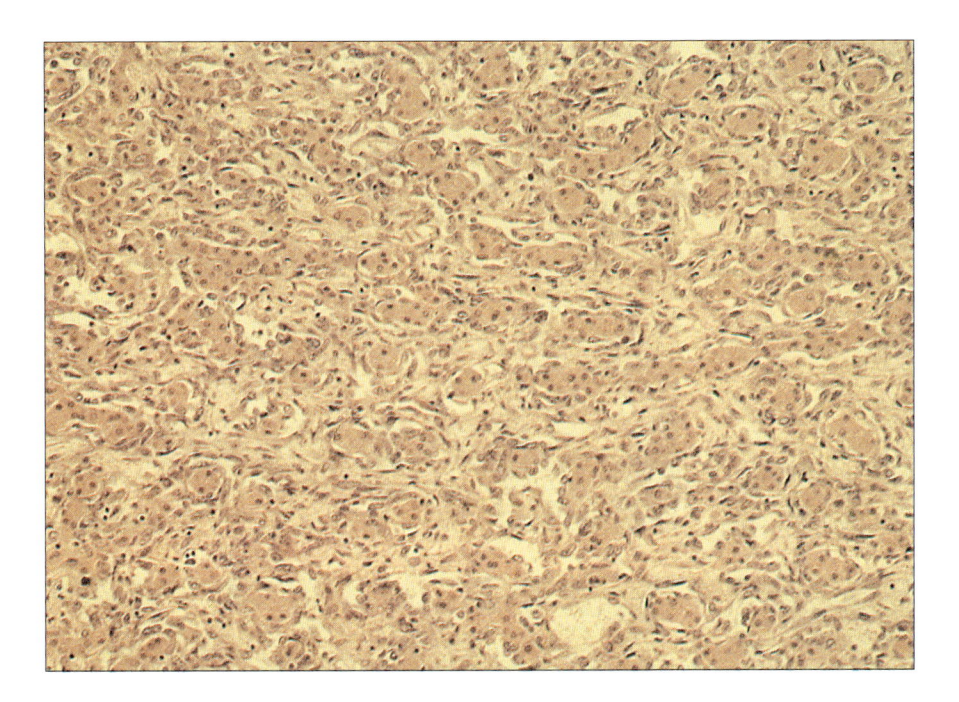

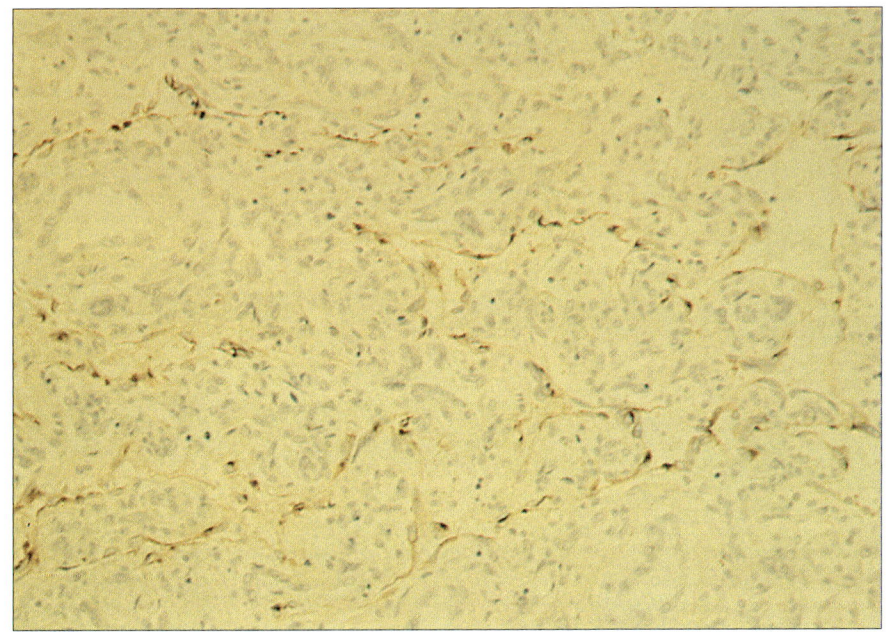

Figs 14.10, 14.11 Capillary haemangioendothelioma. Capillary haemangio-endothelioma are vascular tumours which may be benign or malignant. Histology demonstrates irregular vascular channels lined by atypical endothelial cells with plump nuclei. There are pleomorphic spindle cells lining liver cell plates (**14.10**, top, Haematoxylin and Eosin, ×40), which stain positive for Factor VIII-related antigen (**14.11**, bottom, immunoperoxidase, ×40), confirming endothelial differentiation. Some tumours may respond to steroids, but resection or transplantation may be necessary.

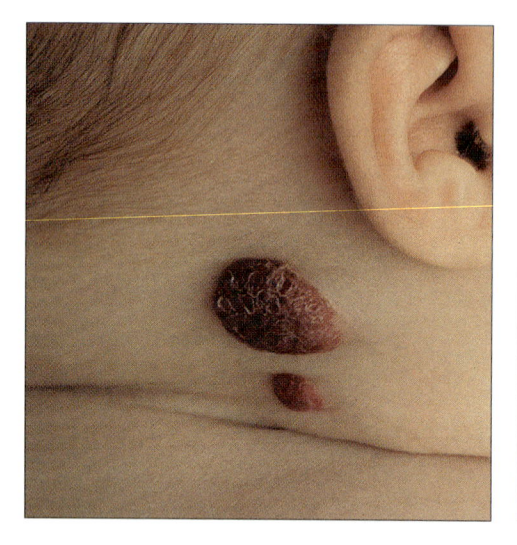

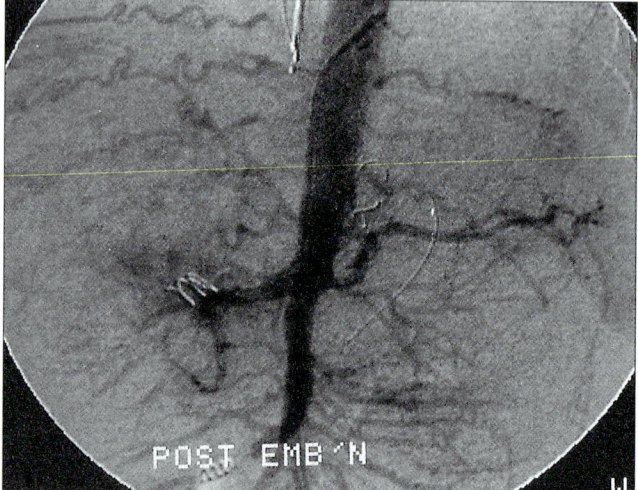

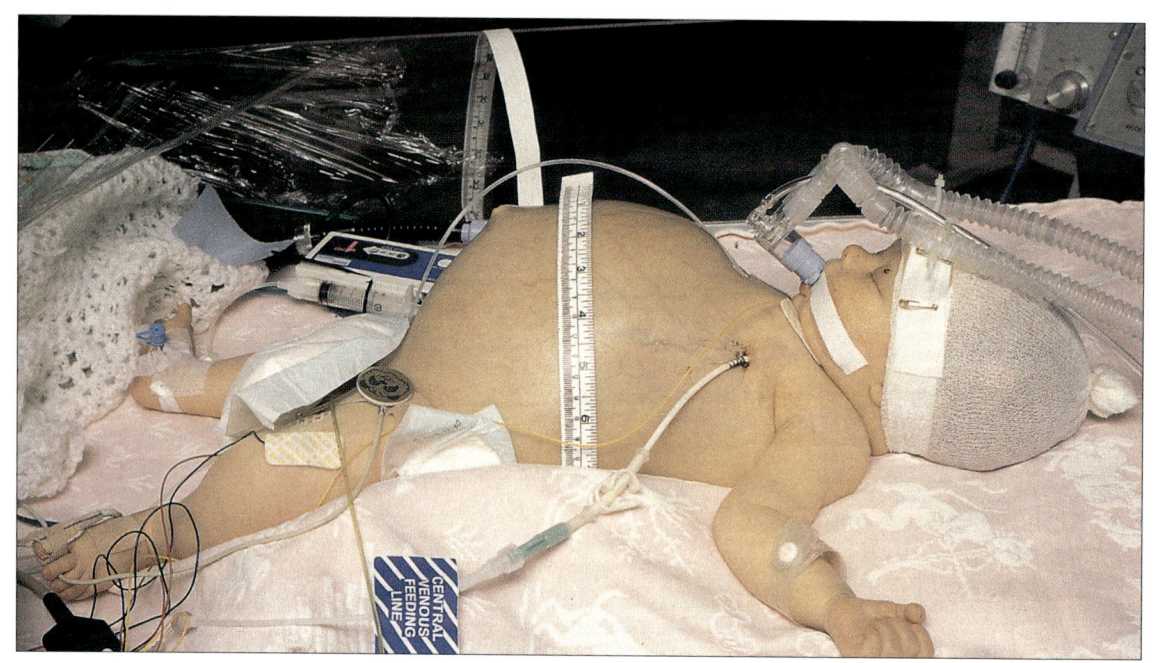

Figs 14.12–14.14 Cavernous haemangiomata. Cavernous haemangiomata may be cutaneous (**14.12**, top left) or hepatic (**14.13**, top right). The diagnosis is established by angiography, which identifies the abnormal vascular supply. Although some tumours regress spontaneously, others may lead to cardiac or hepatic failure (**14.14**, bottom). Embolisation of the haemangiomata may be effective (**14.13**).

15. Acute Liver Disease

INTRODUCTION

Acute liver disease may be secondary to viral hepatitis, autoimmune hepatitis, or metabolic liver disease, or it may be drug-induced. Most children will present with obvious jaundice, anorexia and loss of energy.

ACUTE VIRAL HEPATITIS

All forms of acute viral hepatitis may present in childhood. The diagnosis is usually made by the clinical presentation of jaundice, nausea, and abdominal pain and confirmed by the appropriate serology (hepatitis A, B, C, Epstein–Barr virus). Many children may be asymptomatic or anicteric. Histology is rarely required for diagnosis, unless the presentation is unusual or there is a prolonged cholestatic phase.

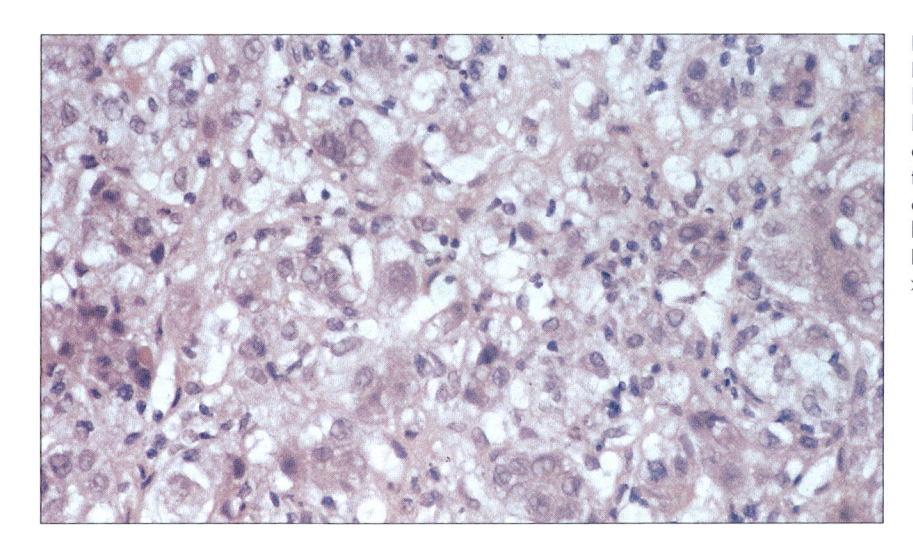

Figs 15.1, 15.2 Histology. The liver histology demonstrates ballooning of hepatocytes and inflammation (**15.1**, top), with lobular disarray and reticulin collapse (**15.2**, bottom). (Haematoxylin and Eosin, ×25; reticulin stain, ×10.)

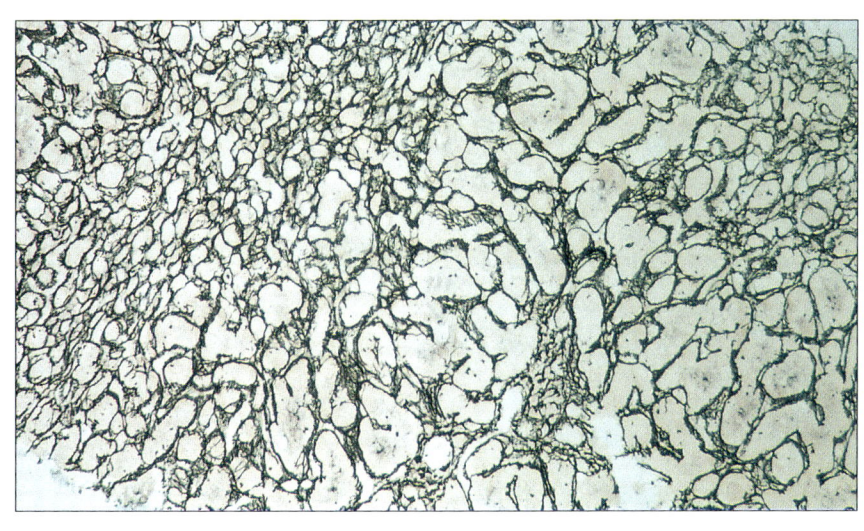

ACUTE LIVER FAILURE

The causes of acute liver failure are listed in **Fig. 15.3**. The clinical features always include encephalopathy and coagulopathy. Jaundice may not be obvious in the early stages. Hepatic transaminases are usually grossly elevated.

Aetiology of acute liver disease	
Cause	**Diagnostic investigations**
Infection Hepatitis A, B, C, undefined, EBV, CMV, Herpes simplex, Echovirus	Viral serology
Drugs Paracetamol Halothane Isoniazide Valproate	Paracetamol level Halothane antibodies Microvesicular fat in liver
Autoimmune hepatitis	Autoimmune screen immunoglobins
Metabolic Wilson's disease Tyrosinaemia type 1 Mitochondrial disorders	Copper, ceruloplasmin Urinary succinylacetone Muscle biopsy/mitochondrial DNA
Reye's syndrome/fatty acid oxidation effects	Microvesicular fat in liver, urinary dicarboxylic acids

Fig. 15.3 Causes of acute liver failure.

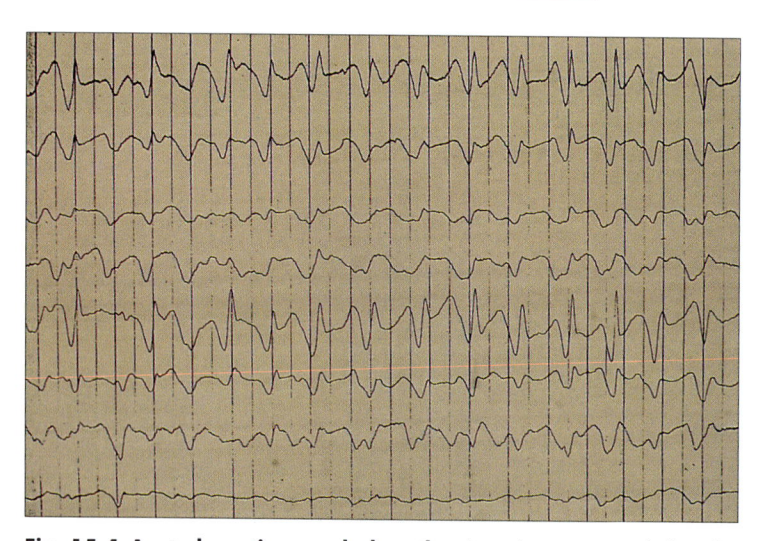

Fig. 15.4 Acute hepatic encephalopathy. Acute hepatic encephalopathy is diagnosed by the clinical features and confirmed by electroencephalography, which indicates a slow rhythm and reduced amplitude with triphasic waves.

Acute Liver Disease

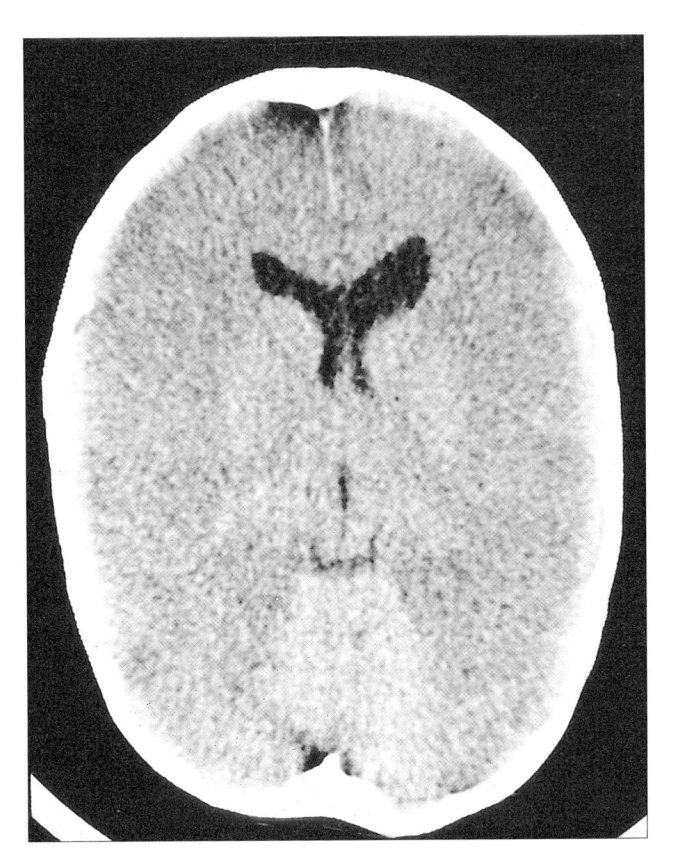

Figs 15.5, 15.6 Cerebral oedema and ischaemia. Cerebral oedema may develop rapidly and is demonstrated by CT scan, which shows slit-like ventricles (**15.5**, top). Cerebral ischaemia is indicated by reversal of grey white matter (**15.6**, bottom). Treatment with mannitol and intracranial pressure monitoring are usually required.

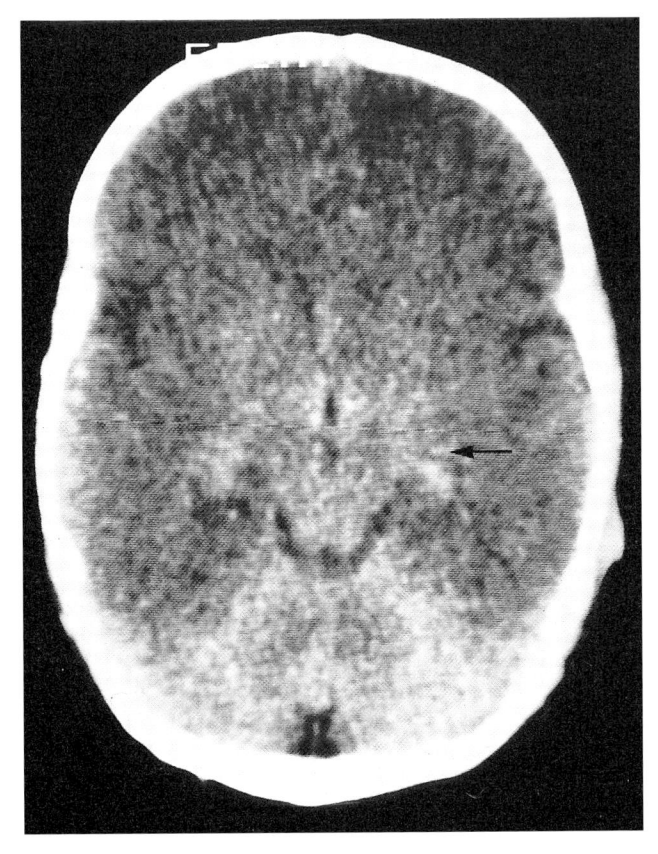

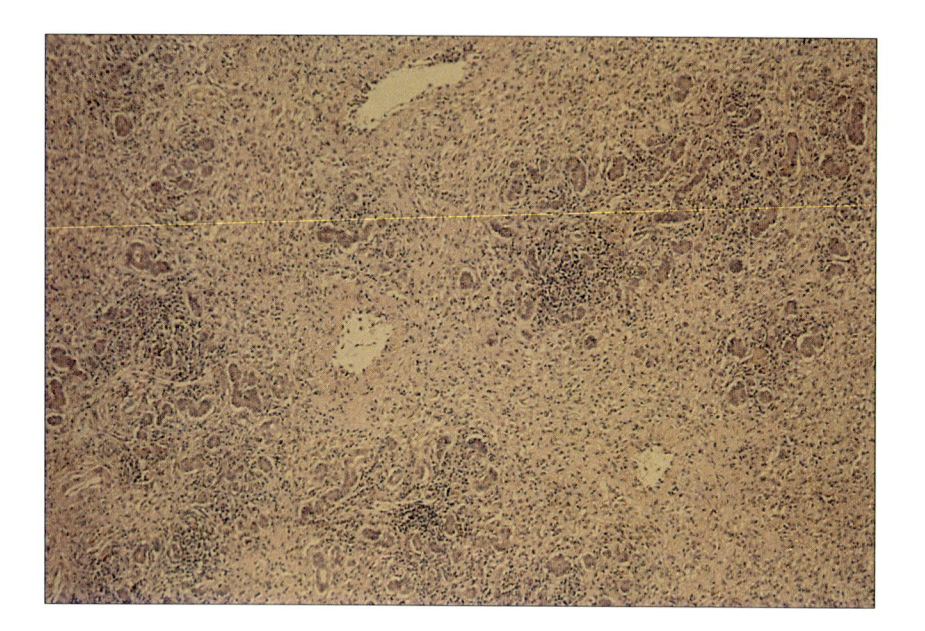

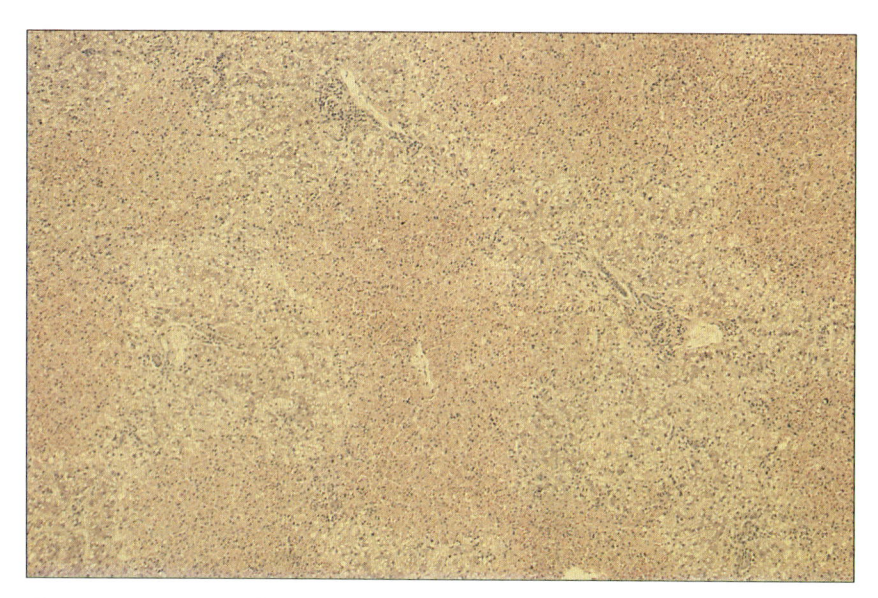

Figs 15.7, 15.8 Viral hepatitis. Severe coagulopathy usually precludes histology, but it is usual to find acute hepatic necrosis with reticulin collapse and biliary reduplication. In viral hepatitis there may be significant inflammation (**15.7**, top) which is absent in paracetamol poisoning (**15.8**, bottom). Survival without liver transplantation may be less than 30%. (Haematoxylin and Eosin, ×25.)

Acute Liver Disease

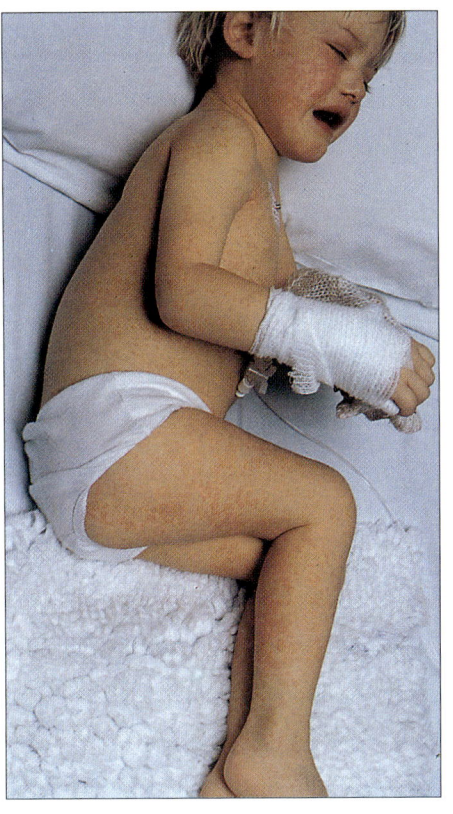

Fig. 15.9 Juvenile chronic arthritis. Juvenile chronic arthritis is occasionally associated with hepatitis. This young girl developed fever, severe arthritis, skin rash, and acute liver failure, which required intensive care support before she responded to high-dose methylprednisolone.

MICROVESICULAR FATTY LIVER

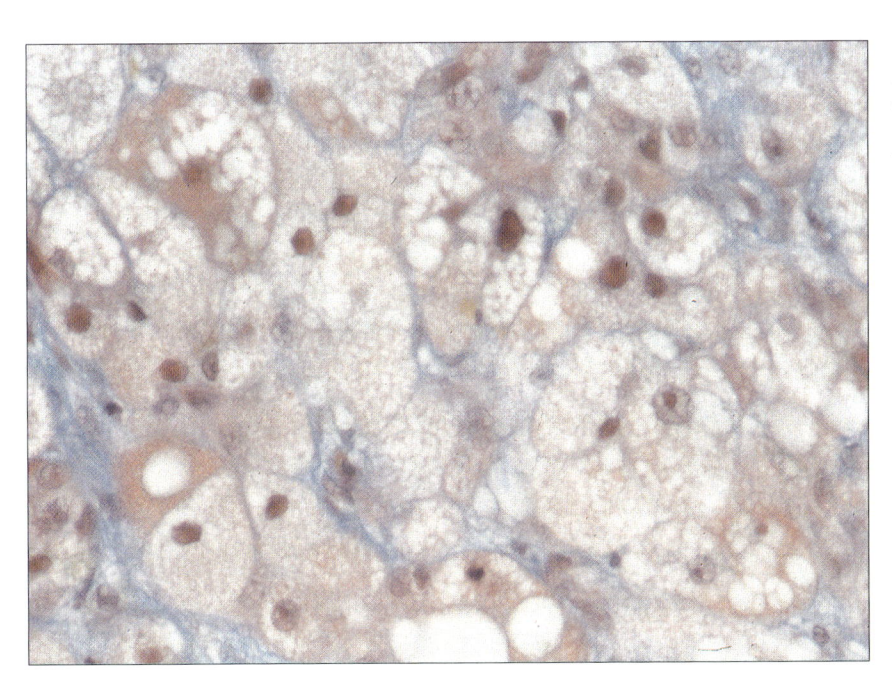

Fig. 15.10 Microvesicular fatty change. Acute liver failure may develop secondary to valproate therapy, Reye's syndrome, mitochondrial disorders, and fatty acid oxidation defects. It is usual to demonstrate microvesicular fatty change in the liver. (Haematoxylin and Eosin, ×40.)

Pediatric Gastroenterology and Hepatology

MITOCHONDRIAL DISORDERS

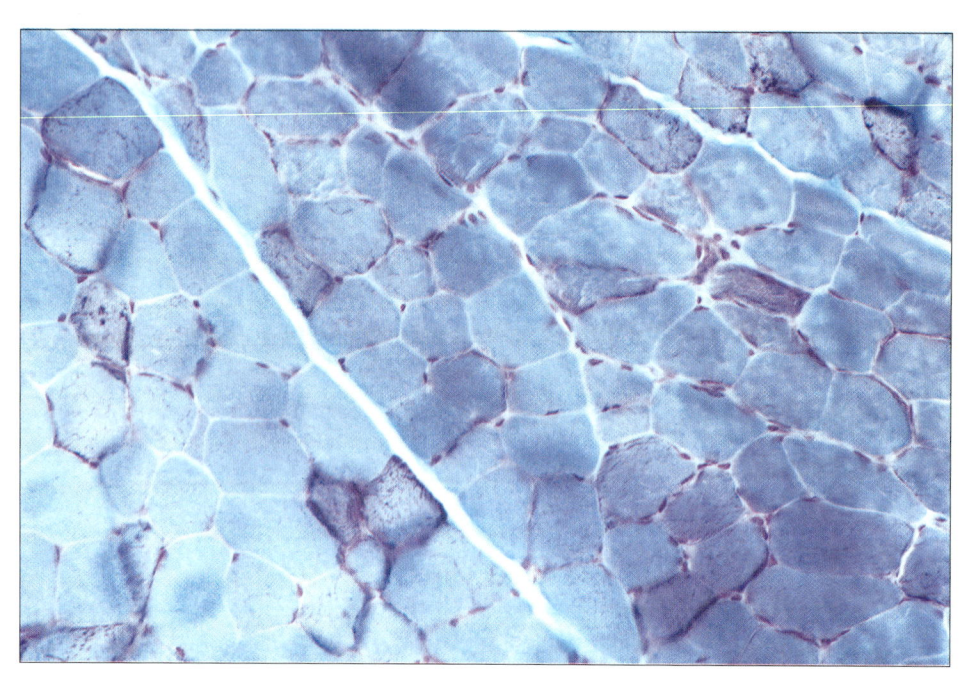

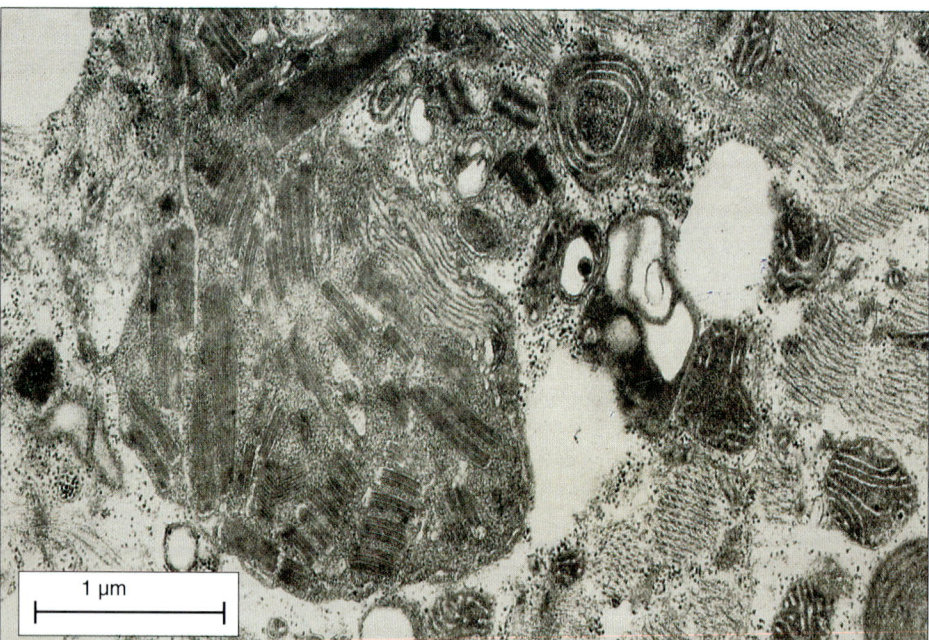

Figs 15.11, 15.12 Mitochondrial disorders. Mitochondrial disorders, such as Alpers' disease, may present with developmental delay, intractable convulsions, and acute liver failure with microvesicular fatty infiltration of the liver. This multisystem disease is not treatable by liver transplantation and thus it is important to identify disease in other organs: a raised cerebrospinal fluid lactate will indicate brain involvement; a muscle biopsy will show ragged red fibres secondary to cytochrome oxidase enzyme deficiency, which should be confirmed enzymatically (**15.11**, top, Gomori's 1-step trichrome, ×25). An electron micrograph of the muscle demonstrates the abnormal mitochondria (**15.12**, bottom).

16. Liver Transplantation

INTRODUCTION

Liver transplantation is indicated for acute or chronic liver failure, metabolic liver disease, and unresectable hepatic tumours without metastases. Current 1-year survival is 90%, with 80% surviving 5 years.

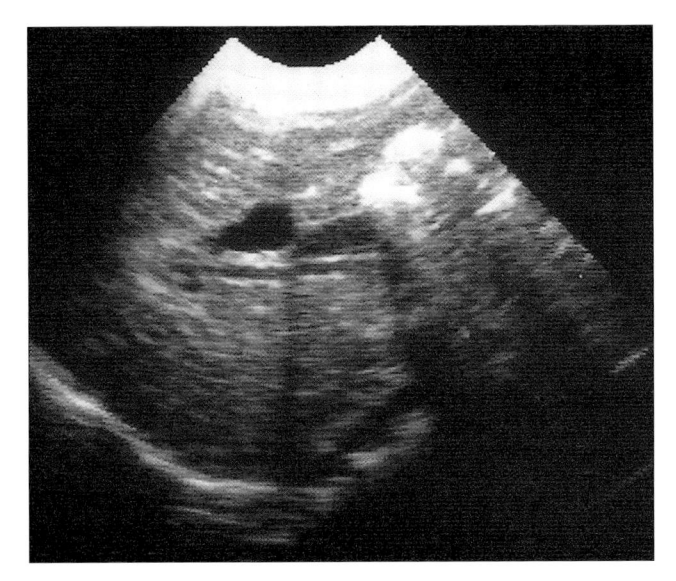

Figs 16.1, 16.2 Technical risks. Assessment for liver transplantation concentrates on establishing the severity and prognosis of the liver disease and whether any extrahepatic disease is reversible post-transplant. It is important to identify conditions which may increase the technical risk, such as hypovascular syndrome in which there is a pre-duodenal portal vein and an absent inferior vena cava (**16.1**, top), or portal vein thrombosis which should be confirmed by angiography to identify alternative vessels. This angiogram demonstrates a blocked portal vein (thick arrow), but good splenic and superior mesenteric vessels (thin arrows) (**16.2**, bottom).

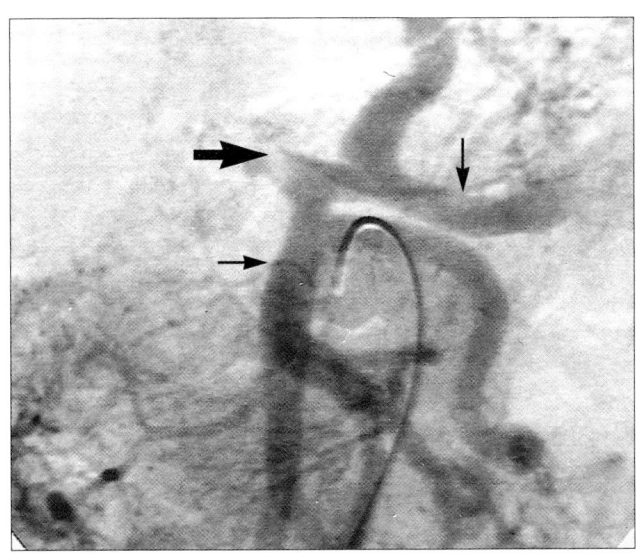

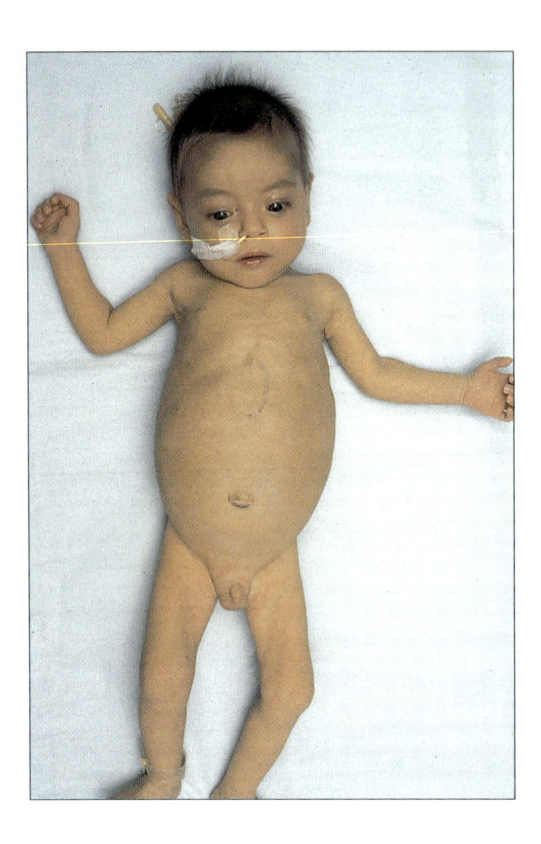

Figs 16.3 Pre-transplant management. Pre-transplant management includes treatment of hepatic complications and reversal of malnutrition. Intensive nutritional support requiring nocturnal enteral feeding is usually required and may have a dramatic effect.

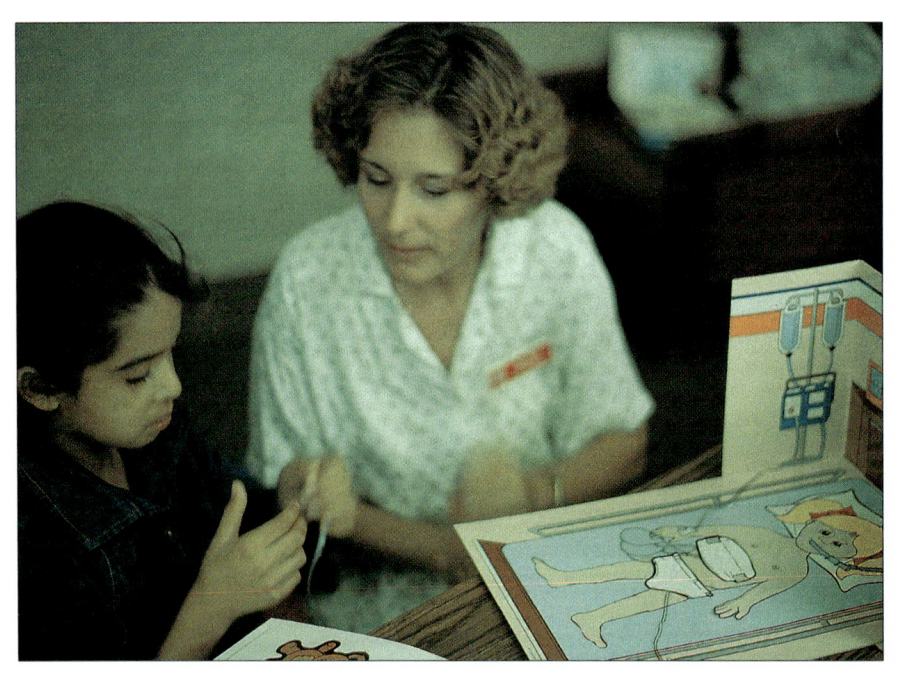

Fig. 16.4 Psychological preparation. It is impossible to underestimate the importance of psychological preparation of both family and child. Children should be prepared for this life-threatening procedure using specialist books and appropriate toys.

Liver Transplantation

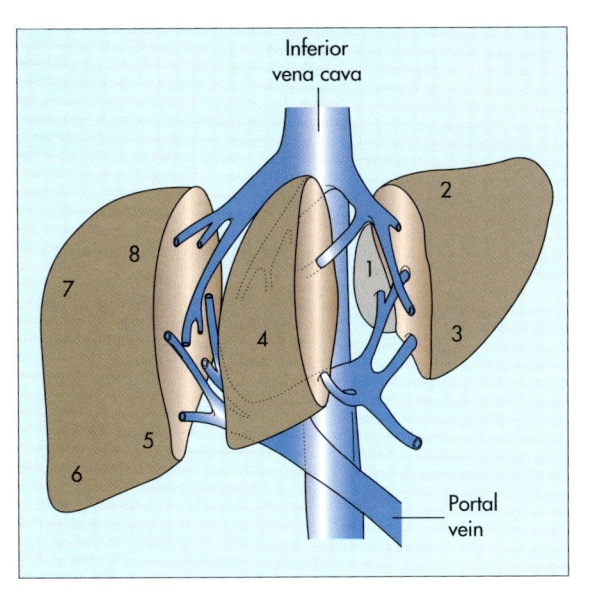

Fig. 16.5 Reduction hepatectomy. The development of reduction hepatectomy (in which segments 2 and 3 of a larger liver are transplanted into a small child) has extended transplantation to the neonatal age group and reduced waiting-list mortality. One-year survival rates are now in excess of 85%. Variants of this technique include split grafts (one liver to two recipients) or living related donation from parent to child.

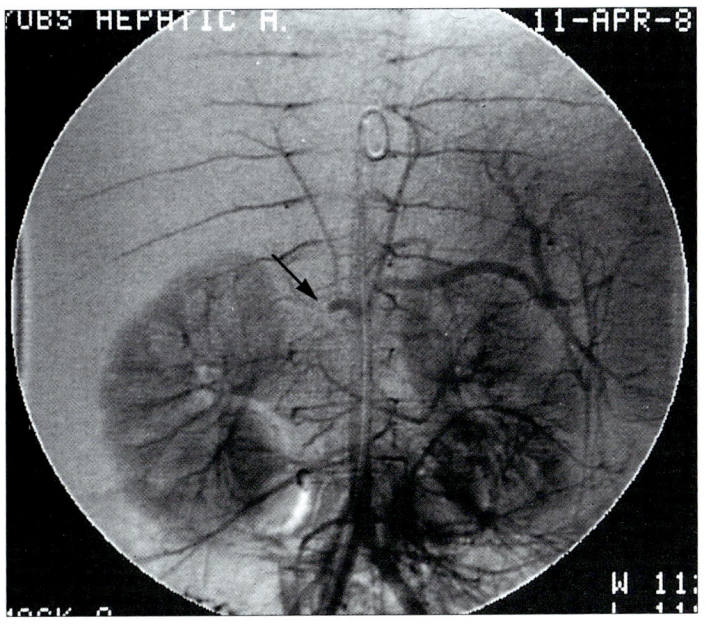

Figs 16.6, 16.7 Hepatic artery thrombosis. Peri-operative morbidity may be high and includes hepatic artery thrombosis, which occurs in 4–10% of children. **16.6** (middle) demonstrates an absent hepatic artery which led to allograft infarction (**16.7**, bottom), acute liver failure, and the necessity for re-transplantation.

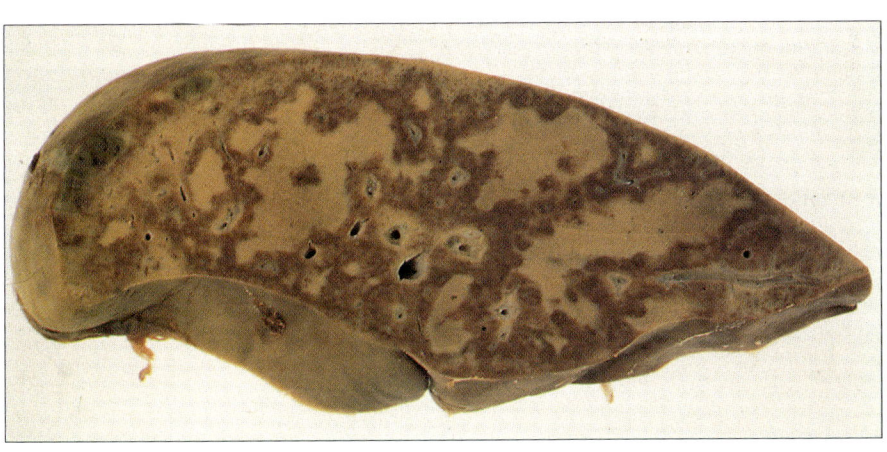

Pediatric Gastroenterology and Hepatology

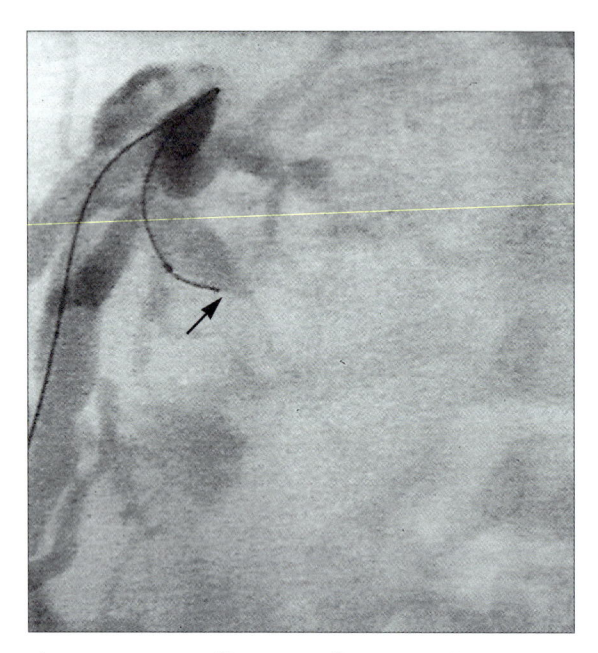

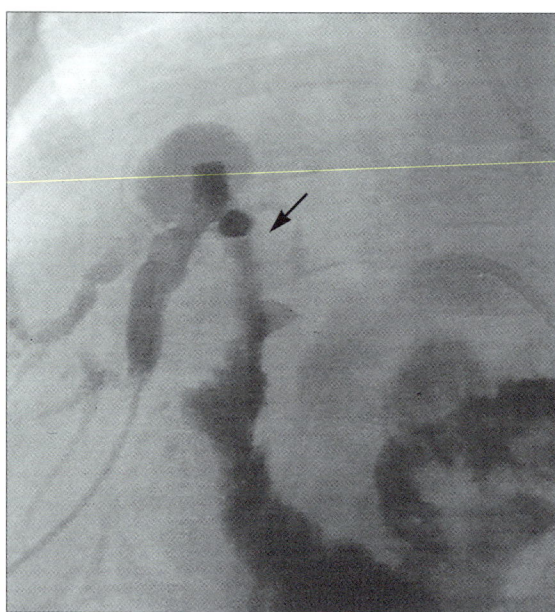

Figs 16.8, 16.9 Biliary complications. Biliary complications occur in 20% of children and include biliary leaks or strictures leading to intrahepatic bile duct dilatation and cholangitis (**16.8**, left). Strictures may be dilated percutaneously (**16.9**, right) or surgically reconstructed.

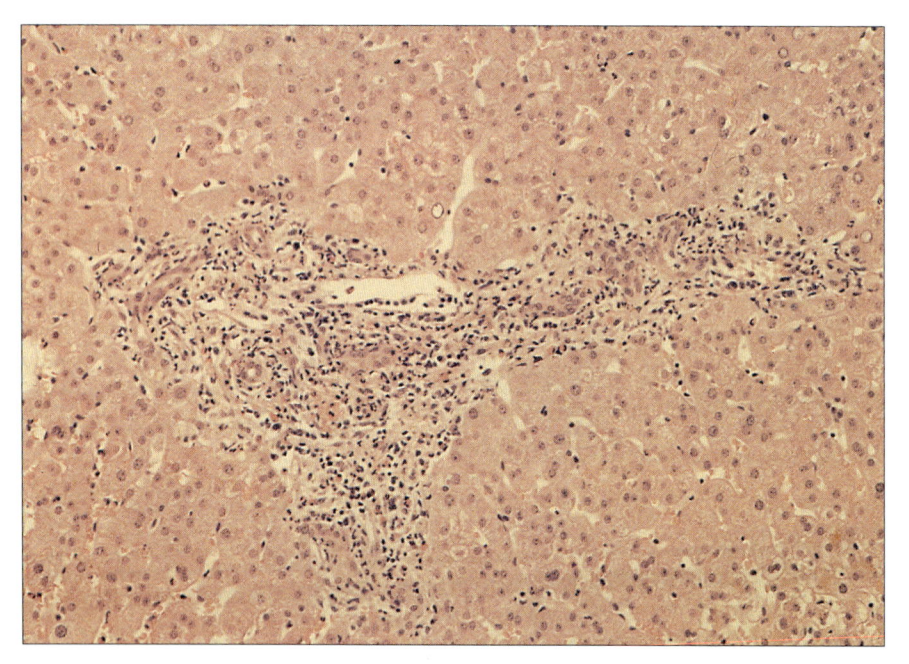

Fig. 16.10 Acute cellular rejection. Acute cellular rejection responsive to increased immunosuppression occurs in 50–80% of children between 7 and 10 days post-transplant; it is less common in children aged under 1 year. The diagnosis is suggested by a fever and rises in bilirubin, alkaline phosphatase, gamma-glutamyl transpeptidase (gamma-GT), and transaminases. Histology indicates a mixed inflammatory infiltrate in the portal tracts, with subendothelial lymphoid infiltration and inflammatory infiltration of bile ducts. (Haematoxylin and Eosin, ×40.)

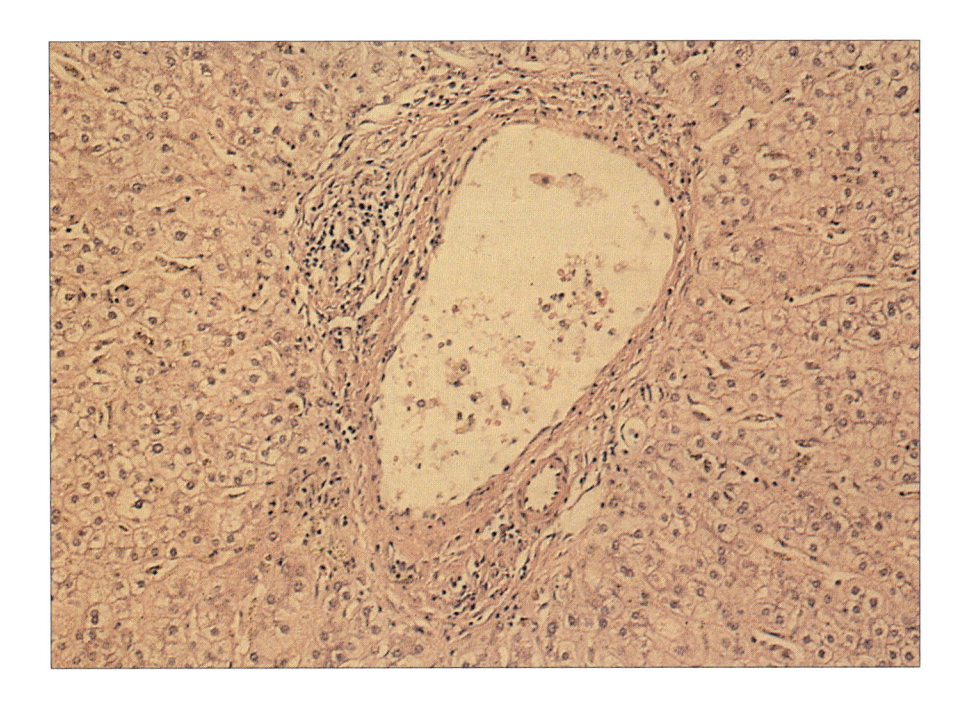

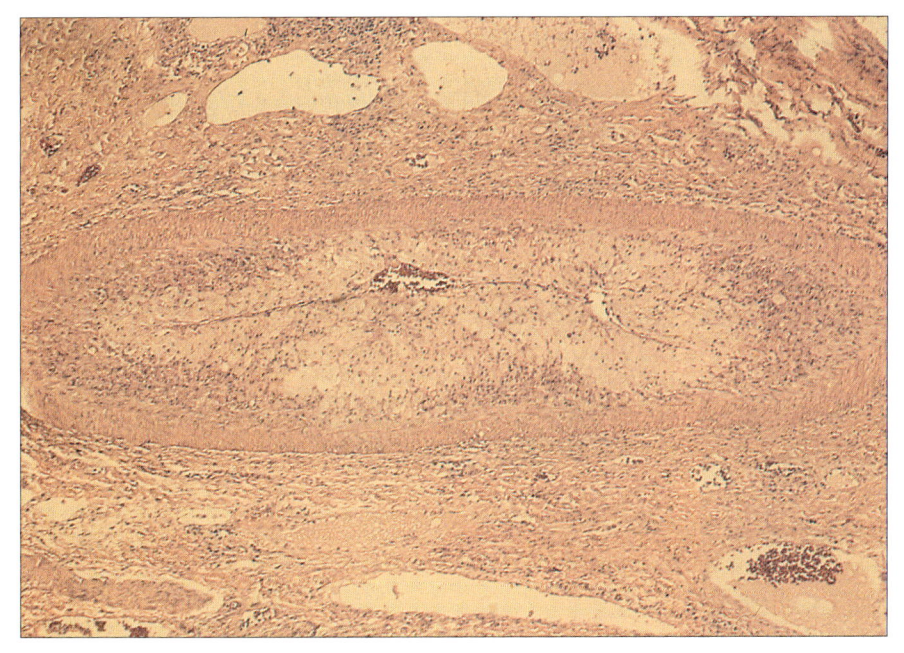

Figs 16.11, 16.12 Chronic rejection. Chronic rejection occurs in less than 10% of children at any time post-transplant. The diagnosis is made by the gradual onset of jaundice and rises in bilirubin, alkaline phosphatase, gamma-GT, and transaminases. Histology demonstrates a vanishing bile duct syndrome. This portal tract (**16.11**, top, Haematoxylin and Eosin, ×40) contains a small arterial branch with no accompanying bile duct. **16.12** (bottom, Haematoxylin and Eosin, ×16) demonstrates a large arterial branch in the hilum with numerous intimal foam cells resulting in luminal obliteration. Some children may respond to increased immunosuppression with tacrolimus, but the majority require re-transplantation.

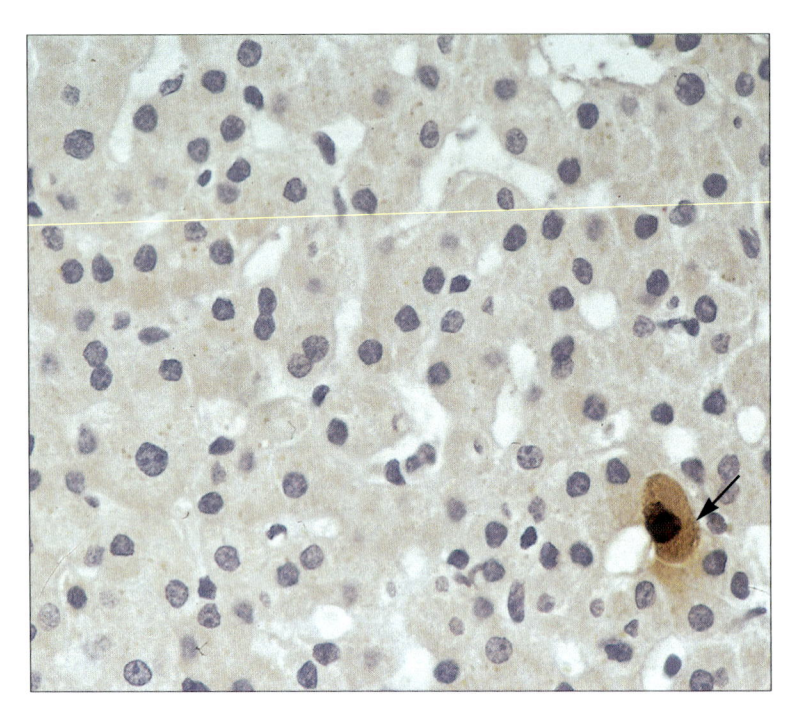

Fig. 16.13 Cytomegalovirus. Late complications include cytomegalovirus (CMV) hepatitis which occurs 6–8 weeks post-transplant, particularly in CMV-negative recipients who have received a CMV-positive graft. Symptoms may be non-specific, with fever, malaise, and abnormal liver function tests. The diagnosis is confirmed by identifying seroconversion to CMV (CMV IgM positive) and by the classic histology which demonstrates CMV inclusion bodies. Treatment with intravenous ganciclovir (DHPG) is effective. (Anti-CMV, ×40.)

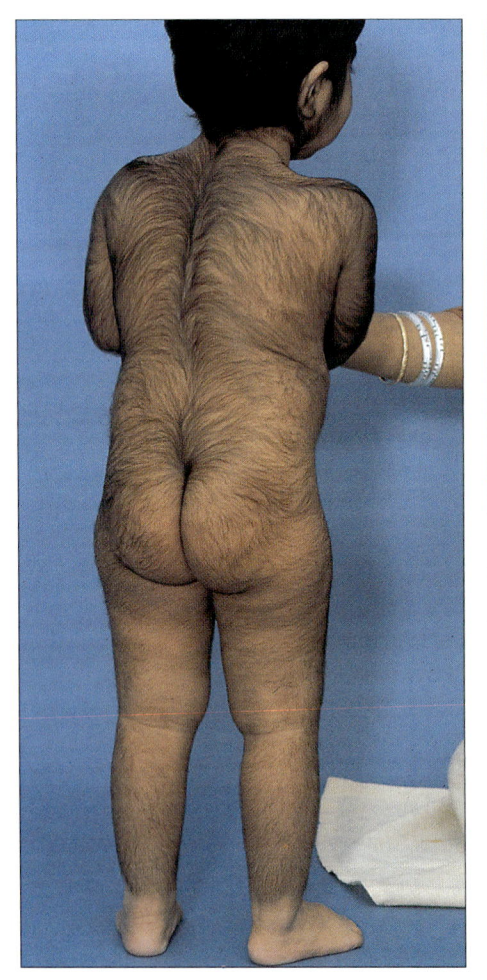

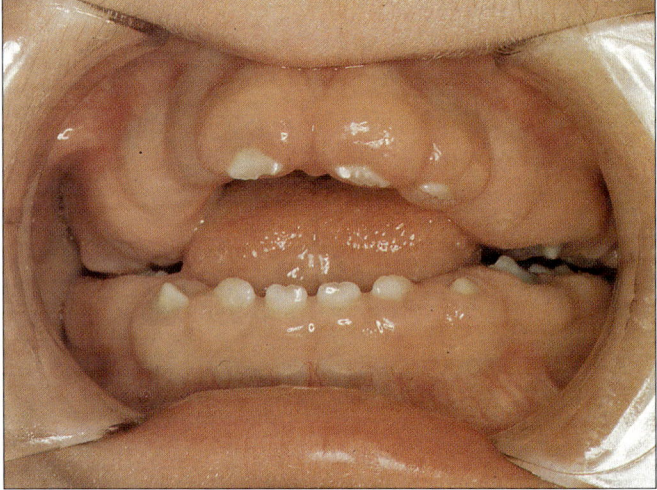

Figs 16.14, 16.15 Long-term complications. Long-term complications are related to the effects of immunosuppression. Early reduction of steroids will prevent stunting, but life-long cyclosporin leads to hirsutism (**16.14**, left), gingival hyperplasia (**16.15**, right), and nephrotoxicity with hypertension.

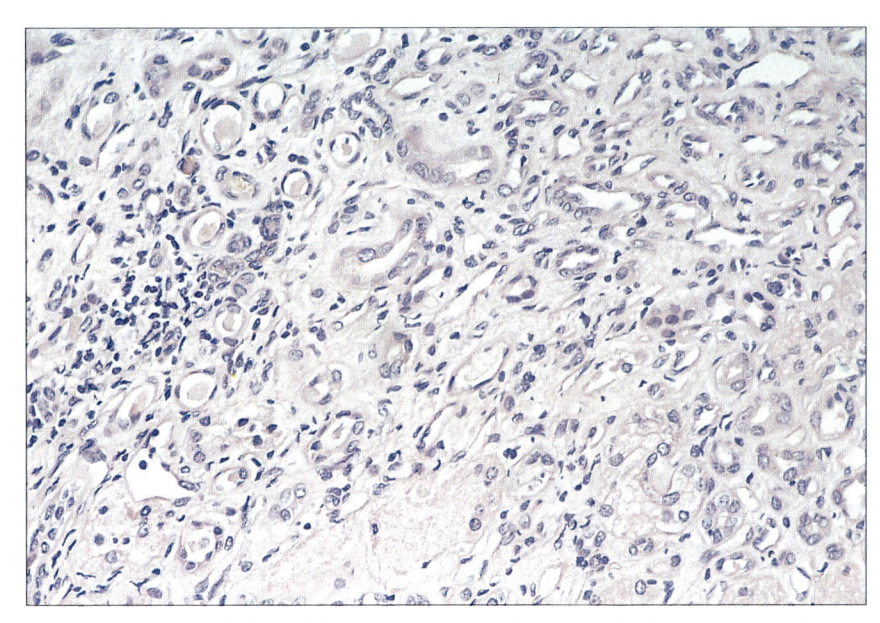

Fig. 16.16 Interstitial nephritis. Cyclosporin nephrotoxicity leads to an interstitial nephritis; here interstitial fibrosis, inflammation, and tubular atrophy are demonstrated. Although both urea and creatinine may be elevated, renal failure is rare. (Haematoxylin and Eosin, ×40.)

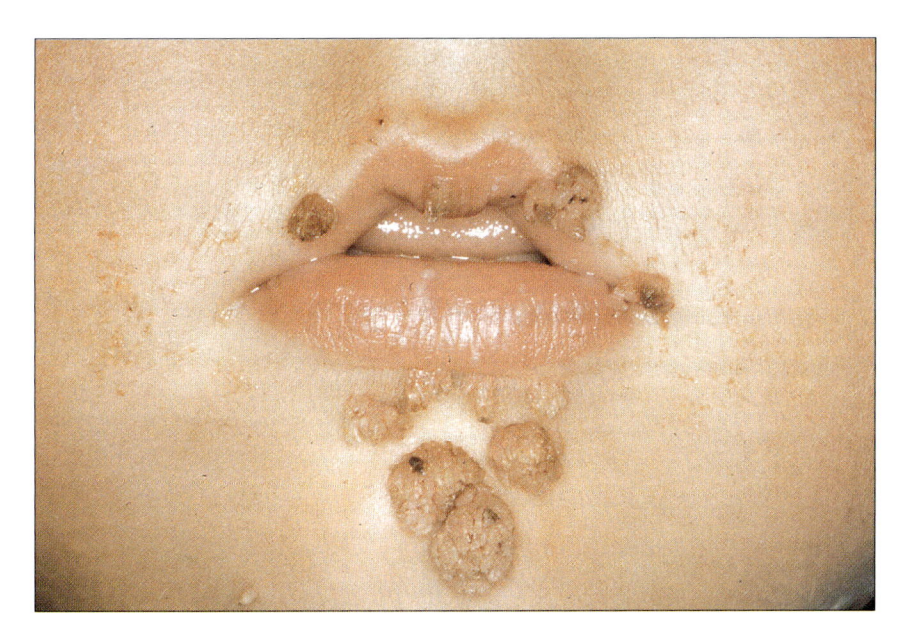

Fig. 16.17 Viral infections. Children on long-term immunosuppression are prone to viral infections, either with herpesviruses (such as herpes labialis (above)) or Epstein–Barr virus (EBV).

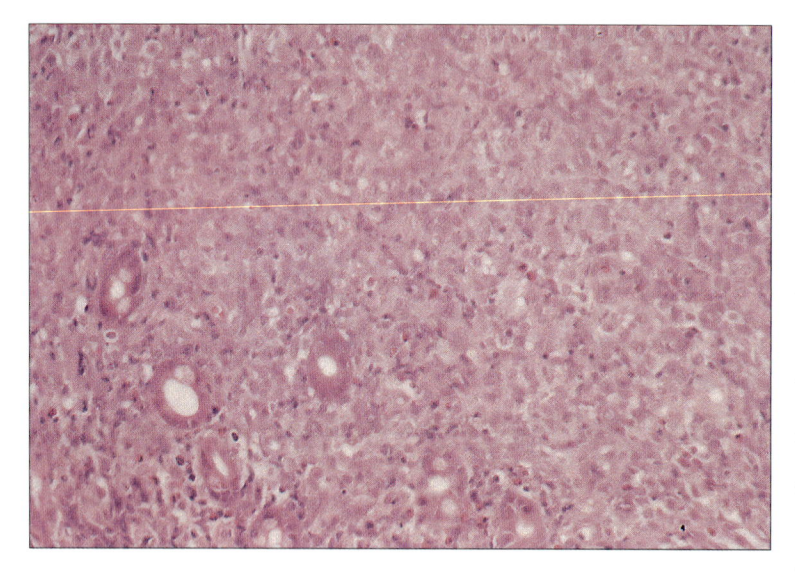

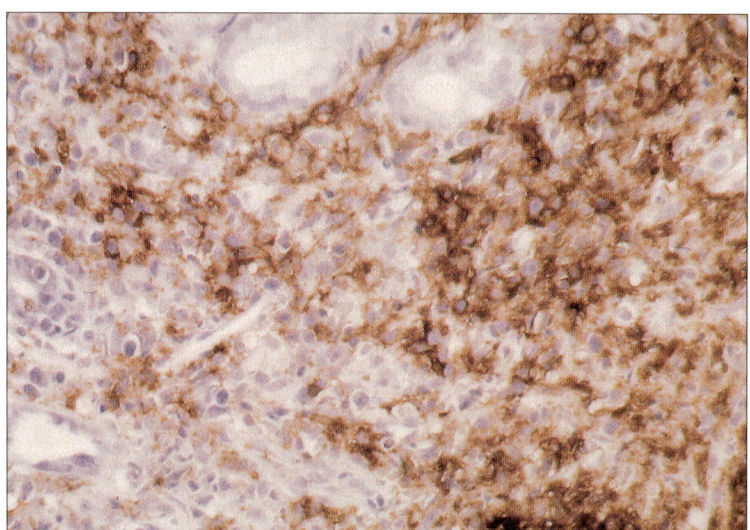

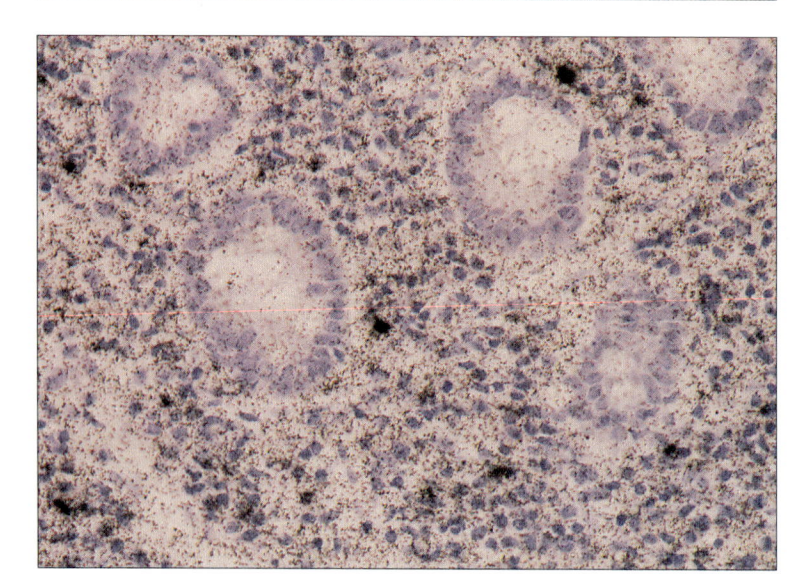

Figs 16.18–16.20 Lymphoproliferative disease of the jejunum. As almost 60% of children are EBV negative pre-transplant, the majority will develop a primary infection within 6 months of the operation. Some may develop lymphoproliferative disease, which usually resolves when immunosuppression is discontinued. This child developed lymphoproliferative disease of the jejunum in which jejunal submucosa was replaced by large pale cells (**16.18**, top, Haemotoxylin and Eosin, ×10), identified as monoclonal B cells (**16.19**, middle, Immunocytochemistry, ×25) using a B cell marker (L26, ×10). In-situ hybridisation for EBV (**16.20**, bottom, Immunocytochemistry, ×25) demonstrated that the cells were infected with EBV.

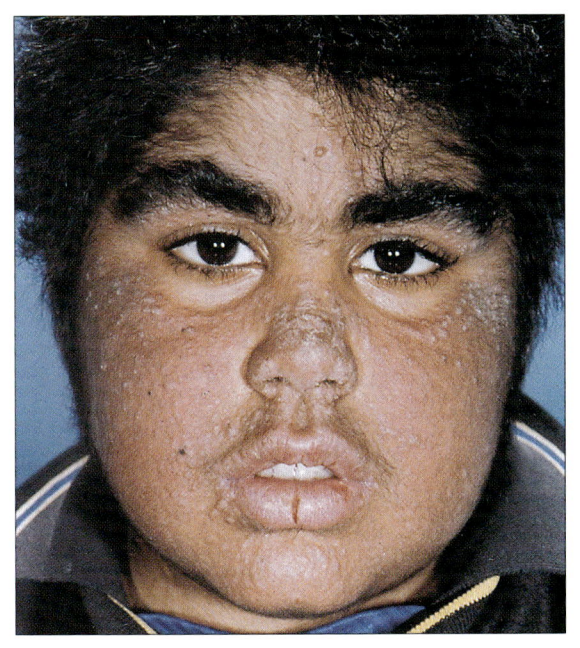

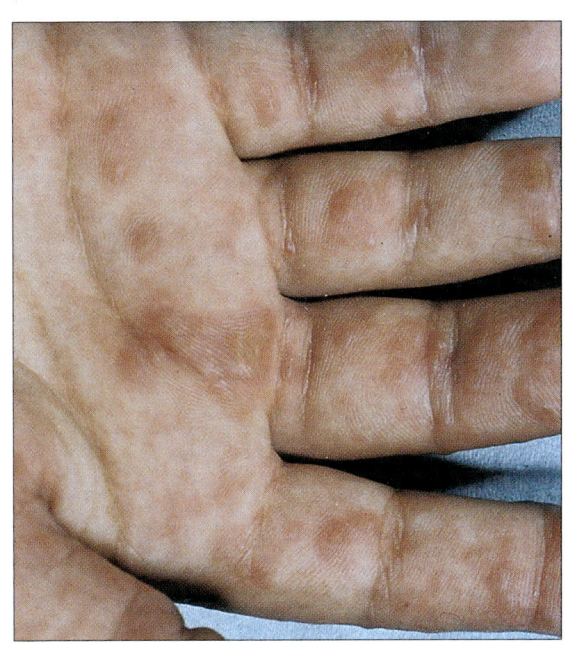

Liver Transplantation

Figs 16.21, 16.22 Hirsutism and a papular skin rash. This 9-year-old boy had extremely high levels of cyclosporin and developed excess hirsutism (**16.21**) and a papular skin rash (**16.22**), secondary to T cell infiltration of the skin. The rash completely resolved when immunosuppression was reduced.

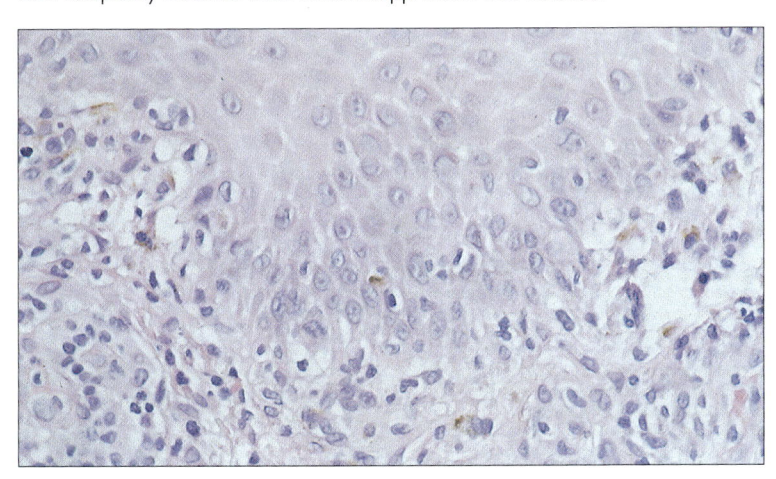

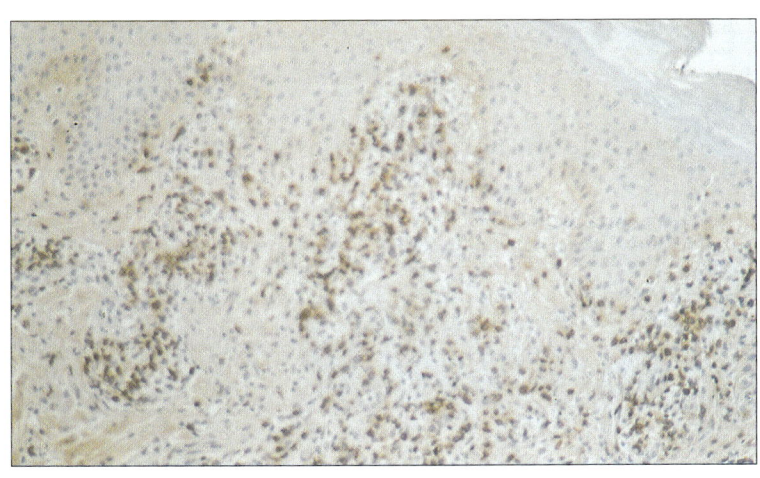

Figs 16.23, 16.24 Papular skin rash. Skin biopsy of the case shown in **Figs 16.21** and **16.22** demonstrated inflammation extending into the epidermis (**16.23**, Haematoxylin and Eosin, ×25), which was due to T cell infiltration (**16.24**, Immunoperoxidase, ×10).

TRANSPLANTATION FOR METABOLIC DISEASE

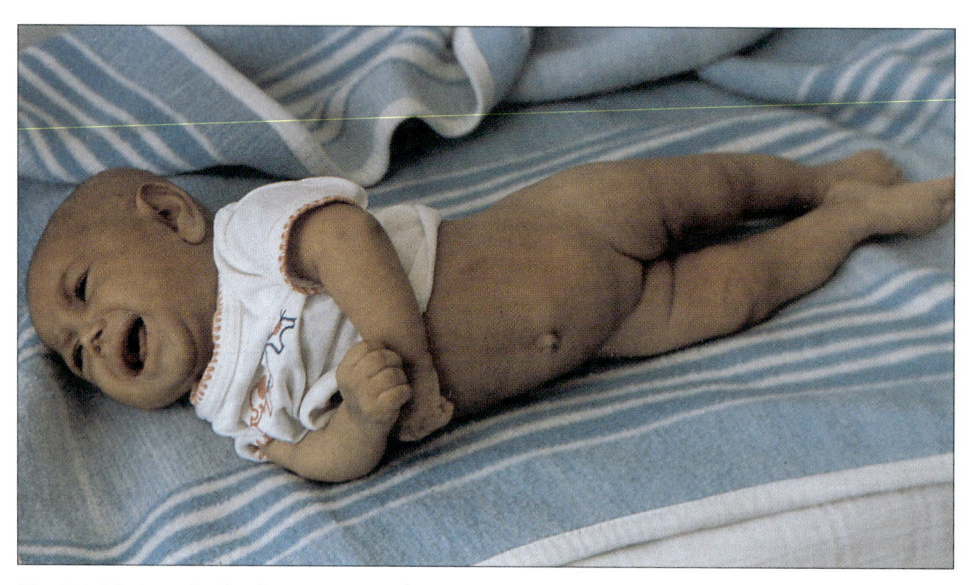

Fig. 16.25 Metabolic disease transplantation. Transplantation may be appropriate for certain metabolic diseases in which the hepatic enzyme deficiency leads to extrahepatic disease. In Crigler–Najjar Type I, the deficiency of bilirubin uridine diphosphoglucuronyl transferase leads to severe unconjugated hyperbilirubinaemia, kernicterus, deafness, opisthotonos, and mental retardation.

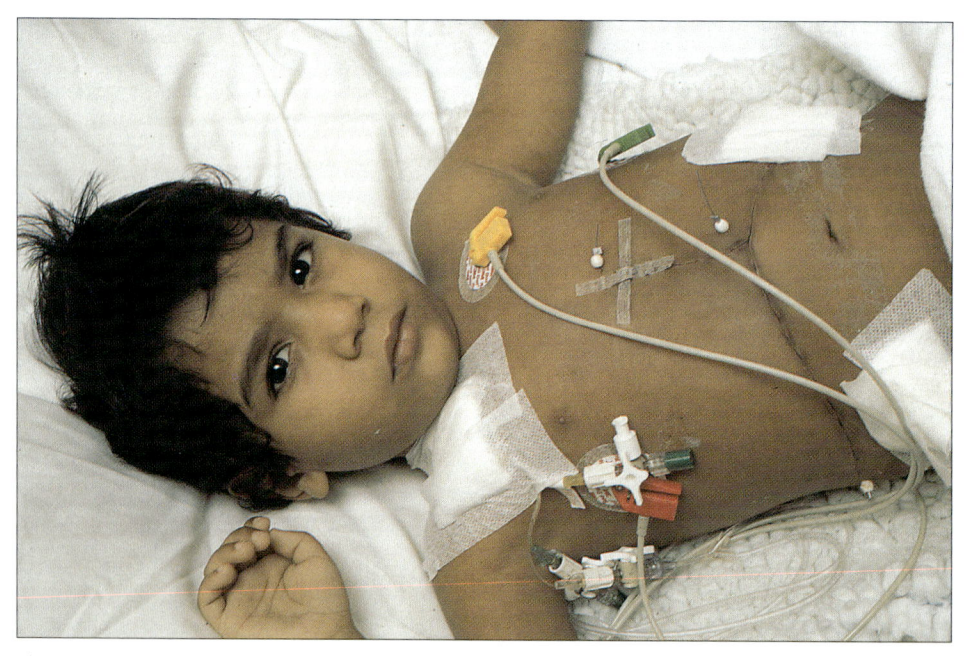

Fig. 16.26 Medical management. Medical management is with phototherapy to reduce levels of unconjugated bilirubin, but the definitive treatment is liver transplantation as in this 3-year-old boy who now leads a normal life.

Liver Transplantation

SMALL BOWEL AND LIVER TRANSPLANTATION

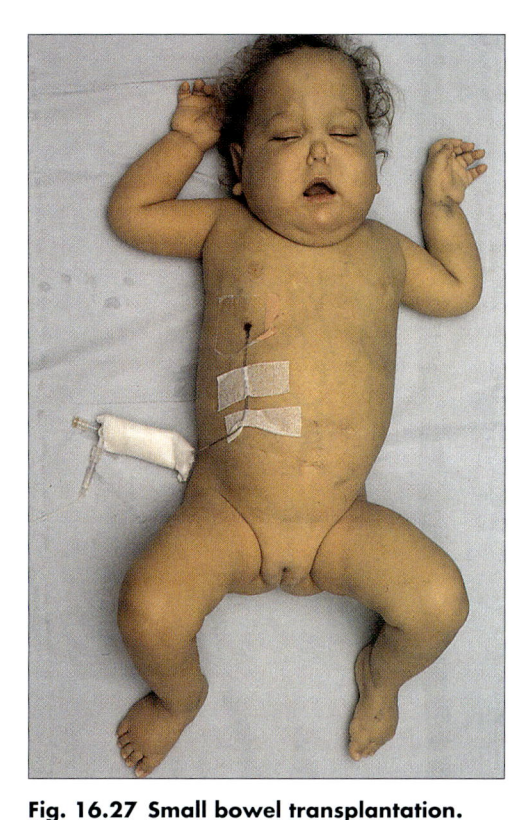

Fig. 16.27 Small bowel transplantation. Small bowel transplantation is indicated in children with intestinal failure who are maintained on long-term parenteral nutrition if they develop either severe liver disease or loss of vascular access. Although this technique is at an early stage of development, it is important that children are referred to a specialist centre early as the shortage of appropriately sized and matched organs means a long pre-operative waiting time and the possibility of dying if no donor is available.

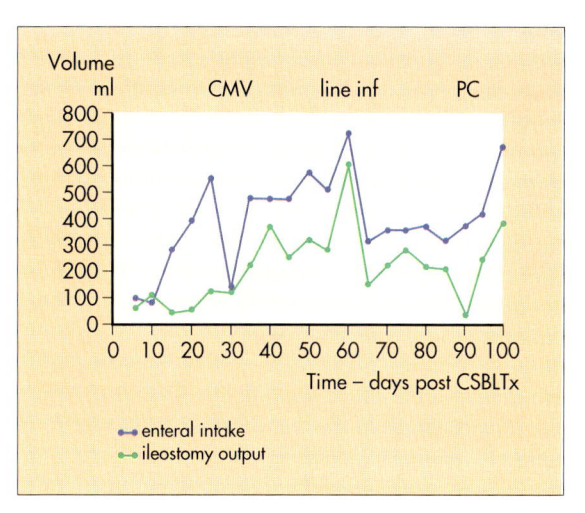

Fig. 16.28 Enteral intake and ileostomy output post-transplant. Following successful combined small bowel and liver transplantation (CSBLTx) intestinal function is rapidly regained. This graph demonstrates enteral intake and ileostomy output post-transplant. There is positive absorption of enteral feeds with a constant ileostomy output until the development of complications (CMV infection, line infection, *Pneumocystis carinii* infection, PC), at which point intestinal function was impaired.

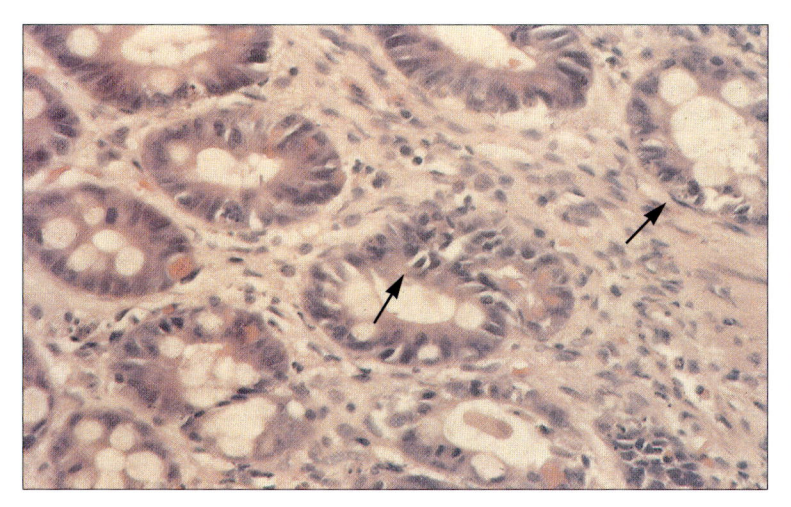

Fig. 16.29 Rejection. Hepatic rejection is unusual in the combined operation, but intestinal rejection is inevitable. Symptoms may be non-specific with fever and increase in stoma output. The histological changes develop much later than the symptoms. This small bowel biopsy demonstrates an inflammatory infiltrate with loss of goblet cells, abnormal nuclei, and apoptopic body and lymphoid cells infiltrating the glands. Increased immunosuppression with prednisolone and tacrolimus is usually effective. (Haematoxylin and Eosin, ×40.)

147

Pediatric Gastroenterology and Hepatology

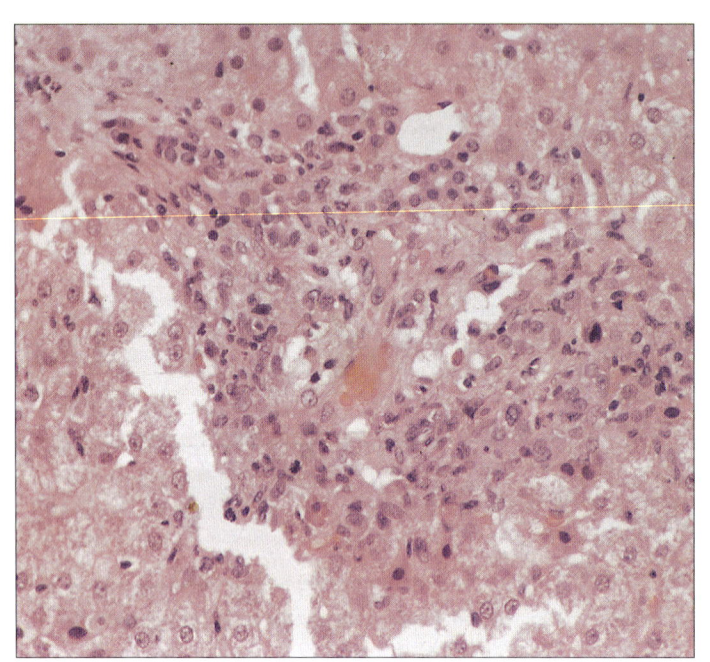

Fig. 16.30 Graft versus host disease. Graft versus host disease is rare after either liver transplantation or small bowel/liver transplantation, but is common following bone marrow transplantation and is often found in association with skin and intestinal involvement (Chapter 4). Shown here is a vanishing bile duct syndrome with an eosinophilic infiltrate. (Haematoxylin and Eosin, ×40.)

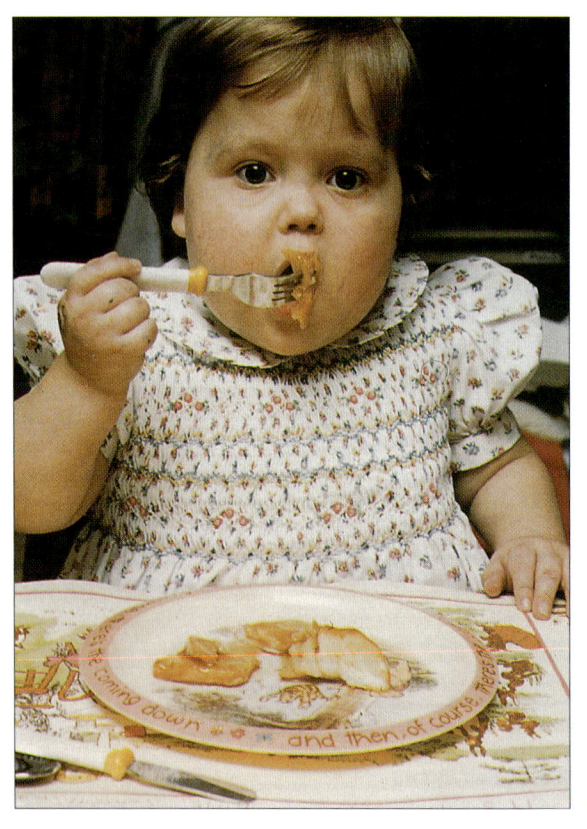

Fig. 16.31 Prognosis of CSBLTx. Although the long-term outcome and prognosis are unknown, approximately 70% of children survive the first year post-transplant; 80% of these are fully enterally fed. Some children find feeding is fun, as for this 2-year-old girl with intestinal failure secondary to gastroschisis, 2 months after a small bowel transplant.

17. Nutrition

INTRODUCTION

The nutritional assessment of children includes the serial measurement of height, weight, triceps skin fold, and mid-arm circumference, and calculation of the mid-arm muscle area. Ideally, this data should be converted into standard deviation scores. Malnutrition is defined as two standard deviations below the mean. Low height for age (stunting) is the result of chronic malnutrition, while low weight for height (wasting) is secondary to acute malnutrition. Triceps skin fold thickness gives an indication of fat stores, while mid-arm muscle area indicates protein stores.

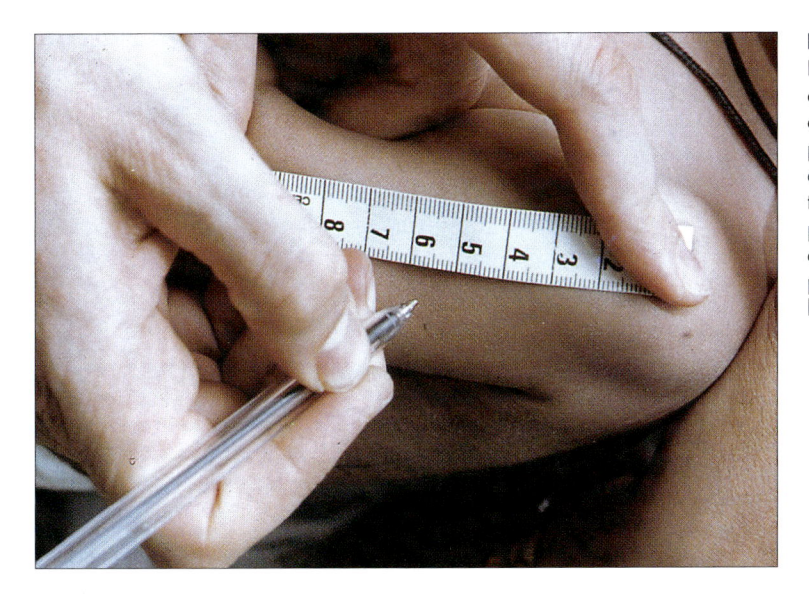

Figs 17.1, 17.2 Anthropometry. In order to maintain the reproducibility of observations, measurements should only be performed by trained personnel. The mid-point of the upper arm is obtained by measuring from the tip of the acromion to the olecranon process (**17.1**, top). Mid-arm circumference is measured at the mid-point, as is the triceps skin fold (**17.2**, bottom).

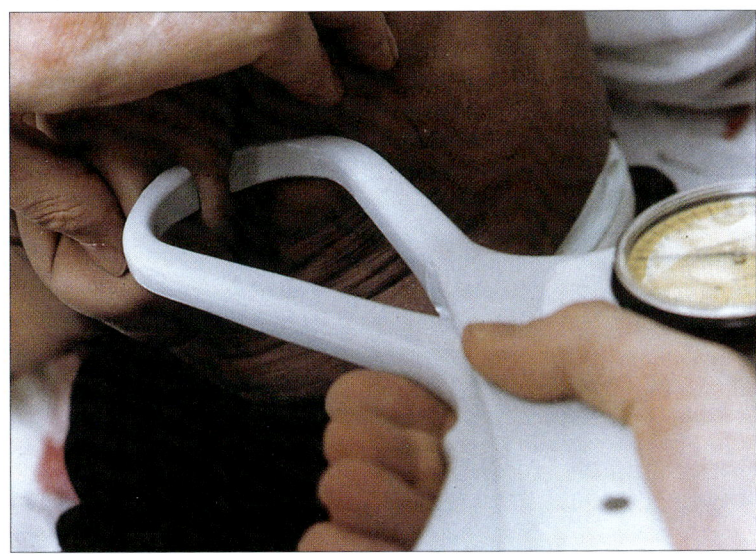

Pediatric Gastroenterology and Hepatology

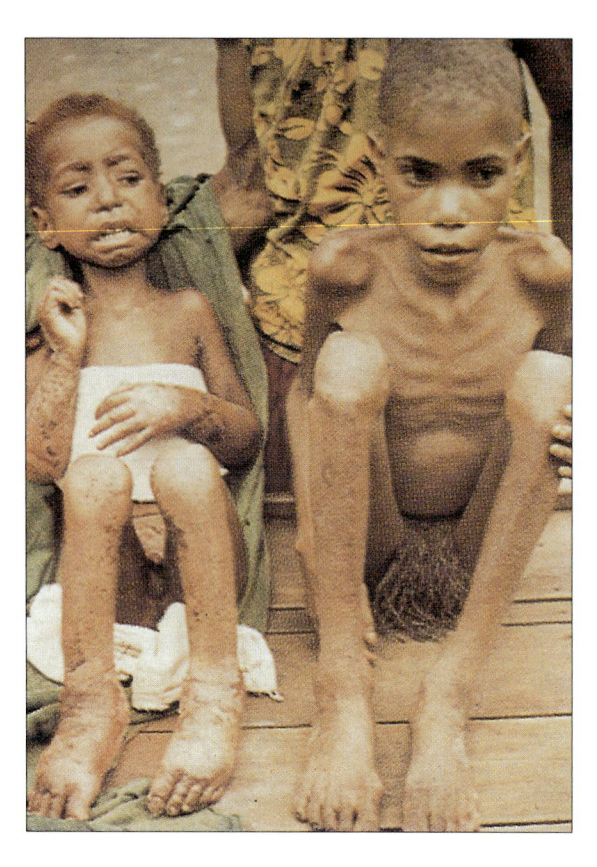

Fig. 17.3 Pathogenesis. The pathogenesis of malnutrition is multifactorial. It may be primary, related to low intake, as in these children in Zimbabwe. The child on the left has kwashiorkor, which is characterised by ascites and peripheral oedema. The child on the right has marasmus.

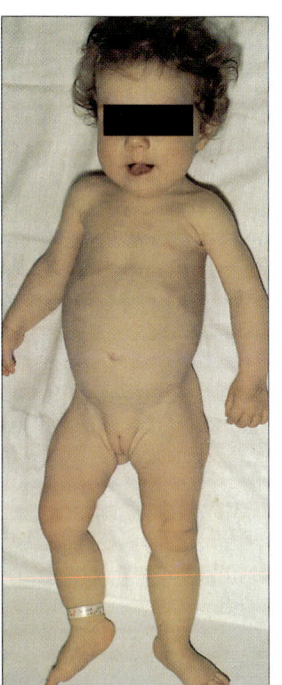

Fig. 17.4 Pathogenesis. Alternatively, reduced intake may be secondary to Munchausen syndrome by proxy. This infant presented with failure to thrive and diarrhoea which proved to be secondary to laxative abuse. Once admitted to hospital the diarrhoea resolved and she rapidly gained weight when fed under supervision.

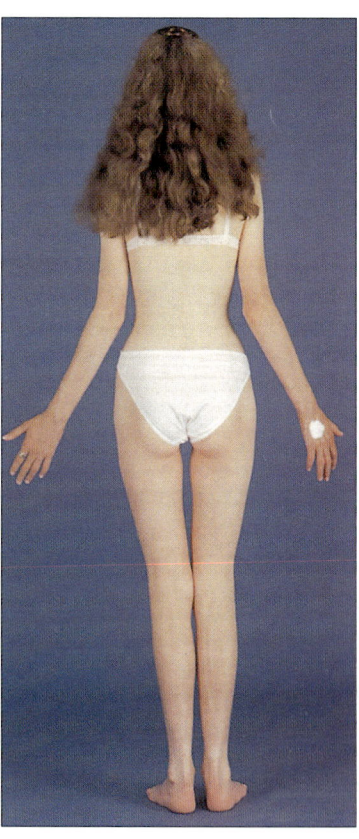

Fig. 17.5 Anorexia nervosa. Anorexia nervosa in adolescent girls may lead to life-threatening malnutrition, as in this girl who lost 25% of her body weight while on a diet.

Nutrition

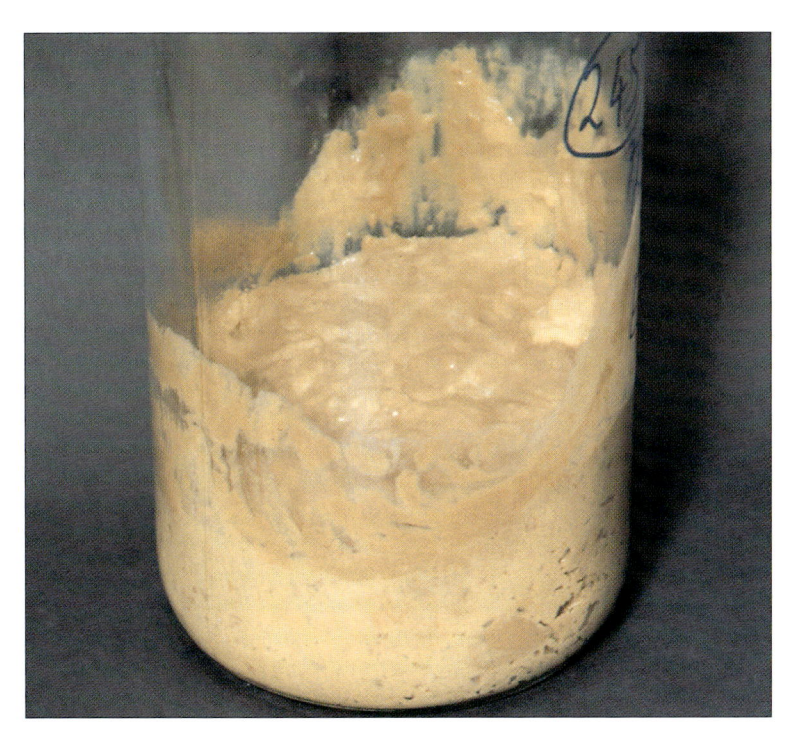

Fig. 17.6 Fat malabsorption. Secondary malnutrition is commonly due to fat malabsorption. Gross steatorrhoea is a feature of many diseases, including cystic fibrosis, coeliac disease, chronic pancreatitis, or cholestatic liver disease. Stools are offensive (parents agree a gas mask is needed to change the baby's nappy), float, and are difficult to flush.

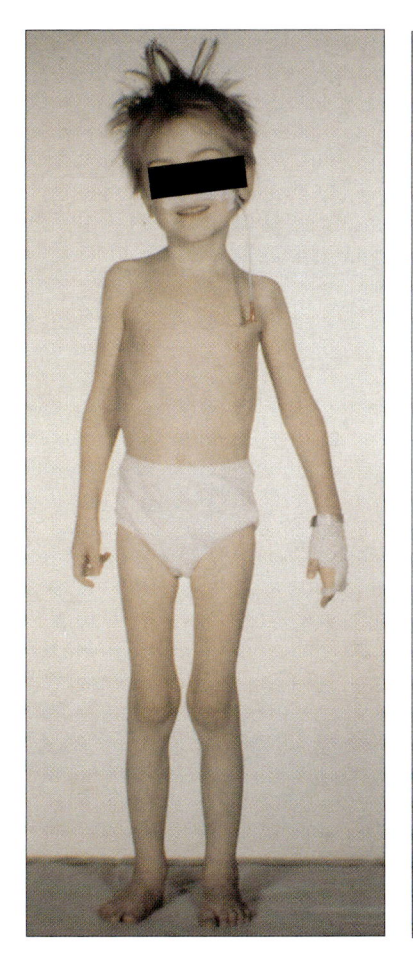

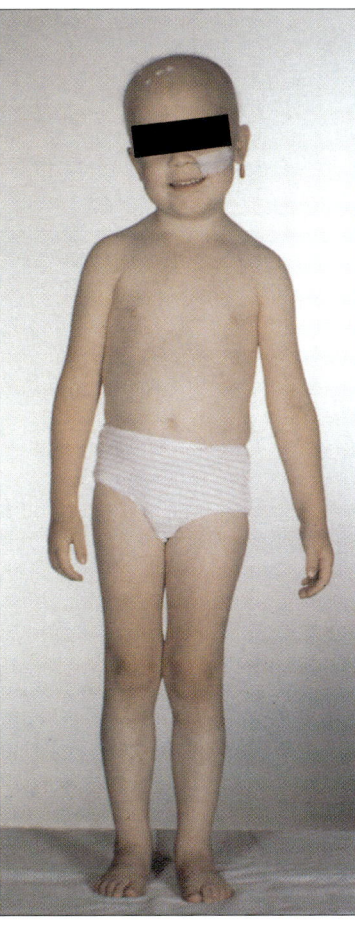

Figs 17.7, 17.8 Chronic diseases. In a number of chronic diseases the increased energy requirements lead to malnutrition, as in this child with non-Hodgkin's lymphoma (**17.7**, left) who was successfully rehabilitated (**17.8**, right) with enteral feeding while being treated with chemotherapy.

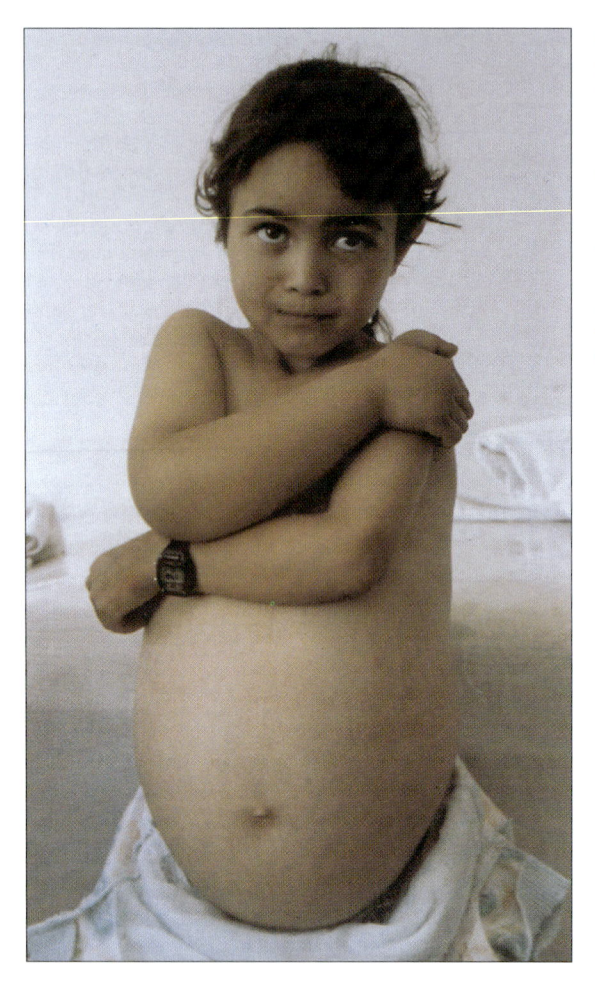

Figs 17.9, 17.10 Intestinal lymphangiectasia. This girl (**17.9**) presented in infancy with peripheral hypoproteinaemic oedema, due to congenital abnormality of the small-intestinal lymphatics (**17.10**, Haematoxylin and Eosin, ×40). Lymph, which is rich in protein, immunoglobulins and lymphocytes, leaks into the intestinal lumen, with consequent deficiencies in the peripheral blood. This girl has marked distension due to ascites (**17.9**). An associated disorder of peripheral lymphatics is causing lymphoedema of her right arm and of the right side of her face. Treatment is with a diet in which long-chain triglycerides are replaced in part by medium-chain triglycerides (not available for this patient in her own country).

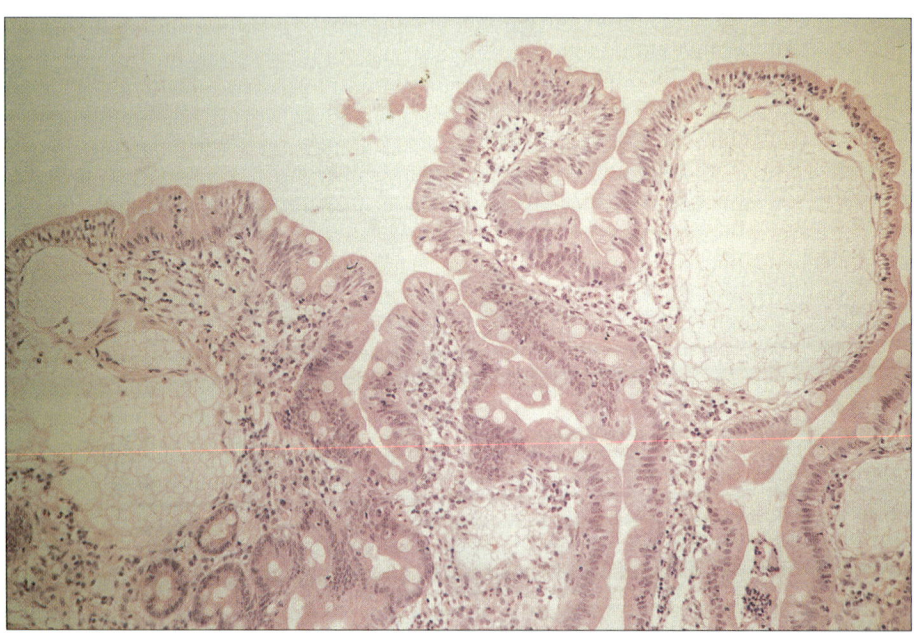

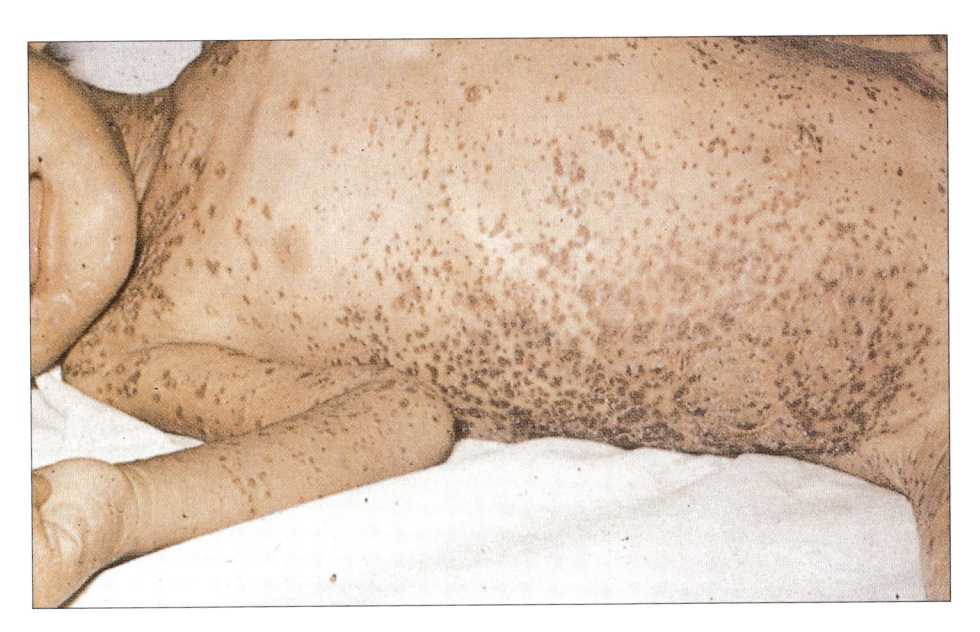

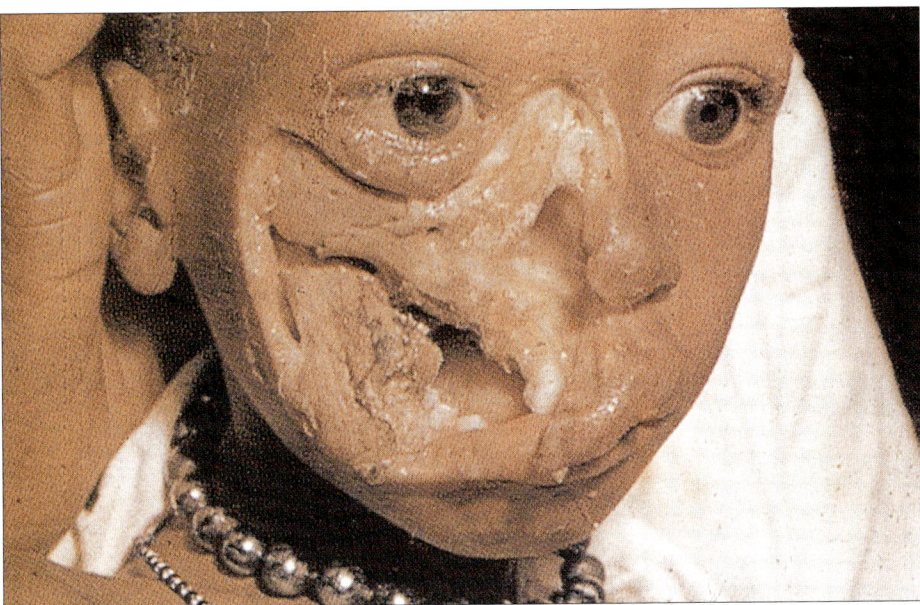

Figs 17.11, 17.12 Infections. Many children with severe malnutrition may be immunosuppressed and have recurrent infections. This child (**17.11**, top) with primary malnutrition has severe measles. Cancrum oris (noma) secondary to primary malnutrition (**17.12**, bottom) tends to occur between 1 and 5 years of age. The causative organisms are thought to be *Borrelia vincentii* and *Fusiformis fusiformis*.

Pediatric Gastroenterology and Hepatology

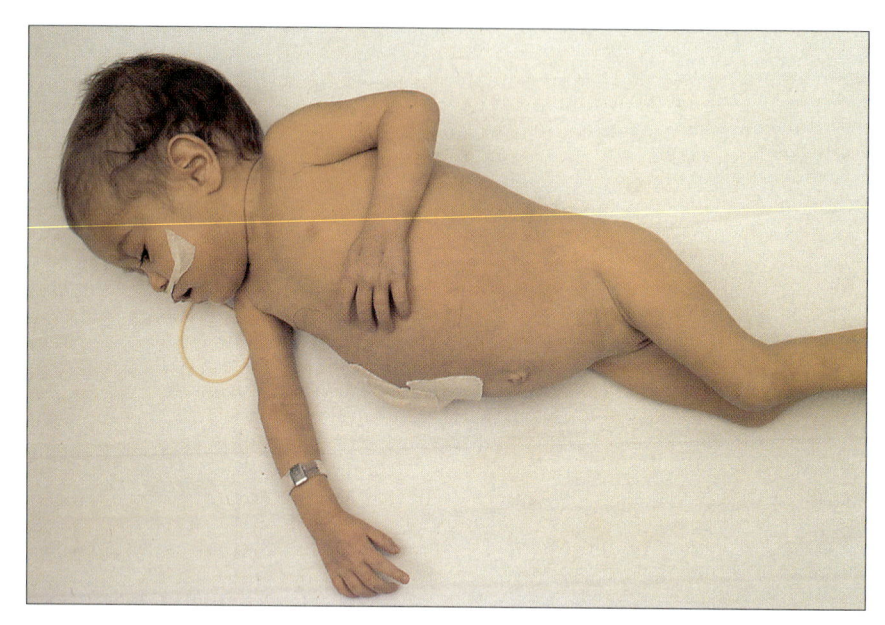

Fig. 17.13 Cholestatic liver disease. Fat malabsorption from any cause leads to loss of fat stores and fat-soluble vitamin deficiency. This may be particularly severe in cholestatic liver disease, as in this 11-month-old baby with biliary atresia and a failed Kasai portoenterostomy, who had severe cholestasis, loss of fat stores, and muscle wasting.

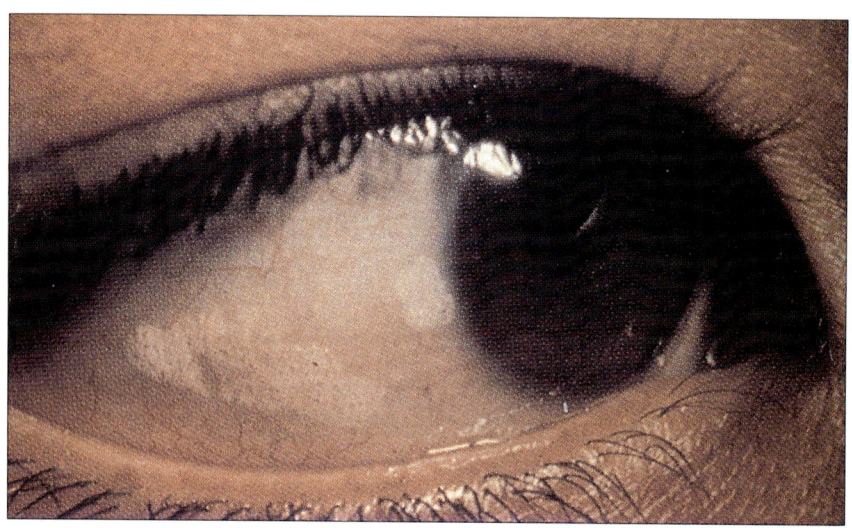

Figs 17.14, 17.15 Vitamin A deficiency. Vitamin A deficiency is the most common cause of blindness in the developing world. Initially, deficiency causes night blindness and conjunctival xerosis (Bitot's spots) (**17.14**, middle). Untreated corneal xerosis and ulceration leads to keratomalacia (**17.15**, bottom). Vitamin A deficiency leading to night blindness is also a feature of severe cholestatic liver disease.

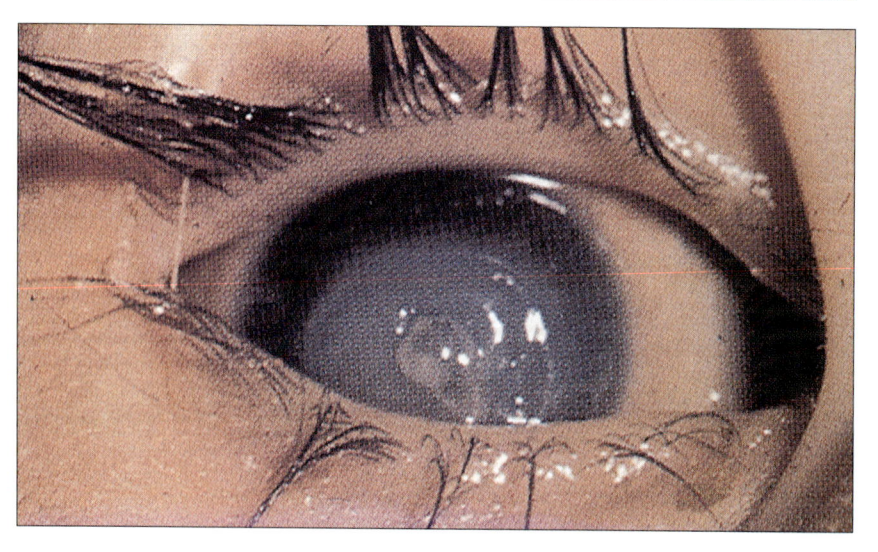

Nutrition

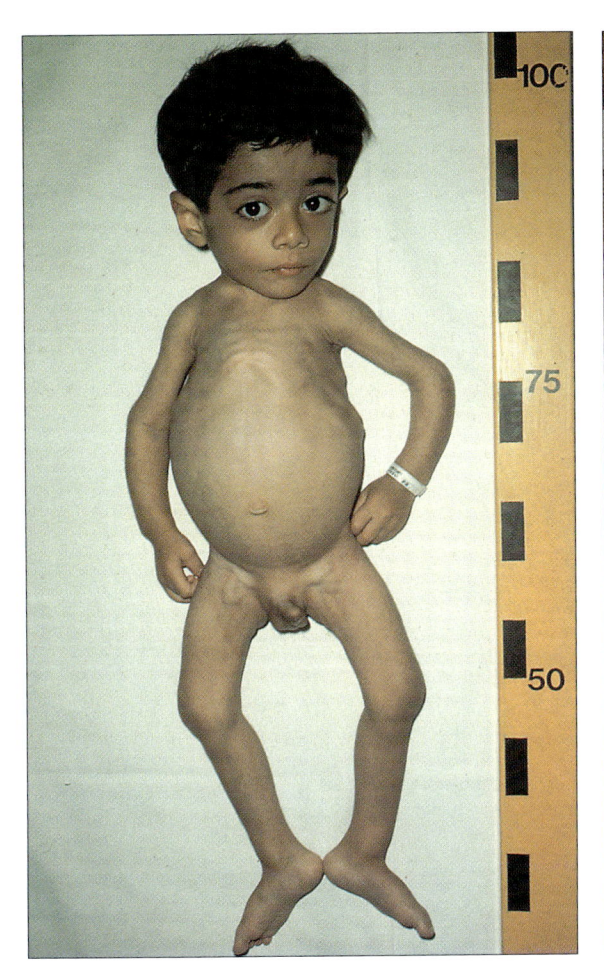

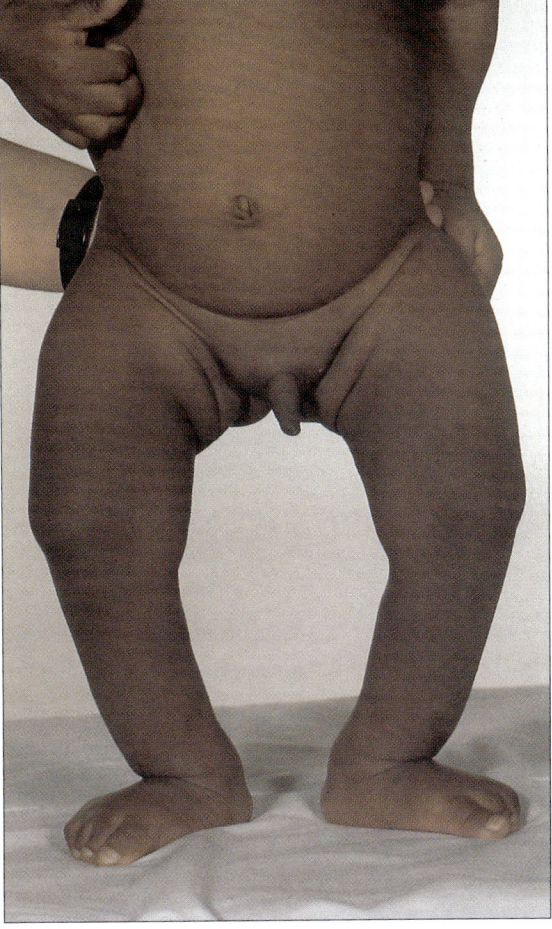

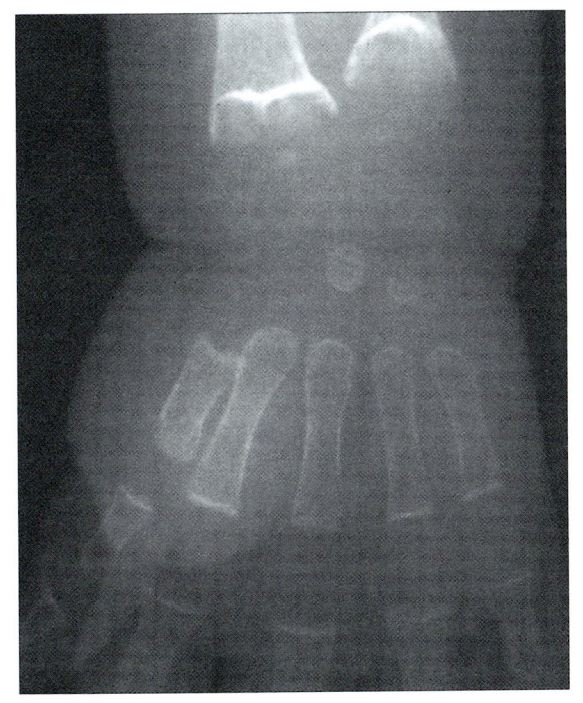

Figs 17.16–17.18 Vitamin D deficiency. Vitamin D deficiency secondary to malabsorption, liver disease, or renal tubular acidosis leads to rickets, with rickety rosary and frontal bossing, Harrison's sulcus (**17.16**, top left) and bowed legs (**17.17**, top right). The radiograph changes are best observed at the wrist, which demonstrates widening and cupping of the metaphyseal plates and osteoporosis (**17.18**, bottom).

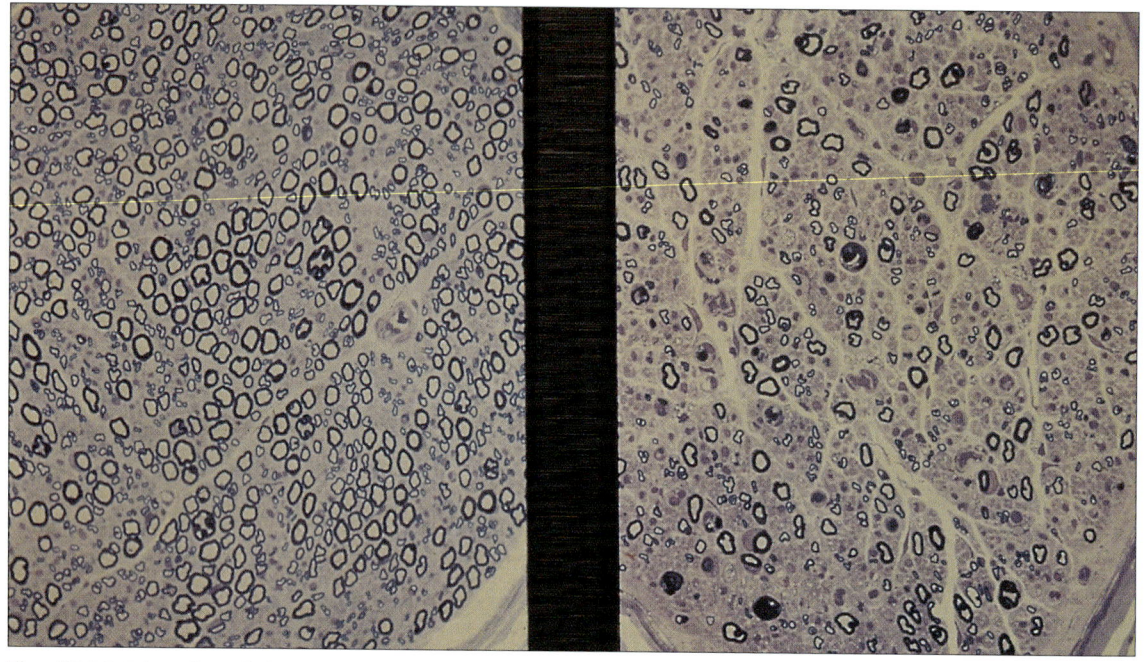

Fig. 17.19 Vitamin E deficiency Vitamin E deficiency is common in cystic fibrosis and cholestatic liver disease, and is especially severe in abetalipoproteinaemia. Deficiency causes a haemolytic anaemia, pigmentary retinopathy, and ataxic neuropathy. Shown here are the reduced numbers of large fibres and dying neurones (right; normal nerve is shown on the left). Axonal degeneration and secondary demyelination are also prominent histological features. Clinically, these changes are associated with ataxia, absent tendon reflexes, delayed motor nerve conduction velocities, pigmentary retinopathy, and abnormal retinal function.

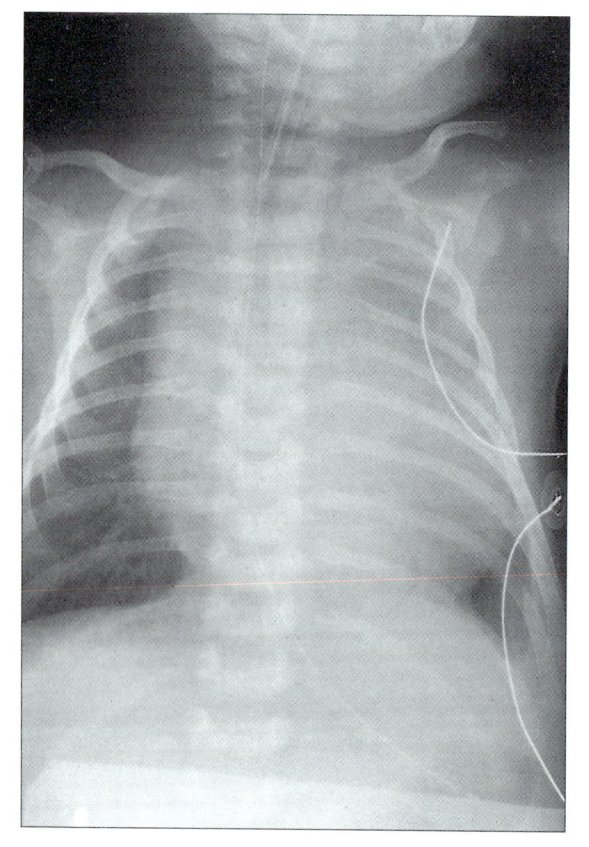

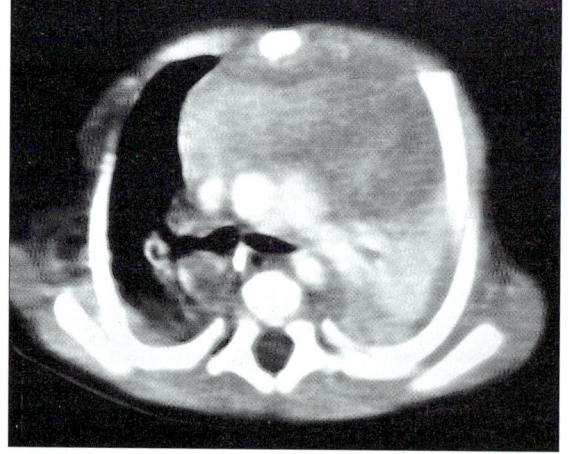

Figs 17.20, 17.21 Vitamin K deficiency. Vitamin K deficiency from fat malabsorption may be exacerbated by underlying liver disease. Clinical symptoms include increased bruising, epistaxis, and intracerebral haemorrhage. Late haemorrhagic disease of the newborn (vitamin K responsive coagulopathy) may develop in breast-fed babies who did not receive prophylactic vitamin K at birth. This 5-week-old baby presented with bruising and sudden collapse secondary to haemorrhage into his thymus gland. The chest radiograph demonstrates the increase in size of the thymus gland (**17.20**, left), while the CT scan confirms that this was due to haemorrhage (**17.21**, right). He was subsequently found to have liver disease from biliary atresia.

Nutrition

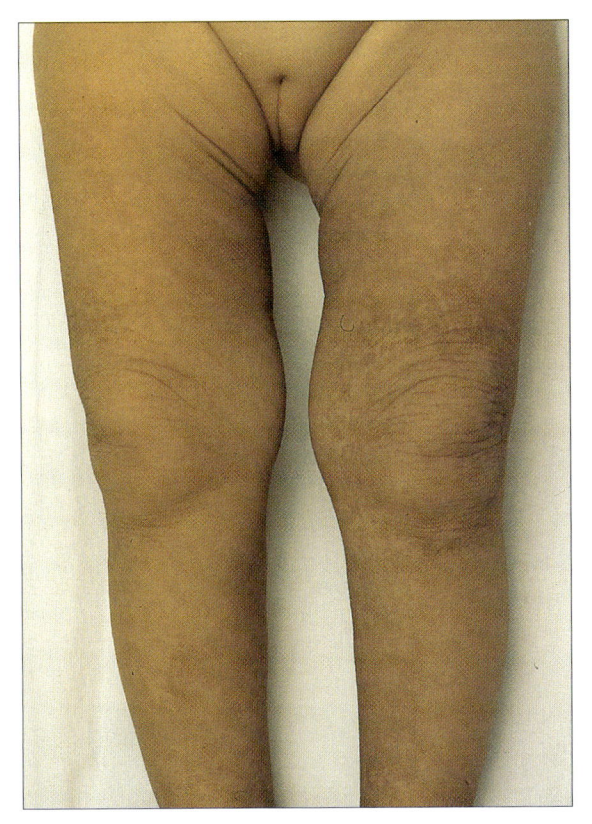

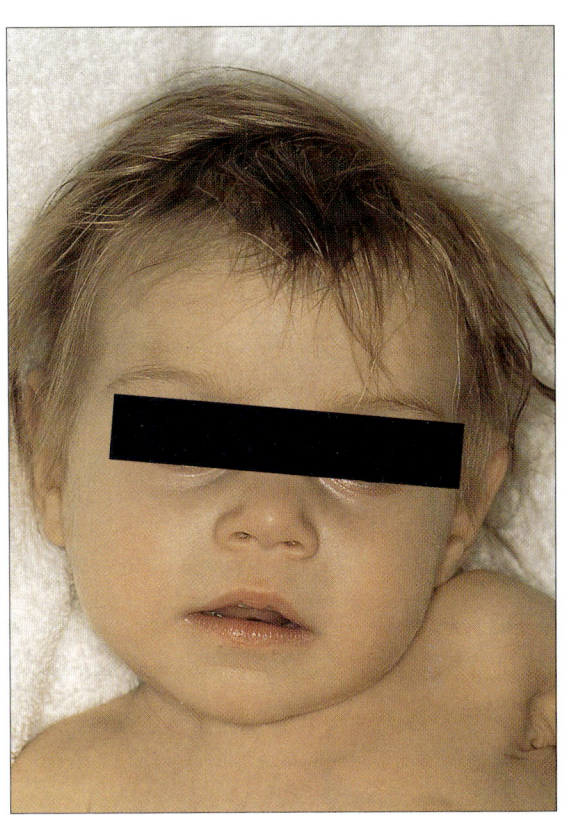

Figs 17.22, 17.23 Essential fatty acid deficiency Essential fatty acid deficiency is common in pre-term babies and children with chronic liver disease. There may be a hyperkeratotic skin rash (**17.22**, left) and brittle hair (**17.23**, right). Both these children with chronic liver disease were fed infant formulas, which contained 80% medium-chain triglyceride, 20% long-chain triglyceride, and an insufficient concentration of essential fatty acids.

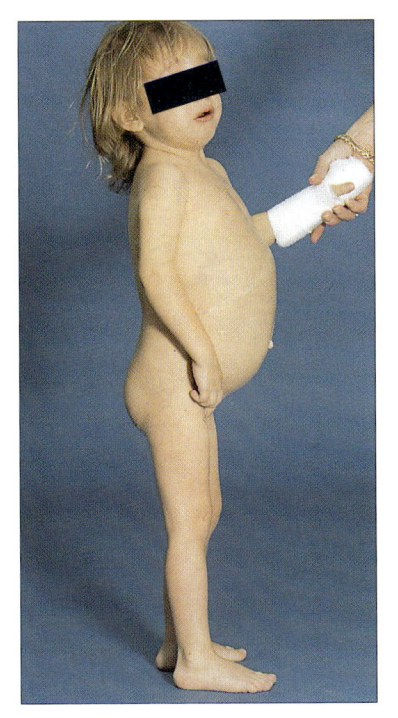

Fig. 17.24 Severe malnutrition. The nutritional status of children with liver disease is difficult to assess because their weight can be increased due to ascites. Severe malnutrition may be present with mild jaundice, as in this 3-year-old girl with biliary atresia and a failed Kasai portoenterostomy. She has obvious abdominal distension secondary to ascites, marked muscle wasting, and loss of fat stores.

Pediatric Gastroenterology and Hepatology

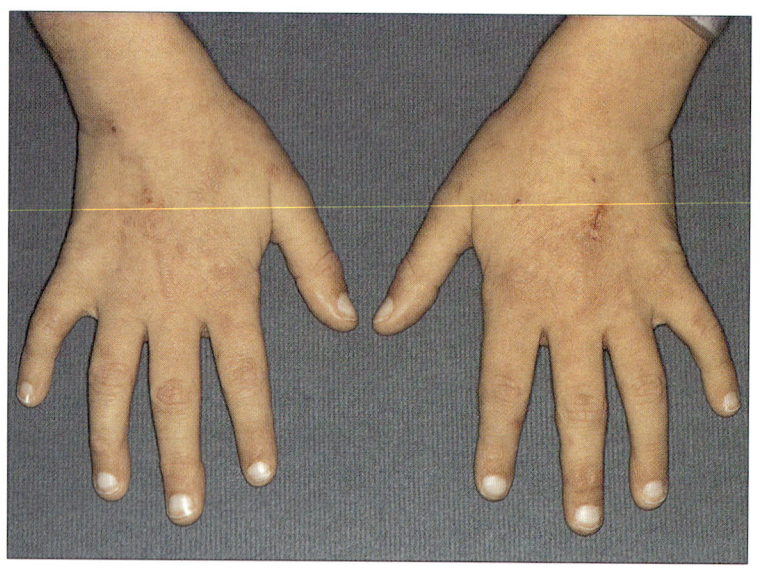

Fig. 17.25 Hypoalbuminaemia. A reduction in hepatic protein synthesis leads to hypoalbuminaemia, which may be indicated by white nails, as in this child with severe cholestasis and pruritus.

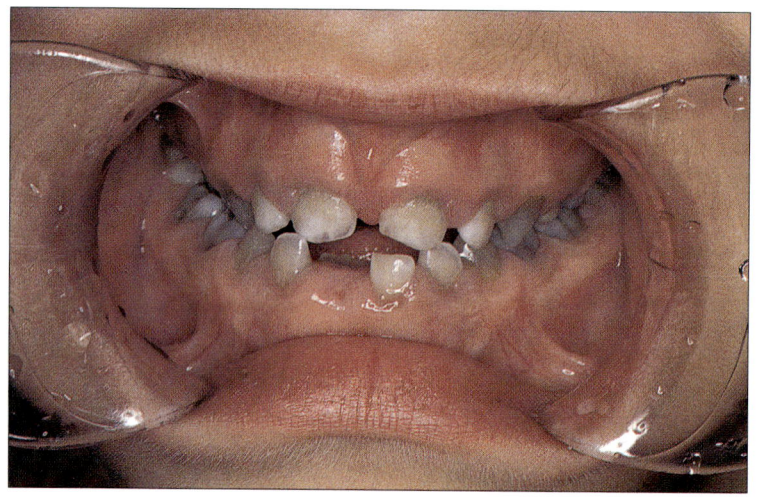

Fig. 17.26 Dysplastic teeth. Children with chronic malnutrition from any cause may have dysplastic teeth, which may be small and abnormal in shape. If associated with a chronic liver disease the teeth can also be green from deposition of bilirubin. Gingival hyperplasia may be secondary to poor hygiene.

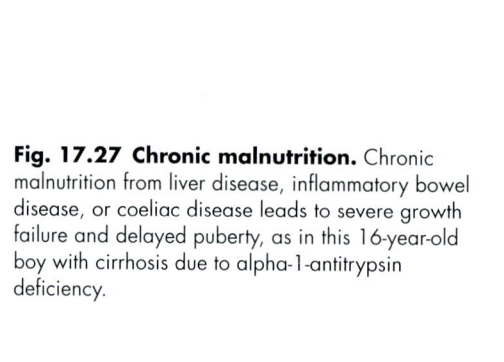

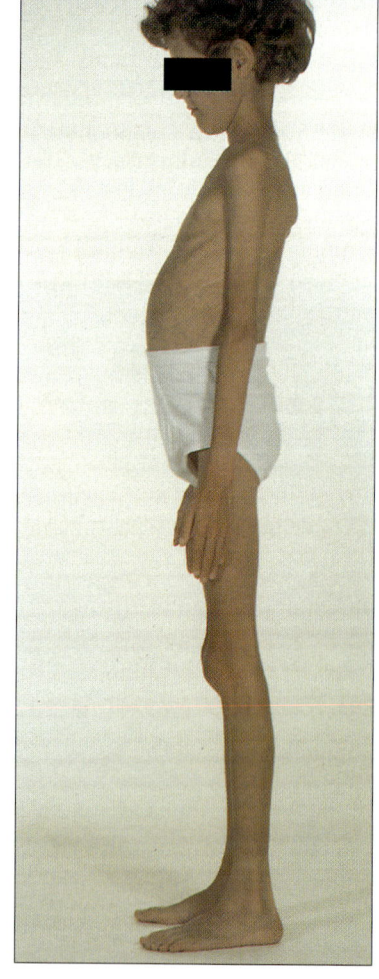

Fig. 17.27 Chronic malnutrition. Chronic malnutrition from liver disease, inflammatory bowel disease, or coeliac disease leads to severe growth failure and delayed puberty, as in this 16-year-old boy with cirrhosis due to alpha-1-antitrypsin deficiency.

WATER SOLUBLE VITAMINS

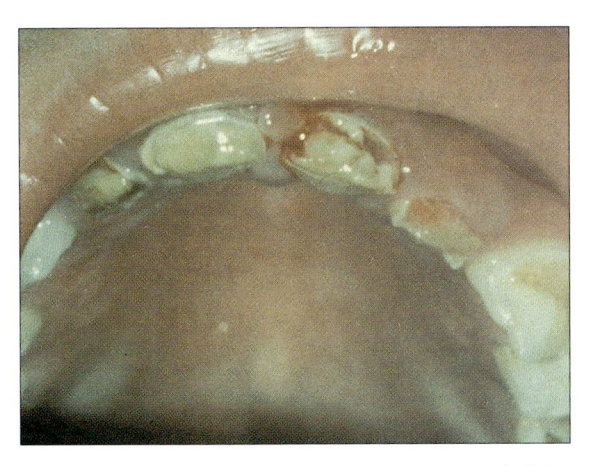

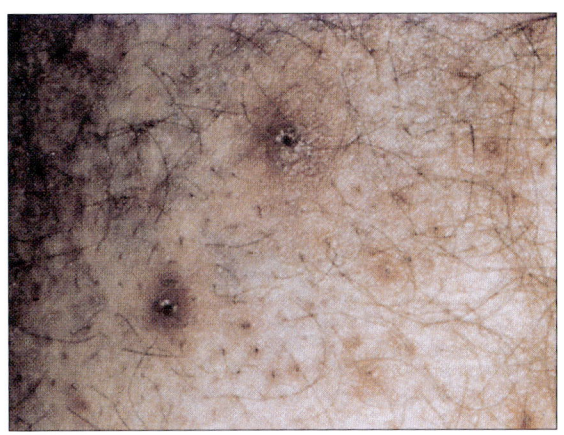

Figs 17.28, 17.29 Ascorbic acid (vitamin C) deficiency. Ascorbic acid (vitamin C) deficiency may occur in pre-term babies fed pooled pasteurised human milk, or in association with severe urban deprivation or food faddism. Clinical features include bleeding at the site of tooth eruption (**17.28**, left), hyperkeratosis of hair follicles, and petechiae (**17.29**, right).

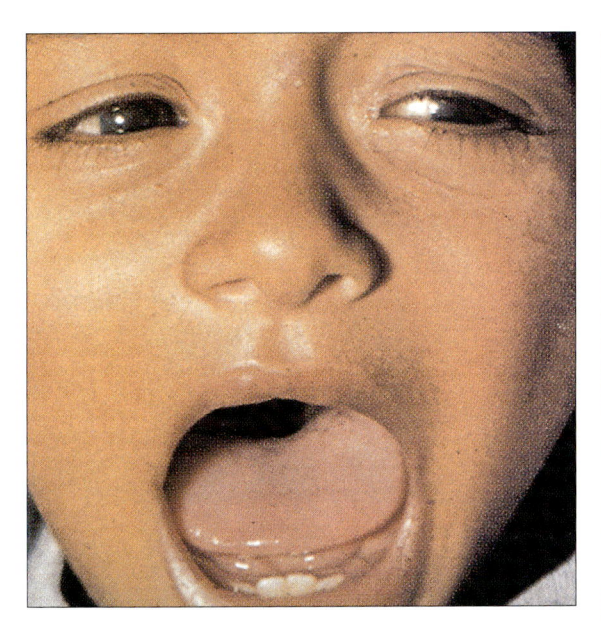

Fig. 17.30 Riboflavin deficiency. Deficiency of riboflavin usually occurs with malnutrition and is associated with deficiencies of other vitamins. Clinical features comprise angular stomatitis and a magenta tongue.

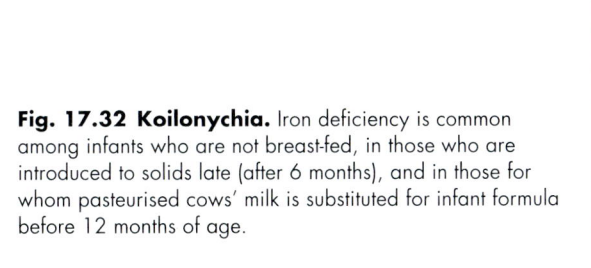

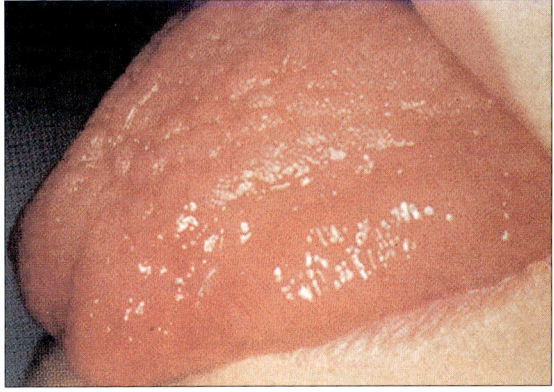

Fig. 17.31 Vitamin B$_{12}$ deficiency. Vitamin B$_{12}$ deficiency presents with a megaloblastic anaemia, angular stomatitis, glossitis, and subacute combined degeneration of the spinal cord.

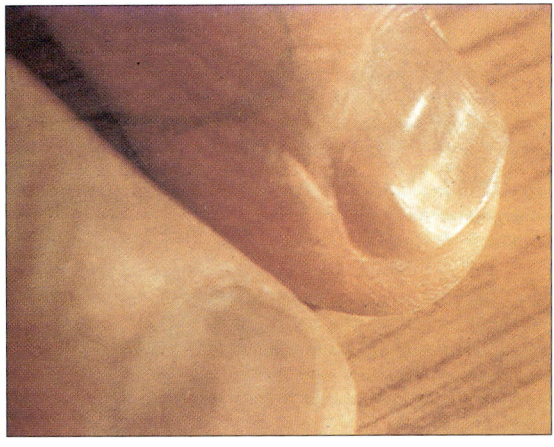

Fig. 17.32 Koilonychia. Iron deficiency is common among infants who are not breast-fed, in those who are introduced to solids late (after 6 months), and in those for whom pasteurised cows' milk is substituted for infant formula before 12 months of age.

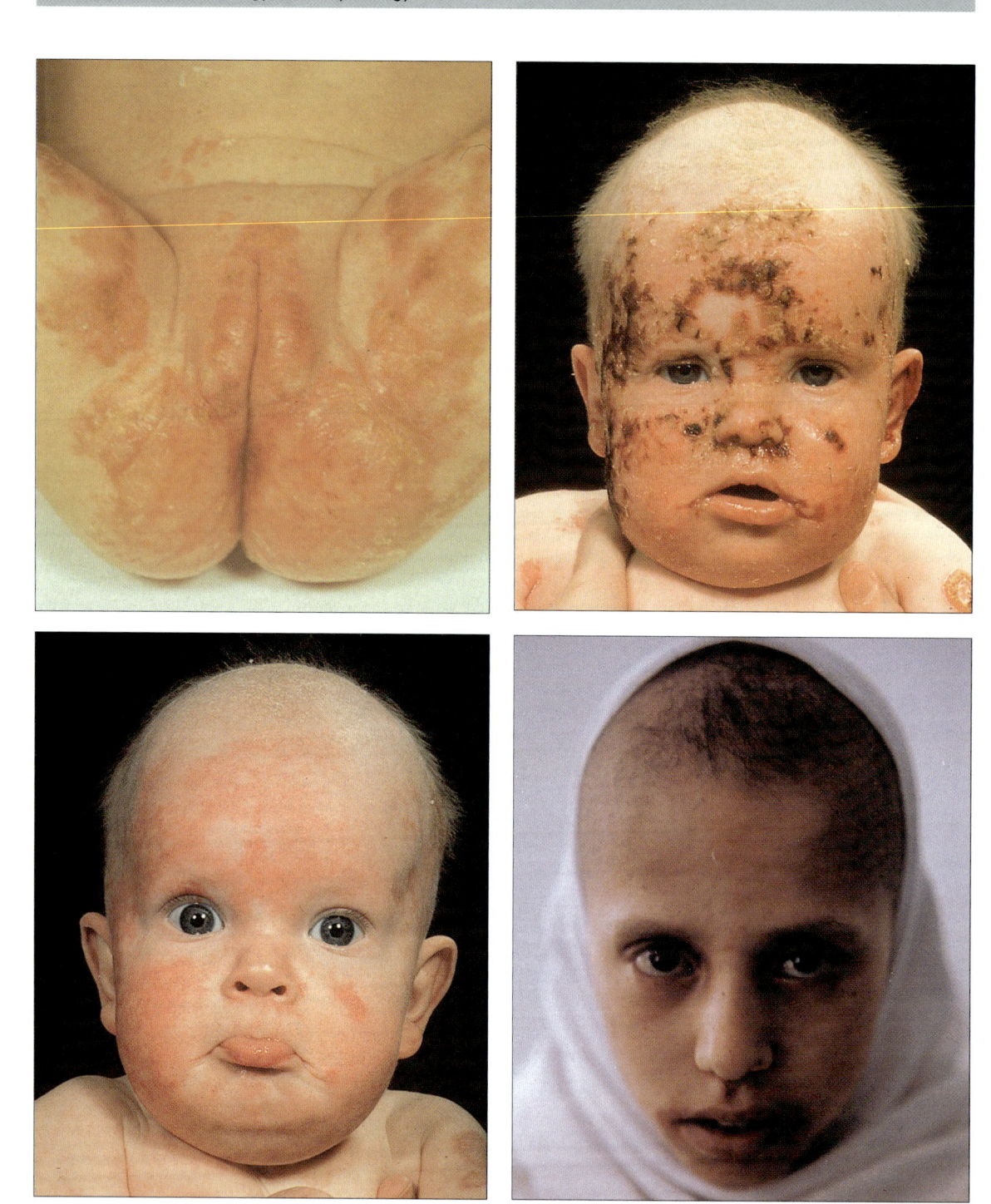

Figs 17.33–17.36 Acrodermatitis enteropathica. This is a recessively inherited specific defect in the intestinal absorption of zinc. It is characterised by the onset in infancy of the features of zinc deficiency. The characteristic skin rash appears in the first few months of life and consists of symmetrical, scaling erythematous lesions around the mouth, perianal area, and elbows (**17.33**, top left). The affected patients develop diarrhoea, alopecia, and failure to thrive. Intercurrent infections are common and over half the children have monilial infection. Dystrophic nails and stomatitis are frequent. Breast-feeding is protective, probably because of a zinc-binding ligand in breast milk. If untreated the disease is usually fatal in later childhood. Plasma zinc is low (less than 6 mmol/litre) and is associated with low plasma alkaline phosphatase activity. Life-long treatment with oral zinc (30–45 mg elemental zinc per day) is curative. This baby showed remarkable improvement after 2 weeks of zinc treatment (**17.34**, top right; **17.35**, bottom left). When the diagnosis is delayed, severe alopecia is a marked feature, as in this 10-year-old who had had diarrhoea and a skin rash from infancy (**17.36**, bottom right).

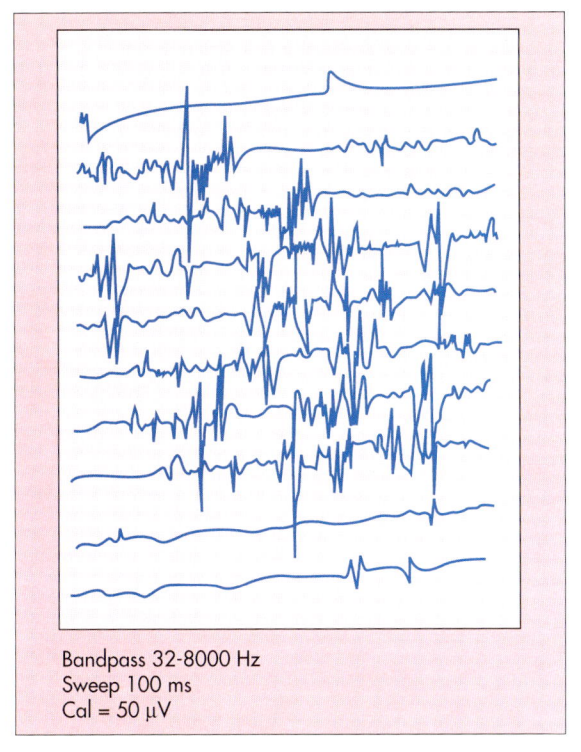

Figs 17.37, 17.38 Selenium deficiency. Selenium is detected in all food, including breast milk. Deficiency states may arise either from poor intake in areas of low soil selenium or secondary to prolonged parenteral or enteral nutrition. This 21-month-old girl developed a tender skeletal myopathy while on home parenteral nutrition. Her electromyogram showed increased polyphasia and reduced amplitude of potentials (**17.37**, top left), while the muscle biopsy (**17.38**, top right) showed a normal fibre-type distribution with non-specific atrophy of Type II fibres. At her age, both Type I and Type II fibres should be uniform in size. Plasma selenium was very low while red blood cell glutathione peroxidase was undetectable. She made a complete recovery following replacement therapy with intravenous sodium selenide.

Fig. 17.39 Taurine deficiency. Children who receive long-term total parenteral nutrition (TPN) seem to be at particular risk of developing clinical taurine deficiency. Abnormal retinograms have been found in association with biochemical taurine deficiency. This electroretinogram shows a delay in the implicit time of the B wave in three parenterally fed children, which was subsequently reversed with appropriate taurine supplementation.

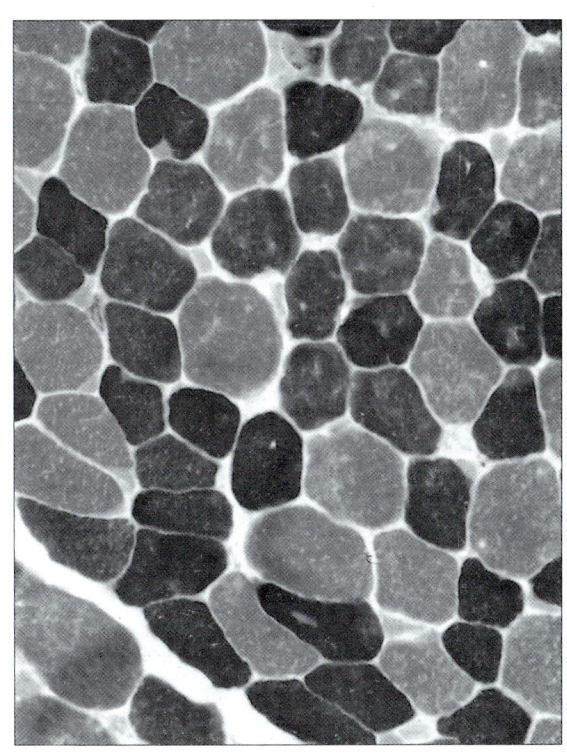

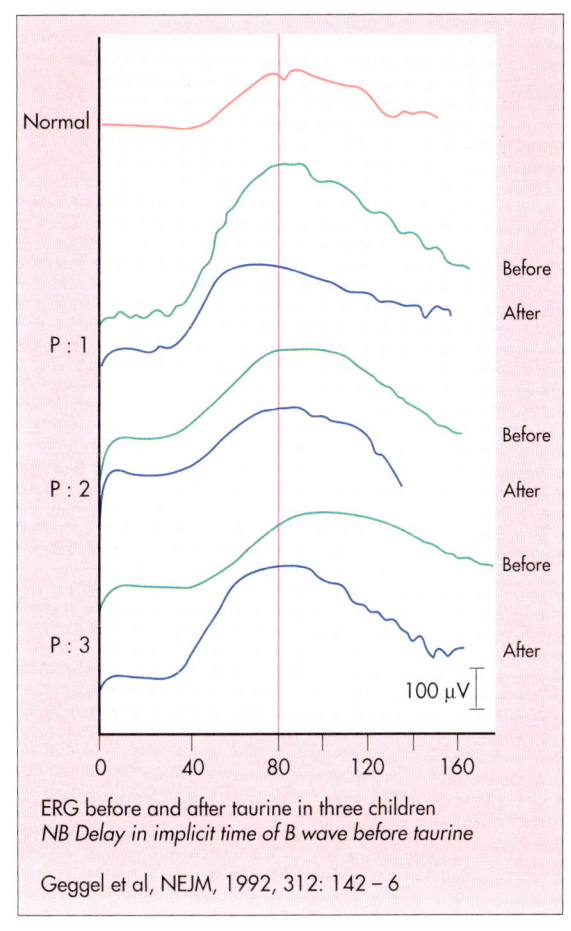

ERG before and after taurine in three children
NB Delay in implicit time of B wave before taurine

Geggel et al, NEJM, 1992, 312: 142 – 6

NUTRITIONAL THERAPY

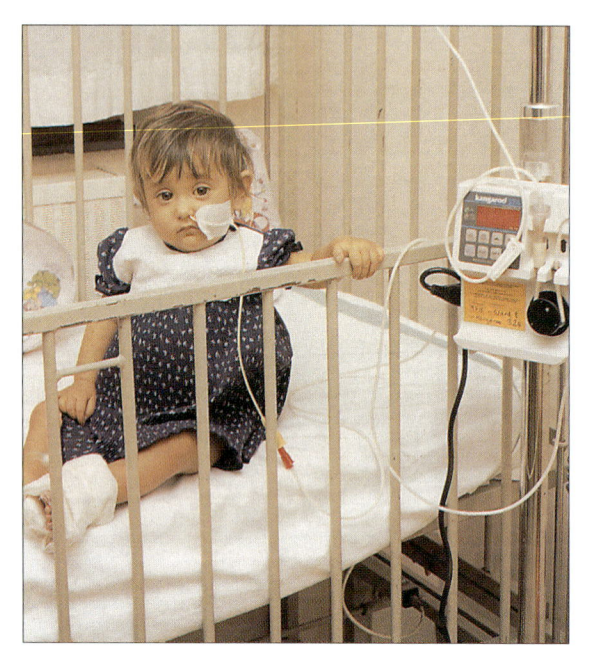

Fig. 17.40 Nutritional therapy. The primary aim of nutritional therapy is not only to provide sufficient energy for basal metabolism, but to provide sufficient intake for catch-up growth and the correction of nutritional deficiency. It is usually possible to treat malnutrition secondary to renal, cardiac, and liver disease and most intestinal disease through enteral feeding.

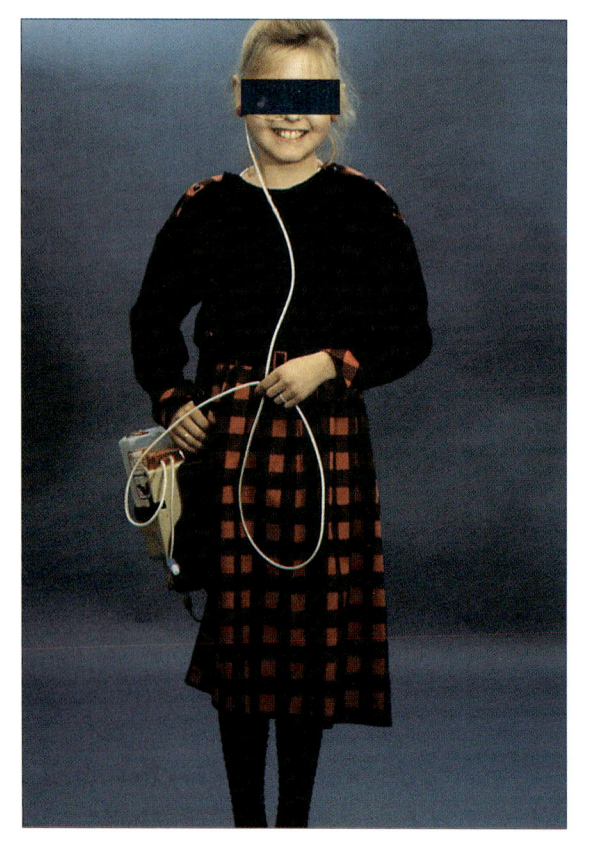

Fig. 17.41 Enteral feeding. Enteral feeding is commonly provided by a nasogastric tube, either as a nocturnal infusion (over 12 hours) supplemented by boluses during the day, or by continuous 24-hour enteral infusion. This is surprisingly well-tolerated and can be administered using portable pumps. Enteral feeding may be successfully managed at home and in the community although it is essential that parents and children are adequately informed and properly trained.

Nutrition

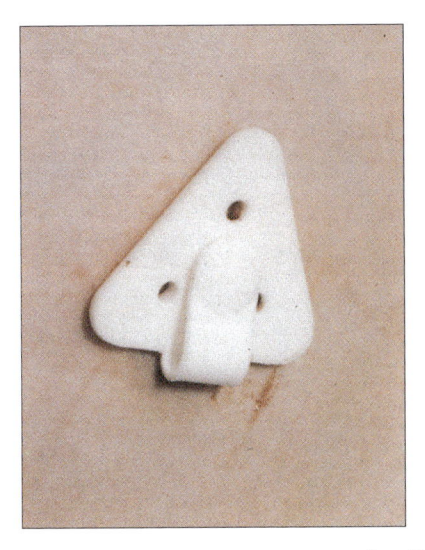

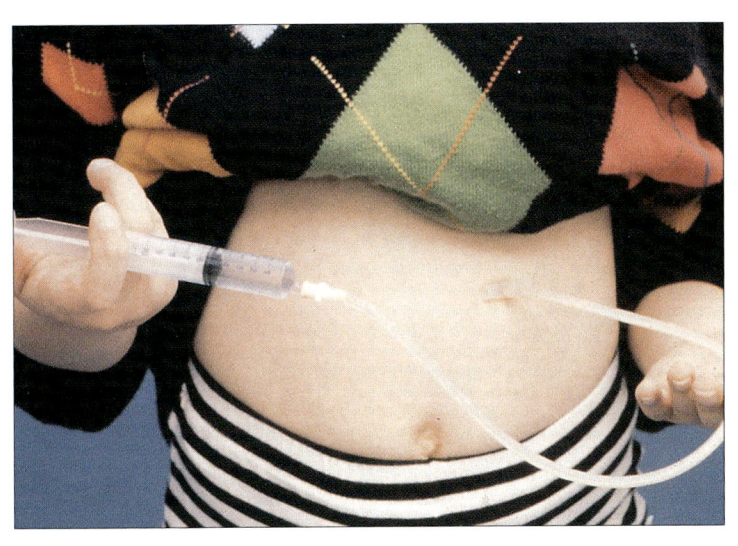

Figs 17.42, 17.43 Gastrostomy feeding. If enteral feeding is likely to be prolonged and there are no specific contraindications, e.g. gastric varices, then gastrostomy feeding is preferred. Shown here is a button gastrostomy which has been endoscopically placed (**17.42**, left). The young girl in **17.43** (right) manages her own feeds.

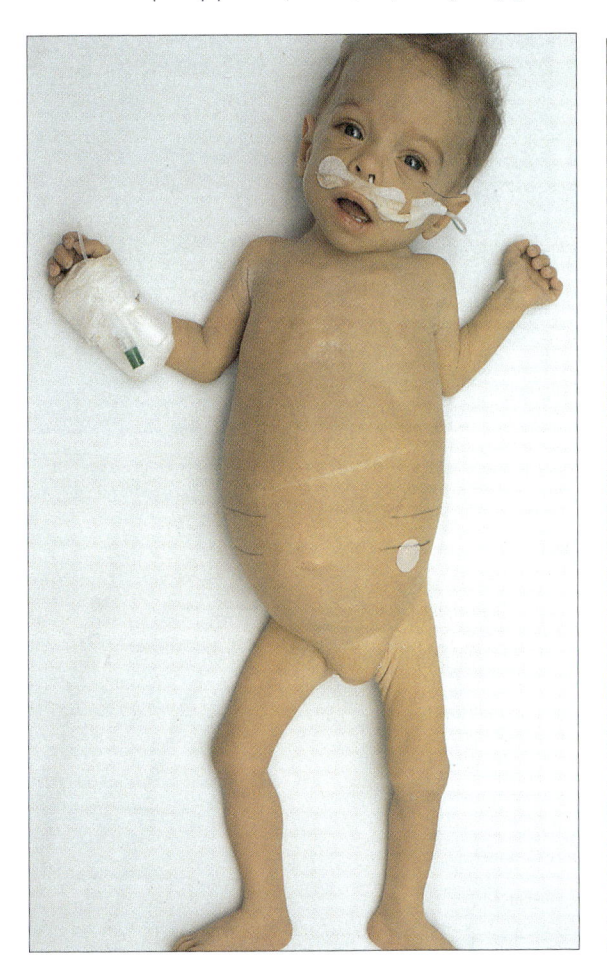

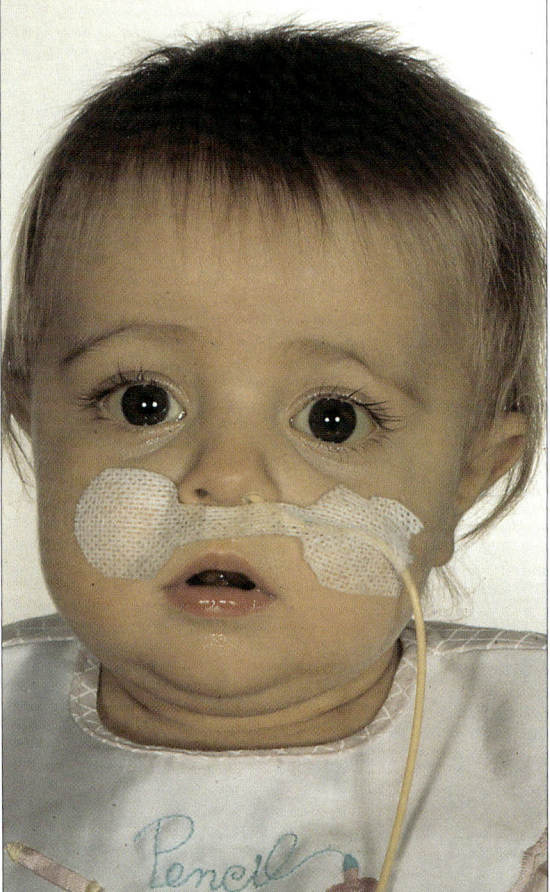

Figs 17.44, 17.45 Results. The results of enteral feeding may be dramatic. This baby with severe liver disease (**17.44**, left) was successfully rehabilitated using nocturnal enteral feeding with a modified formula containing a low salt protein with 50/50 medium-chain and long-chain triglycerides and a high energy intake (**17.45**, right).

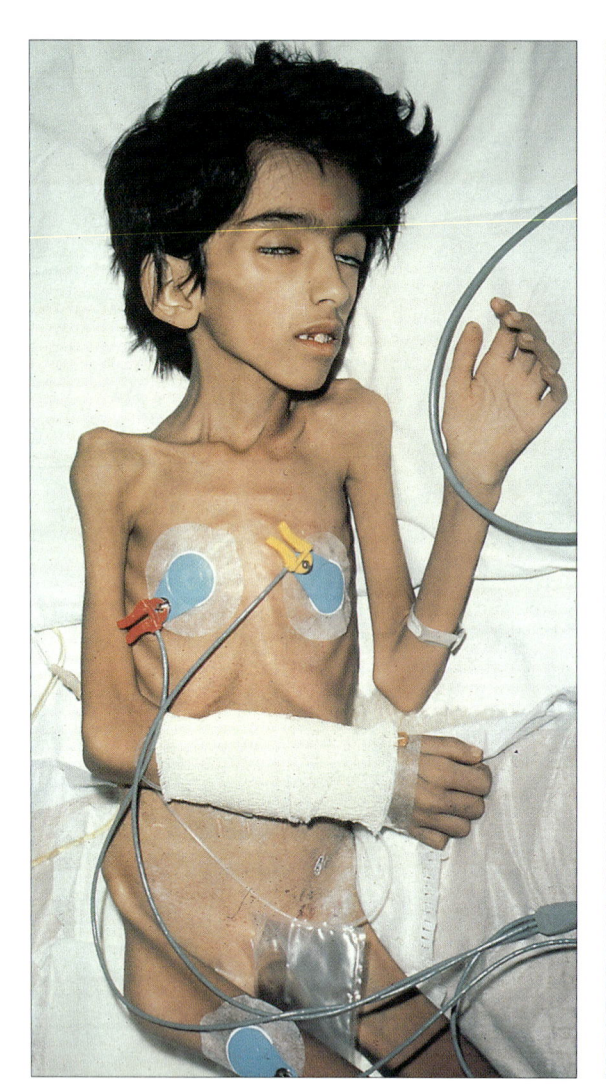

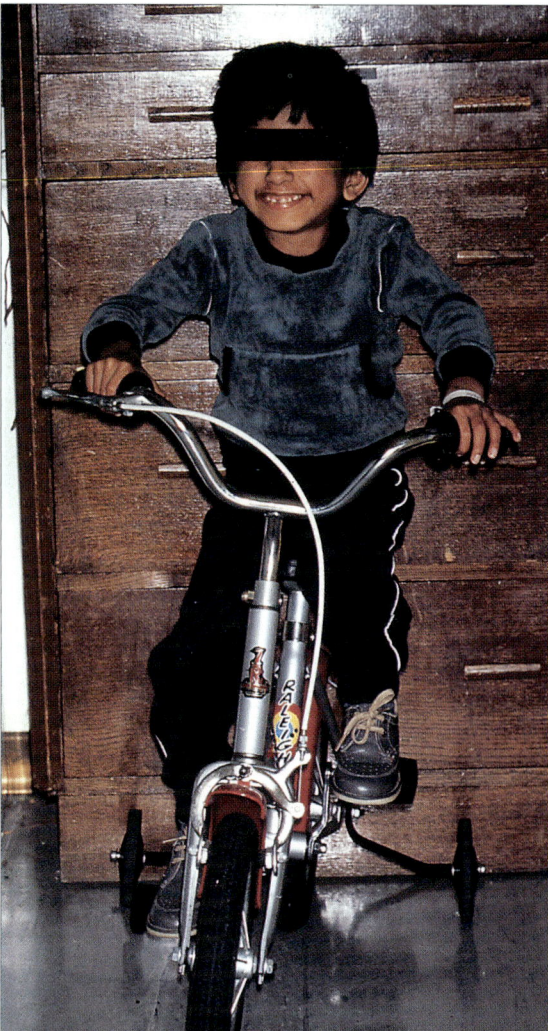

Figs 17.46, 17.47 Parenteral nutrition. The successful development of parenteral nutrition (PN) has dramatically transformed the management of severe malnutrition, as in this boy with intestinal failure seen here before treatment (**17.46**, left) and 4 months later (**17.47**, right).

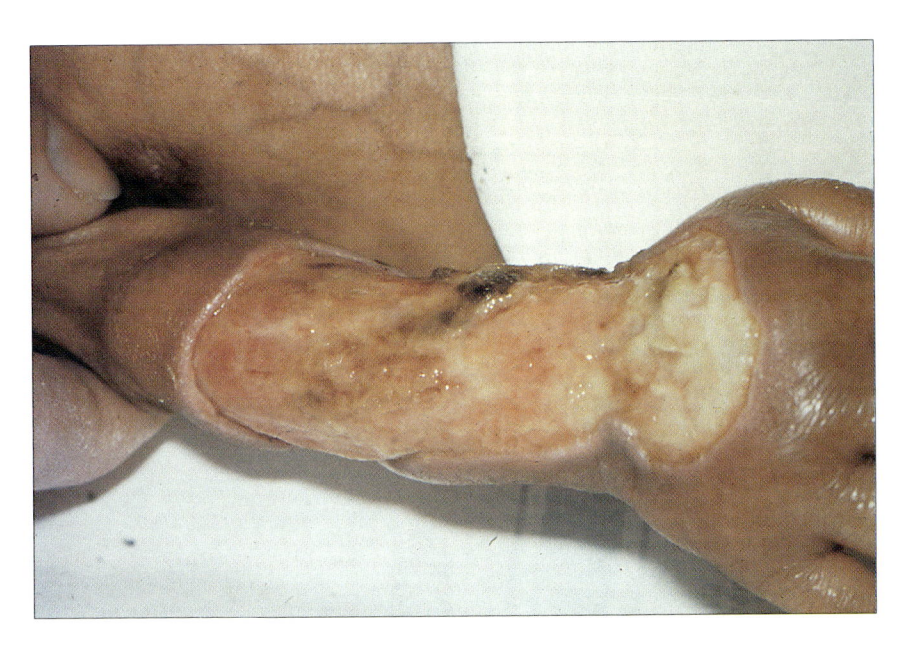

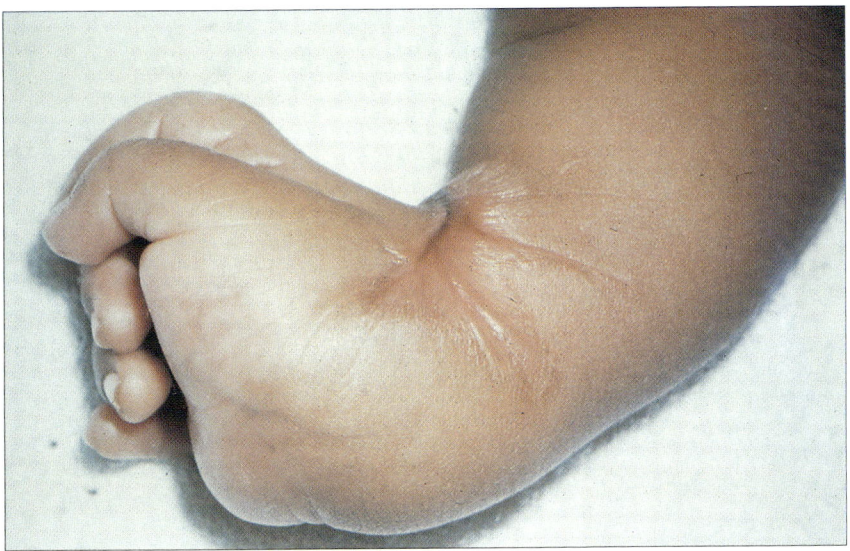

Figs 17.48, 17.49 Peripheral vein PN complications. It is preferable to use a central vein to deliver PN in order to provide sufficient calories. Here are shown the results of extravasation of PN from a peripheral vein, causing necrosis of the subcutaneous tissue and muscle (**17.48**, top) leading to a severe extension deformity (**17.49**, bottom).

Pediatric Gastroenterology and Hepatology

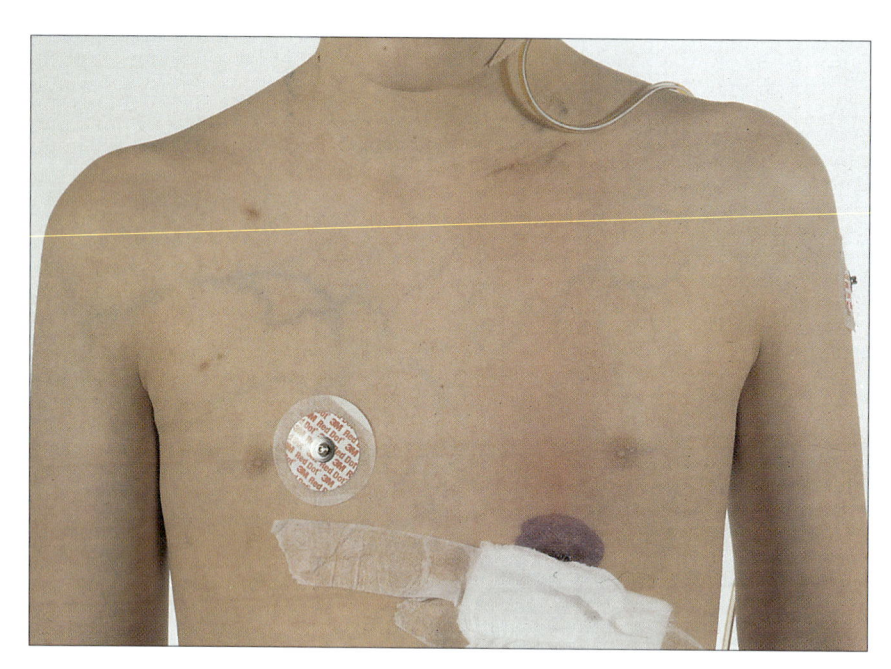

Fig. 17.50 Cellulitis. Despite the many benefits of PN there are significant complications, such as this cellulitis around a tunnelled line. In contrast to infection in the intravascular part of the catheter, sepsis in the tunnel almost invariably fails to respond to antibiotic treatment. Lines infected in this way frequently need removal.

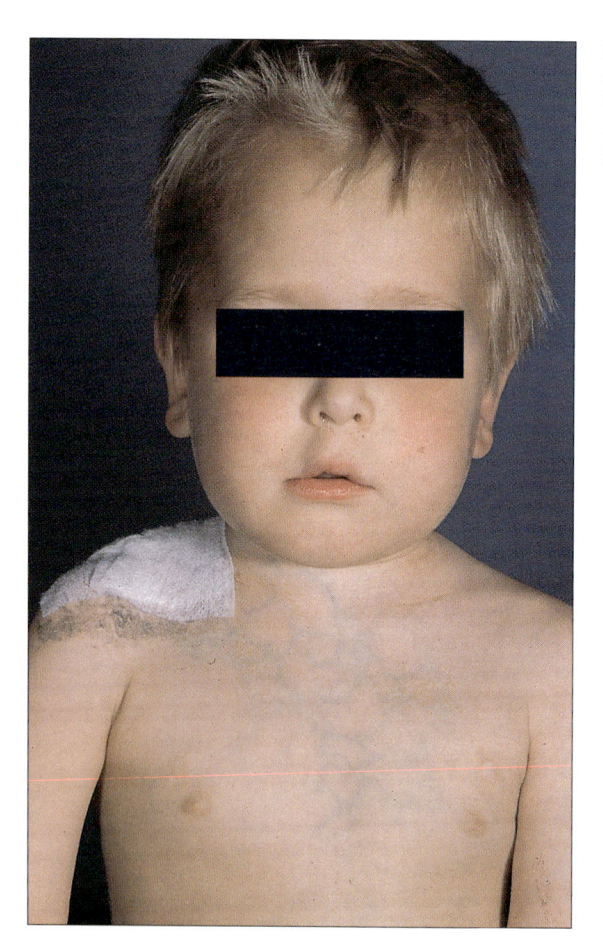

Fig. 17.51 Thrombosis. There is a significant incidence of thrombosis of the central veins. This boy with intestinal failure secondary to short-gut syndrome developed superior vena caval (SVC) obstruction which necessitated removal of the line.

Nutrition

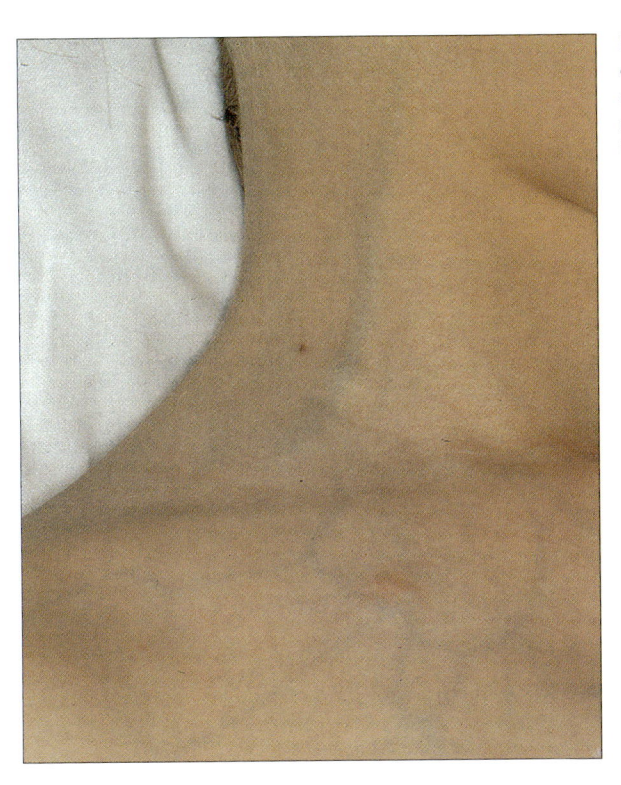

Figs 17.52, 17.53 Superior vena caval obstruction. The local signs of SVC obstruction are dilated veins (**17.52**, top) which may be confirmed radiologically (**17.53**, bottom) using contrast medium injected into the central line.

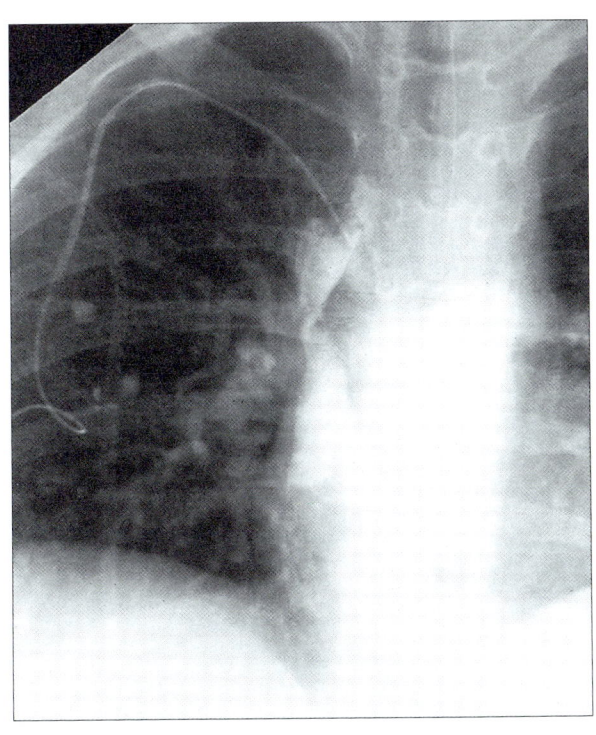

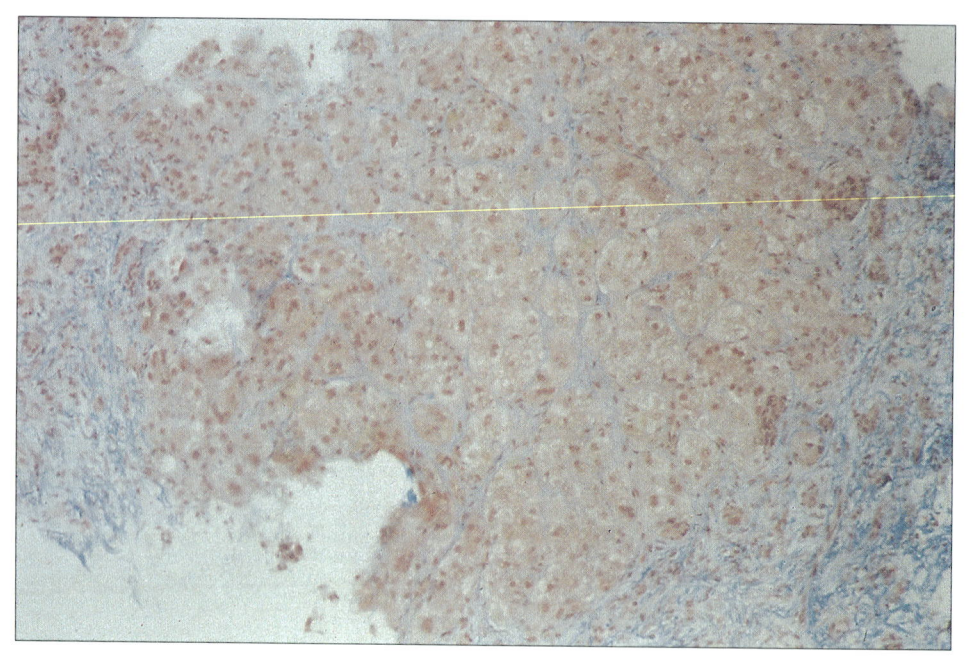

Fig. 17.54 Total parenteral nutrition (TPN) liver disease. TPN liver disease is almost inevitable and occurs in more than 40% of children who are parenterally fed for more than 2 years. The aetiology of TPN cholestasis is unknown, but the incidence is highest in pre-term babies who are maintained on TPN because of gut resection or difficulties in enteral feeding and who have recurrent episodes of sepsis. Biochemical features reflect conjugated hyperbilirubinaemia with transaminitis and a high alkaline phosphatase. The liver histology demonstrates fatty change, cholestasis with bile plugs, pseudorosettes, regression of portal tract fibrosis, and expansion with a lymphocytic inflammatory infiltrate. Bile duct re-duplication may be present. Histological and clinical changes are reversible once TPN has stopped and normal enteral feeding is resumed. Progressive TPN liver disease is an indication for liver and small bowel transplantation. (Masson Trichrome, ×10.)

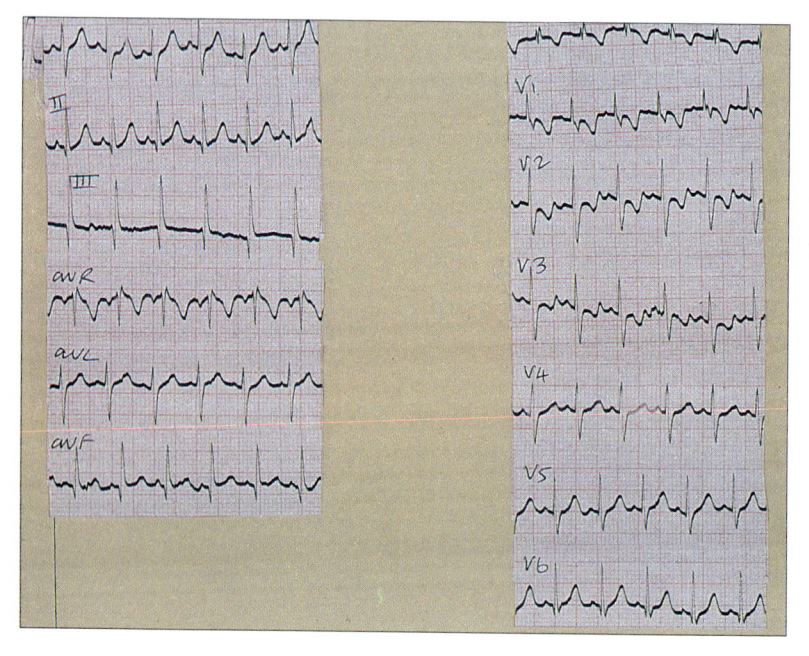

Fig. 17.55 Pulmonary embolism. Pulmonary embolism is the most recently described complication of PN and has led to sudden death in a number of children on long-term PN. The features of pulmonary embolism are demonstrated in this electrocardiogram, which has a prominent S wave in lead 1 (>1.5 mm), a Q wave in lead III, and a T wave inversion. Echocardiography may indicate right ventricular strain with an increase in end-diastolic diameter.

Nutrition

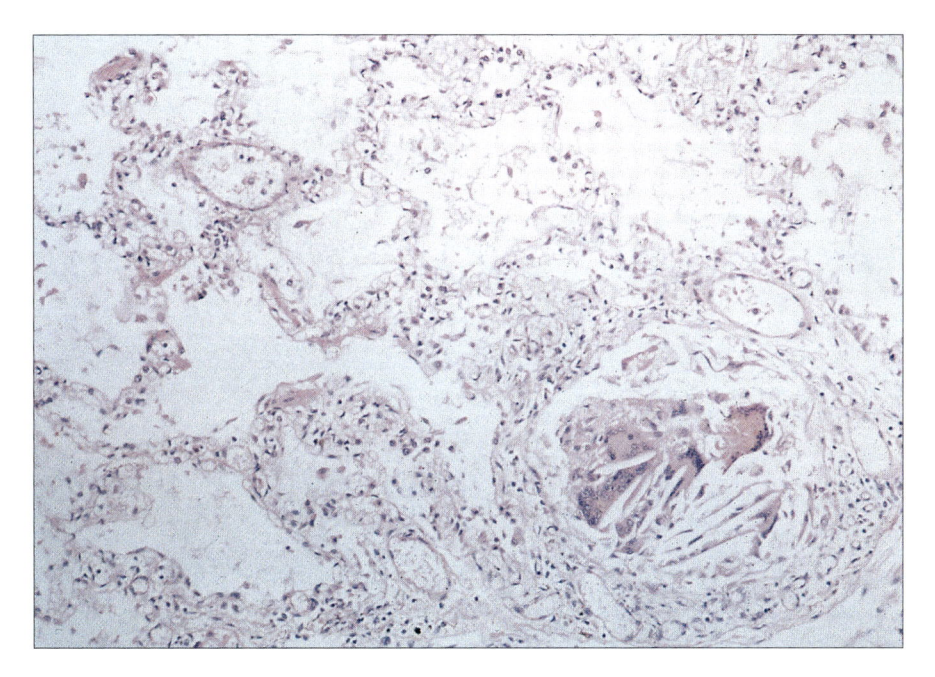

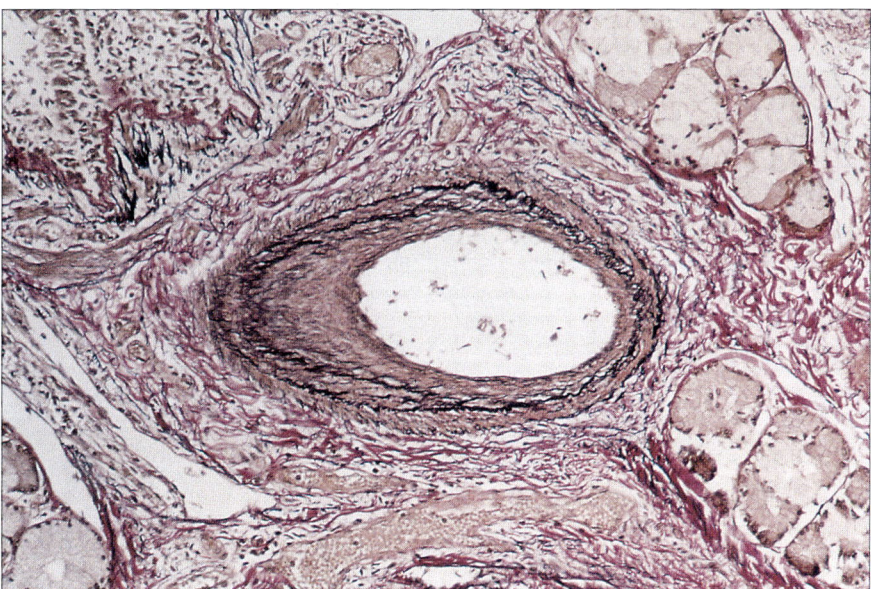

Figs 17.56, 17.57 Pulmonary thromboembolism. This child with intestinal failure and long-term PN died following a respiratory illness. Post-mortem sections of the lung showed multiple lipid emboli with residual cholesterol clefts (**17.56**, top, Haematoxylin and Eosin, ×25), pulmonary vascular muscular hypertrophy consistent with mild pulmonary hypertension, and intimal proliferation in large blood vessels indicating recurrent pulmonary thromboembolism (**17.57**, bottom, Haematoxylin and Eosin, ×40).

Pediatric Gastroenterology and Hepatology

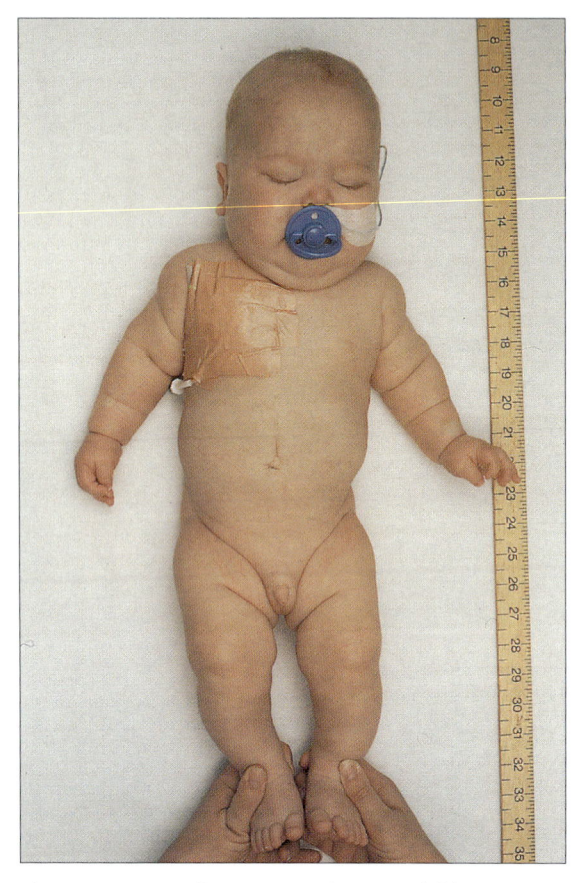

Fig. 17.58 Poor linear growth. Many children on PN have a rapid growth of fat and muscle, but little linear growth, as in this child with short-gut syndrome who was parenterally fed from birth. The reasons for poor linear growth are uncertain, but may include rickets and phosphate or aluminium toxicity.

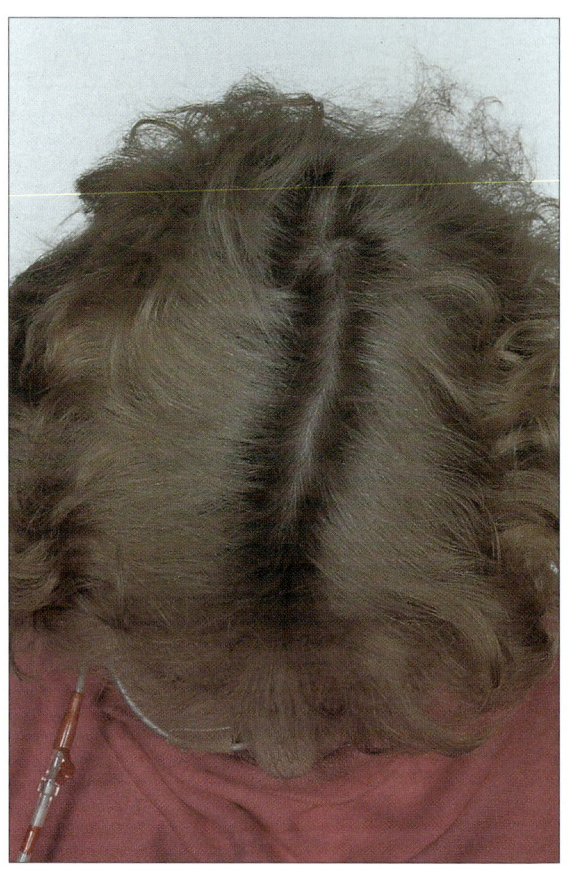

Fig. 17.59 The 'flag' sign. As malnutrition improves, the 'flag' sign may be seen. Here the dark normal hair is growing from the roots and replacing the older depigmented hair.

Index

Abdominal distension
  air swallowing 71
  coeliac disease 33, 36
  congenital secretory diarrhoea 41
  cows' milk intolerance 36
  cystic fibrosis 83
  Hirschsprung's disease 15
  malnutrition 157
  mesenteric cyst 13
  peritoneal mesothelioma 78
  VIP-secreting ganglioneuroblastoma 76
Abdominal pain, recurrent 73–74
  pancreatitis 80, 81
Abetalipoproteinaemia 42–43
Acetylcholinesterase staining 14
N-Acetylcysteine 83
Achalasia 20
Acrodermatitis enteropathica 160
Adenocarcinoma, small intestine 76
Adenoviruses 52
Air swallowing 71
Alagille's syndrome 103–105
Alopecia 160
Alper's disease (progressive neuronal degeneration with liver disease) 112, 136
Alpha-1-antitrypsin deficiency 99–100
Alphafetoprotein 101
Amylo-1,6-glucosidase deficiency 111
Anderson's disease 47
Angular cheilitis 58
Angular stomatitis 159
Ankyloglossia 72
Ankylosing spondylitis 61
Anorexia nervosa 150
Anthropometry 149
Arthritis, juvenile chronic 135
Ascites
  cirrhosis 121
  intestinal lymphangiectasia 152
  peritoneal mesothelioma 78
Ascorbic acid deficiency 159
Aspirin 29
Atresia
  biliary see Biliary atresia
  duodenal 10
  jejunal 11
  oesophageal 19
  rectal 12
Autoimmune enteropathy 43
Autoimmune hepatitis 114–115

Azathioprine 115

Bacterial infectionssmall intestine 53
Barrett's oesophagus 25
Bassen–Kornsweig syndrome 43
Beckwith's syndrome 9
Behçet's disease 68
Bile acid metabolism, inborn errors 106–107
Bile ducts
  cystic fibrosis 84
  paucity of interlobular 103, 106
  spontaneous perforation 79
  vanishing bile duct syndrome 148
Biliary atresia 89–92
  versus neonatal hepatitis 94
Biliary hypoplasia, intrahepatic 103–106
Biliary peritonitis 79
Biliary tree, dilated intrahepatic 79, 81, 117, 140
Bilirubin uridine diphosphoglucuronyl transferase deficiency 146
Bitot's spots (conjunctival xerosis) 154
Blindness 154
Borrelia vincentii 153
Brain
  ischaemia 133
  oedema 133
  tumours 73
Bruising 120
Brushfield's spots 107
Bulbar palsy (Möbius syndrome) 73
Buttock wasting 33
Bylers' disease 106

Campylobacter jejuni 54
Cancrum oris (noma) 153
Candidiasis
  oesophageal 26
  oral 49
  perineal 49
Capillary haemangioendothelioma 129
Carbohydrate intolerance, testing 46
Cardiac cirrhosis 118
Cardiomyopathy, hypertrophic 101
Caroli's disease (intrahepatic biliary dilatation) 79, 81, 117, 140
Cavernous haemangiomata 130
Cellular hyperplasia 24
Cellulitis 166
Central venous thrombosis 166
Cerebral ischaemia 133

Cerebral oedema 133
Cerebral tumour 73
Chenodeoxycholic acid 106
Cholangiogram
    operative 92
    percutaneous transhepatic 93
Cholangitis 140
    primary sclerosing 116
Choledochal cysts 92–93
Cholestasis, progressive fibrosing intrahepatic 106
Cholestatic liver disease 154
Cholesterol catabolism 105
Cholic acid 106
Chylomicron retention disease (Anderson's disease) 47
Cirrhosis
    cardiac 118
    and portal hypertension 119–124
Cisapride 26, 69
Clinitest 46
Clostridium difficile 74
Clubbing
    cirrhosis 120
    Crohn's disease 60
Coagulopathy, vitamin K responsive 156
Codeine 51
Coeliac disease 33–36
Colitis
    Crohn's 57–63
    pseudomembranous 74
    ulcerative 64–68
Colonic strictures 18
Combined small bowel and liver transplantation (CSBLTx) 147–148
Conjunctival xerosis 154
Constipation, severe 70
Copper 102–103
Cows' milk intolerance 36–37
Crigler–Najjar Type I 146
Crohn's disease 57–63
Cryptosporidiosis 53–54
Cushingoid appearance
    steroid-responsive enterocolitis 45
    ulcerative colitis 67
Cyclosporin
    hirsutism 142, 145
    nephrotoxicity 142–143
Cystic fibrosis 82–85
    neonatal hepatitis 102
Cytochrome oxidase enzyme deficiency 136
Cytomegalovirus hepatitis 97
    post-transplant 142
Cytomegalovirus infection 31

Dehydration 50–51
Dermatitis herpetiformis 34
Dextrocardia 90

Diaphragmatic hernia 11
Diarrhoea
    congenital secretory 41
    modular feeds 46
    parenteral nutrition 47
    stool testing 46
Diazoxide 101
Diphenoxylate 51
Down's syndrome 96
Duodenal atresia 10
Duodenal ulcers 29, 30
    perforation 32
Dysphagia 19

Elemental diet 63
Embryotoxin, posterior 103
Encephalopathy, hepatic 121, 132
Endoscopic retrograde cholangiopancreatography (ERCP) 79, 93
Enteral feeding 138, 162–163
Enterocolitis
    Hirschsprung's disease 15
    necrotising 17–18
    steroid-responsive 45
Eosinophilic gastroenteritis 48
Eosinophils 25
Epstein–Barr virus 143–144
Erythema
    nodosum 61
    palmar 119
    plantar 119
Erythromycin 54
Escherichia coli 53
Essential fatty acid deficiency 157
Exomphalos 9

Faecal impaction 70
Familial adenomatous polyposis 77
Fast atom bombardment ionisation mass spectrometry (FAB–MS) 106
Fat malabsorption 151, 154
Fatty acids
    deficiency 157
    oxidation defects 112, 135
Fatty liver, microvesicular 135
Fibrolamellar hepatocellular carcinoma 128
Fibropolycystic disease 117
Finger clubbing *see* Clubbing
Fissures, perianal 62
Fistulas
    perianal 62
    rectovesical 12
    tracheo-oesophageal 19
Flag sign 170
Foamy storage cells 107
Foreign bodies 28
Fructose intolerance 109

Index

Fumarylacetoacetase deficiency 100
Fundoplication 26
Fusiformis fusiformis 153

Galactosaemia 109
Gallbladder 91
Gallstones 79
  cystic fibrosis 84
Ganciclovir 142
Ganglioneuroblastoma 74
  VIP–secreting 75–76
Ganglionic biopsy 14
Gardner's syndrome 77
Gastric carcinoma 32
Gastric lymphoma 32
Gastric ulcers 29, 32
Gastric varices 122
Gastritis 30
Gastro-oesophageal reflux 21–23
  treatment 26
Gastroenteritis
  Campylobacter 54
  dehydration 50–51
  eosinophilic 48
  infective 50–56
Gastrograffin enema 83
Gastropathy, hypertrophic 31
Gastroschisis 9
Gastrostomy feeding 163
Gaucher's disease 108
Genital Crohn's disease 60
Genu valgum 87
Giardia lamblia 53
Gingival hyperplasia 142, 158
Glioblastoma multiforme 77
Glossitis 159
Glucose-6-phosphatase deficiency 110–111
Gluten withdrawal 36
Glycogen storage disease 110–111
Goats' milk 38
Graft versus host disease 44, 148
Growth failure
  coeliac disease 34
  Crohn's disease 63
  malnutrition 158
  severe hepatic dysfunction 123

H_2-antagonists 26, 29, 30
Haemangioendothelioma, capillary 129
Haemangiomata, cavernous 130
Haematemesis 122
Haemochromatosis, neonatal 112
Haemorrhagic disease of the newborn (vitamin K responsive coagulopathy) 156
Hair
  brittle 157
  hirsutism 142, 145
  loss (alopecia) 160
  swallowed 28
Harrison's sulcus 82, 155
Helicobacter pylori infection 30–31
Hemihypertrophy 125
Henoch–Schönlein purpura 71
Hepatectomy, reduction 139
Hepatic artery thrombosis 139
Hepatic encephalopathy 121, 132
Hepatic storage cells 107
Hepatitis
  acute viral 131
  autoimmune 114–115
  chronic viral 113–114
  cytomegalovirus 97, 142
  granulomatous 116
  neonatal 94–98, 102
  rubella 97
  viral 134
Hepatitis B 113
Hepatitis C 114
Hepatoblastoma 125, 128
Hepatocellular carcinoma 101, 125, 128
Hernias
  diaphragmatic 11
  hiatus 21
  inguinal 12
  umbilical 13
Herpes virus 143
Hiatus hernia, sliding 21
Hirschsprung's disease 14–15
Hirsutism 142, 145
Hydronephrosis 73
Hyperinsulinism 101
Hypertrophic gastropathy 31
Hypoalbuminaemia 34, 158
Hypoglycaemia 101
Hypotonia 121
Hypovascular syndrome 90, 137

Ileal pouch 67
Ileocolic anastomotic bleeding 15
Ileus 51
  meconium 82–83
Immunological disorders 43–44
Immunosuppression 115
  complications 142
  rejection 140–141, 147
  viral infections 143
Infant feeds 38
Infections
  bacterial 53
  cytomegalovirus 31
  gastroenteritis 50–56
  Helicobacter pylori 30–31
  malnutrition 153
  viral 143

Inferior vena cava, absent 90
Inguinal hernia 12
Interferon-α 113
Interstitial nephritis 143
Intestinal lymphangiectasia 152
Intestinal non-rotation 11
Intestinal obstruction
    congenital anomalies 10–11
    distal intestinal obstruction syndrome 83
    Hirschsprung's disease 14–15
    meconium ileus 82–83
Intestinal pseudo-obstruction 69
Intestinal resection, sequelae 45–48
Intrahepatic biliary dilatation (Caroli's disease) 79, 81, 117, 140
Intramural gas 17
Intussusception 28
Iron deficiency 159
Ischaemia, cerebral 133
Isolated lipase deficiency 87

Jaundice, obstructive 79
Jejunal biopsy
    abetalipoproteinaemia 42
    coeliac disease 34
    cows' milk intolerance 37
    microvillus inclusion disease 39–40
Jejunum
    atresia 11
    coeliac disease 35
    lymphoproliferative disease 144
    normal mucosa 35
Johanson Blizzard syndrome 87
Juvenile chronic arthritis 135
Juvenile polyps 78

Kasai portoenterostomy 92
Kayser–Fleischer rings 102
Keratomalacia 154
Koilonychia 159
Kwashiorkor 150

Lactulose 121
Ladd's bands 10
Lead poisoning 73
Lipase deficiency 87
Liver disease
    acute 131–136
    cholestatic 154
    chronic 113–124
    cystic fibrosis 83
    neonatal 89–98
    Schwachman's syndrome 86
    total parenteral nutrition–associated 168
Liver failure, acute 132–135
Liver function tests 94
Liver transplantation 137–148

Liver tumours 125–130
Loperamide 51
Lungs
    Crohn's disease 62
    see also Pulmonary entries
Lymphangiectasia, intestinal 152
Lymphoma
    gastric 32
    non-Hodgkin's 76, 151
Lymphoproliferative disease of the jejunum 144

Magenta tongue 159
Malabsorption, fat 151, 154
Malnutrition 149–158
Malrotation 10
    and intestinal pseudo-obstruction 69
Mannitol 133
Marasmus 150
Measles 153
Meckel's diverticulum 16
Meconium ileus 82–83
Megacolon *see* Toxic megacolon
Megarectum 70
Ménétrièr's disease (hypertrophic gastropathy) 31
Mesenteric cyst 13
Mesotheliomas, peritoneal 78
Metabolic disease 146
Metaphyseal dysostosis 86
Methylprednisolone 135
Metronidazole 53
Microvesicular fatty liver 135
Microvillus inclusion disease (microvillus atrophy) 39–40
Midgut infarction 10
Mitochondrial disorders 136
Möbius syndrome 73
Morphine infusion 69
Munchausen syndrome by proxy 72, 150
Myopathy 111

Nails
    koilonychia 159
    white 158
Necrotising enterocolitis 17–18
Neonatal short gut syndrome *see* Short bowel syndrome
Nephritis, interstitial 143
Nephrotoxicity, cyclosporin 142–143
Neuronal storage 108
Neutrophils 25
Niemann–Pick disease type C 107–108
Night blindness 154
Noma 153
Non-Hodgkin's lymphoma 76, 151
Non–steroidal anti-inflammatory agents 29
Norwalk virus 52
NTBC 100, 101

Nutrition
　elemental diet 63
　enteral feeding 138, 162–163
　gastrostomy feeding 163
　infant feeds 38
　malnutrition 149–158
　nutritional therapy 162
　parenteral 47, 69, 164–170
　total parenteral 161, 168
Obstructive jaundice 79
Oedema
　cerebral 133
　hypoalbuminaemic 34
　peripheral hypoproteinaemic 152
Oesophagus
　atresia 19
　Barrett's 25
　candidiasis 26
　pH 23
　varices 122, 123
　vascular ring 19
　web 19
Oesophagitis 24–25
Ophthalmoplegia, supranuclear 108
Opioids 51
Oral candidiasis 49
Oral rehydration therapy 51
Oral ulceration 59, 68
Orofacial granulomatosis 60
Osteoporosis 155

Palmar erythema 119
Pancreatic duct, congenital abnormalities 80
Pancreatic rest 32
Pancreatin 87
Pancreatitis 80–81
Paracetamol poisoning 134
Parenteral nutrition 47, 69, 164–170
Patent processus vaginalis 12
Paucity of interlobular bile ducts (PIBD) 103, 106
Penicillamine 102
Percutaneous transhepatic cholangiogram 93
Perianal abnormalities 62
Pericarditis, chronic tuberculous constrictive 118
Peripheral pulmonary stenosis 104, 105
Peritonitis, biliary 79
Peutz–Jeghers syndrome 75
pH, oesophageal 23
Phototherapy 146
Plantar erythema 119
Plummer–Vinson syndrome 19
Pneumatosis intestinalis (intramural gas) 17
Poisoning
　lead 73
　paracetamol 134
Polyhydramnios 41
Polyps
　familial adenomatous polyposis 77
　inflammatory (pseudopolyps) 65
　juvenile 78
Portal cavernoma 124
Portal hypertension 119–124
Portal vein
　extrahepatic obstruction 124
　thrombosis 137
Portoenterostomy 92
Posterior embryotoxin 103
Prednisolone 115, 147
Primary sclerosing cholangitis 116
Proctocolectomy with ileal reservoir and anal anastomosis 67
Progressive neuronal degeneration with liver disease (Alper's disease) 112, 136
Projectile vomiting 27
Prokinetic agents 26
Proton pump inhibitors 26, 29, 30
Pseudocyst, pancreatic 80
Pseudomembranous colitis 74
Pseudo-obstruction 69
Pseudopolyps 65
Psychological preparation 138
Puberty, delayed 158
Pulmonary aspiration 21–22
Pulmonary embolism 168
Pulmonary hypoplasia 11
Pulmonary stenosis, peripheral 104, 105
Pulmonary thromboembolism 169
Purpura, Henoch–Schönlein 71
Pyloric stenosis 27
Pyoderma gangrenosum 67
Pyrexia 61

Rectal atresia 12
Rectal biopsy 44
Rectal prolapse 72
Rectovesical fistula 12
Reduction hepatectomy 139
Rejection 140–141, 147
Renal tubular acidosis 101, 105
Reye's syndrome 135
Ribbon stool 70
Riboflavin deficiency 159
Rickets 87, 101, 155
Rotavirus 52
Rubella hepatitis 97

Sacroiliitis 61
Sandifer's syndrome 22
Schwachman's syndrome 85–87
Selenium deficiency 161
Seminoma 74
Severe combined immunodeficiency 44
Short bowel syndrome (neonatal short gut syndrome) 45

and pseudo–obstruction 69
Skeletal abnormalities 104
Skin
   cavernous haemangiomata 130
   Crohn's disease 62
   hyperkeratotic rash 157
   papular rash 145
   prick tests 37
   tags 62
Small bowel
   adenocarcinoma 76
   infections 53
   transplantation 147–148
Sodium valproate 112, 135
Soya formulas 38
Spider naevi 120
Spiramycin 98
Steatorrhoea 87, 151
Steroid-responsive enterocolitis 45
Stomatitis, angular 159
Stool collection
   secretory diarrhoea 46
   VIP-secreting ganglioneuroblastoma 76
Stools
   biliary atresia 90
   ribbon stool 70
   tests 46
Stress ulceration 29
Striae 115
Stunting 149
Succinylacetone 100
Superior vena caval obstruction 166–167
Supranuclear ophthalmoplegia 108

Tacrolimus 141, 147
Taurine deficiency 161
Technetium BIDA liver scan 91, 93, 95
Technetium HMPAO-labelled white-cell scan 68
Technetium labelled red-cell scan 74
Technetium Meckel's scan 16
Teeth, dysplastic 158
Telangiectasia, facial 119
Testicular feminisation syndrome 12
Thrombosis
   central venous 166
   hepatic artery 139
   portal vein 137
Tissue necrosis 50
Tongue
   magenta 159
   tie (ankyloglossia) 72
Total parenteral nutrition 161
   liver disease 168
Toxic megacolon
   Crohn's disease 58
   ulcerative colitis 66

Toxoplasmosis 98
Tracheo-oesophageal fistula 19
Transjugular intrahepatic portal systemic shunting (TIPS) 123
Transplantation 137–148
Triceps skin fold measurement 149
Trichotillomania 28
Tuberculosis, intestinal 55
Tumours
   cerebral 73
   liver 125–130
Turcot's syndrome 77
Tyrosinaemia type I 100–101

Ulceration
   Behçet's disease 68
   Crohn's disease 58–59
   duodenal *see* Duodenal ulcers
   gastric 29, 32
   oral 59, 68
   perianal 62
   stress 29
Ulcerative colitis 64–68
Umbilical hernia 13

Vanishing bile duct syndrome 148
Varices 122
   bleeding 123
Vasoactive intestinal peptide (VIP) secreting ganglioneuroblastoma 75–76
Viral infections 143
Vitamin A deficiency 154
Vitamin B12 deficiency 159
Vitamin C (ascorbic acid) deficiency 159
Vitamin D deficiency 155
Vitamin E
   abetalipoproteinaemia 42–43
   deficiency 156
Vitamin K
   alpha-1-antitrypsin deficiency 99
   deficiency 156
Volvulus 10
Vomiting, projectile 27

Wasting 149
   buttocks 33
Weight charts 89
Wilson's disease 102–103

Xanthomata 105
Xerosis, conjunctival 154

Yersinia enterocolitica 56

Zellweger's syndrome 107
Zinc deficiency 160